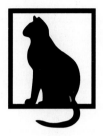

THE FELINE PATIENT

Essentials of Diagnosis and Treatment

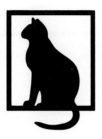

THE FELINE PATIENT
Essentials of Diagnosis and Treatment

Gary D. Norsworthy, DVM
Diplomate, ABVP
Acres North Animal Hospital
Alamo Veterinary Referral Center
San Antonio, Texas

Mitchell A. Crystal, DVM
Diplomate, ACVIM
North Florida Veterinary Specialists
Jacksonville, Florida

Sharon K. Fooshee, MS, DVM
Diplomate, ABVP, ACVIM
Animal Health Center of Franklin
Franklin, Tennessee

Larry P. Tilley, DVM
Diplomate, ACVIM
VetMedFax Consultation Services
Veterinary Specialty Referral Center
Santa Fe, New Mexico

Editor: Carroll C. Cann
Managing Editor:
Marketing Manager: Diane M. Harnish
Development Editor:
Production Coordinator: Peter J. Carley
Project Editor: Jennifer D. Weir
Designer: Circa 86
Illustration Planner: Wayne Hubbel
Cover Designer: Circa 86
Typesetter and Digitized Illustrations: Peirce Graphic Services, Inc.
Printer/Binder: RR Donnelly & Sons Company

351 West Camden Street
Baltimore, Maryland 21201-2436 USA

Rose Tree Corporate Center
1400 North Providence Road
Building II, Suite 5025
Media, Pennsylvania 19063-2043 USA

Accurate indications, adverse reactions and dosage schedules for drugs are provided in this book, but it is possible that they may change. The reader is urged to review the package information data of the manufacturers of the medications mentioned.

Printed in the United States of America

Library of Congress Cataloging-in-Publication Data
The feline patient : essentials of diagnosis and treatment / Gary D.
    Norsworthy . . . [et al.].
        p.   cm.
    Includes bibliographical references and index.
    ISBN 0-683-06556-4
    1. Cats—Diseases.   I. Norsworthy, Gary D.
SF985.F46   1997
636.8′089—dc21

                                97-13122
                                CIP

The publishers have made every effort to trace the copyright holders for borrowed material. If they have inadvertently overlooked any, they will be pleased to make the necessary arrangements at the first opportunity.

To purchase additional copies of this book, call our customer service department at **(800) 638-0672** or fax orders to **(800) 447-8438.** For other book services, including chapter reprints and large quantity sales, ask for the Special Sales department.
Canadian customers should call **(800) 665-1148,** or fax **(800) 665-0103.** For all other calls originating outside of the United States, please call **(410) 528-4223** or fax us at **(410) 528-8550.**

Visit Williams & Wilkins on the Internet: *http://www.wwilkins.com* or contact our customer service department at ***custserv@wwilkins.com.*** Williams & Wilkins customer service representatives are available form 8:30 am to 6:00 pm, EST, Monday through Friday, for telephone access.

                                        97 98 99 00
                                        2 3 4 5 6 7 8 9 10

T his book is dedicated to my fellow primary-care private practitioners. You have supported me for the last 20 years when I have lectured and published. It is for you that this book is prepared. I sincerely hope that it addresses the issues in feline medicine that you need on a daily basis.

The leaders in diagnostic and therapeutic thought are now the veterinary referral specialists. However, it is, and probably always will be, the primary-care practitioner who will deliver health care to the vast majority of the world's pet cats and dogs. Although the primary-care practitioner seems to be relegated to a place at the bottom of the health care chain, in reality, he or she is the person to whom Mr. and Ms. Client will turn for advice and care for 95% of their veterinary needs.

I have traveled North America extensively, and I am constantly impressed with the personal integrity and dedication of the primary-care private practitioner. I am proud to be one of you.

Gary D. Norsworthy

In loving memory of my parents,
Joel and Janie Fooshee,
and friends,
Mary Reinmuth and David H. Jones

Sharon K. Fooshee

To my wife, Tedisue Suthers Crystal:
I simply love you more than life itself

Mitchell A. Crystal

To my wife, Jeri,
and my son, Kyle,
and to all students of feline medicine,
for whom this book is written

Larry P. Tilley

Preface

The purpose of this book is to give you, the private practitioner, rapid access to the important information needed in the daily practice of feline medicine. As a practitioner myself, I know that clients want to know four things: the diagnosis, the way in which treatment is to be accomplished, the likely outcome, and the cost. You should be able to access the first three of the four answers to your client's questions with this book. And, because your client wants those answers NOW, you should be able to do so quickly.

Your feedback to my success in providing this information is appreciated.

Gary D. Norsworthy

Contributors

John-Karl Goodwin, DVM
Veterinary Heart Institute
3601 Southwest 2nd Ave.
Suite X
Gainesville, FL 32607

Mark G. Papich, DVM
College of Veterinary Medicine
School of Veterinary Medicine
North Carolina State University
Raleigh, North Carolina

Contents

PART THREE **APPENDICES**

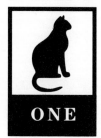

ONE

SYNDROMES

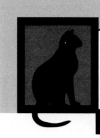

CHAPTER 1

Alopecia of the Trunk

Gary D. Norsworthy

Overview

T
runcal alopecia is typically bilateral and symmetrical. It occurs most commonly on the ventral abdomen; the next most likely site is the posterior aspects of the rear legs, especially above the hocks. Other areas include the area just cranial to the tail head and the flanks. In some cats, all of these areas are affected and may coalesce, resulting in alopecia of the entire caudal half of the trunk. One of the most important aspects of the diagnostic workup is determining if pruritus is present. The owner should be asked if the cat has been engaged in licking, scratching, chewing, or excessive grooming. A negative response does not rule out pruritus or self-induced alopecia, however, because many cats are "closet lickers."

 D i a g n o s i s

Differential Diagnoses: Pruritic or Self-Induced

- Atopy
- Flea-allergic dermatitis
- Psychogenic
- Food allergy
- Dermatophytosis
- *Cheyletiella* infection
- Demodicidosis
- Anal sac impaction
- *Sarcoptes*
- Truncal ear mites

Differential Diagnoses: Non–self-Induced

- Stress: surgery, systemic illness, fever
- Anagen defluxion
- Telogen defluxion
- Hyperadrenocorticism
- Hyperthyroidism
- "Endocrine-deficiency alopecia"

Primary Diagnostics

- **History:** The determination of self-induced (including pruritus) versus non–self-induced alopecia is critical to the rest of the diagnostic workup.
- **Trichogram:** This is a microscopic examination of the distal ends of hair within the area of alopecia. Broken tips indicate that the hair loss is self induced. See Appendix F.
- **Steroid response:** Cats that have response to steroids can be presumed to be pruritic. If so, these diseases should be considered: atopy, flea allergic dermatitis, *Cheyletiella* infection, demodicidosis, *Sarcoptes*, and truncal ear mites. Cats with food allergy may have a short response (a few days) to a long-acting steroid injection.
- **Intradermal skin test for flea reaction or strict flea control:** These tests are used to document flea allergic dermatitis.
- **Intradermal skin test antigens:** This test is for atopy.
- **Fungus culture:** Dermatophytosis can create skin lesions and hair loss with many different clinical appearances.
- **Food elimination trial:** A food that the cat has never eaten should be fed exclusively for at least 4 weeks and preferably for 8 weeks. The protein source is the portion of the food that is most likely to be antigenic, so a new protein source is critical.
- **Cellophane tape preparation:** This microscopic examination is to detect *Cheyletiella*.
- **Ivermectin injection:** If the cellophane tape test is negative, this should be considered, especially for kittens from multicat facilities.
- **Skin scraping:** This test is to detect *Demodex*, *Sarcoptes*, and ear mites.
- **Anal sac expression:** Feline anal sacs rarely abscess. Impaction may cause the cat to lick excessively near the perineal area.
- **Serum total T4 or T3 suppression test:** Hyperthyroidism should be eliminated, especially in cats over 10 years of age. See Appendix F.

Diagnostic Notes

- Response to steroids should be considered a diagnostic, not therapeutic, procedure unless a thorough diagnostic workup eliminates a specific diagnosis.

- Endocrine-deficiency alopecia is unlikely to be a true disease of cats. The use of this term is discouraged.

 T r e a t m e n t

Primary Therapeutics

- Truncal hair loss is not life threatening. If pruritus is not present, the hair loss is more a cosmetic problem than a medical problem.
- It is important to identify a primary disease, if at all possible, and treat accordingly.

Secondary Therapeutics: Psychogenic Alopecia

- This is a disease that occurs in some cats; however, there is no test for it. It is a diagnosis of exclusion.
- In the author's opinion, there is a psychogenic component that complicates many pruritus-associated causes of truncal alopecia. Without addressing it,

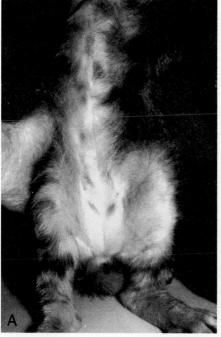 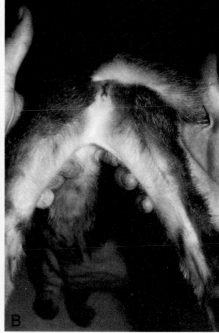

FIGURE 1.1. Alopecia of the trunk: The ventral aspects of the abdomen (*A*) and the caudal aspects of the rear legs (*B*) are the areas most commonly affected.

these cats may not respond to the relief of pruritus alone. Therefore, it is suggested that phenobarbital (1/4 gr. PO BID) be given to cats with truncal alopecia in addition to whatever therapy is appropriate for relief of pruritus.

Prognosis

The prognosis will depend upon a proper diagnosis and treatment for an underlying disease. However, this is not a life-threatening condition.

Suggested Readings

Merchant SR. The skin: diseases of unknown or multiple etiology. In: Norsworthy GD, ed. Feline practice. Philadelphia: JB Lippincott, 1993;532–539.

Moriello KA. Diseases of the skin. In: Sherding RG, ed. The cat: Diseases and clinical management, 2nd ed. Philadelphia: WB Saunders, 1994;1907–1968.

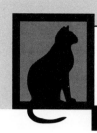

CHAPTER 2
Anemia
Sharon K. Fooshee

Overview

Anemia, which is defined as a reduction below normal in the number of circulating red blood cells and hemoglobin, may have numerous causes in the cat. It should be noted that the cat's RBC count is normally lower than that of dogs. An orderly approach to evaluation of the anemic cat is required.

Depending on the chronicity of the anemia, the history may indicate decreased activity or tolerance for exercise. Physical examination of anemic cats may reveal pale mucous membranes, increased ventilatory effort (especially with stress), a soft systolic heart murmur, and tachycardia. Particular attention should be given to the size of the peripheral lymph nodes and the spleen.

It is important to first determine whether the anemia is regenerative or nonregenerative. Reticulocytes, or immature red blood cells, should be counted whenever the hematocrit is less than 20% so that the bone marrow response to the anemia can be evaluated. Generally, regenerative anemias are associated with two main categories of causes: blood loss or hemolysis. Nonregenerative anemias are caused by decreased production of erythrocytes; the underlying cause may be a disease of the bone marrow or may be secondary to an extramedullary disorder.

The cat is unique in that two types of reticulocytes may be present. Aggregate reticulocytes are more reflective of a recent regenerative response and contain numerous dark-staining clumps of ribosomes, whereas the punctate reticulocytes contain small clumps of ribosomal material. The presence of aggregate reticulocytes is the most reliable indicator of a regenerative response.

 D i a g n o s i s

Differential Diagnoses
- **Regenerative**

Hemolysis

Erythrocyte parasites: *Hemobartonella felis*, *Cytauxzoon felis*, *Babesia* spp.

Immune-mediated destruction

Heinz-body hemolytic anemia

Oxidative injury: methylene blue, acetaminophen, benzocaine, phenazopyridine

Neonatal isoerythrolysis

Blood Loss

Trauma or surgical loss

Chronic flea infestation

• **Nonregenerative**

Intramedullary

Hematopoietic neoplasia with or without feline leukemia virus (FeLV) feline immunodeficiency virus (FIV)

Lymphoproliferative

Myeloproliferative

Red blood cell aplasia

Extramedullary

Chronic renal disease

Chronic inflammatory disease (e.g., fungal disease, etc.)

Neoplasia

Poor nutrition or starvation

Primary Diagnostics

• **CBC:** A complete blood count should be performed if anemia is suspected. Diagnosis of anemia requires identification of erythrocyte numbers or a hematocrit lower than normal for the individual laboratory. The blood smear should be evaluated for the presence of red blood cell parasites, Heinz bodies, and morphologic changes. Because of the small size of feline erythrocytes, spherocytosis (indicative of immune-mediated destruction) is not detectable on the smear.

• **Reticulocyte count:** Equal parts of ethylenediaminetetra-acetic acid (EDTA)-anticoagulated blood and new methylene blue stain are gently mixed and the solution allowed to incubate at room temperature for 10 to 15 minutes. A smear is made, and the percentage of the first 1000 erythrocytes that are aggregate and punctate reticulocytes is recorded. After 5 to 6 days and with sufficient anemia to stimulate erythrocyte production, the percentage of reticulocytes should be 2 to 5%. The feline regenerative response is much less than that of the dog with a comparable anemia. Additionally, some peculiarities of the feline erythron occasionally make it difficult to interpret the significance of a response; a veterinary clinical pathologist should be consulted. The reticulocyte count should be corrected for the hematocrit (HCT):

$$\text{Corrected reticulocyte count} = \frac{\text{Measured reticulocyte count (\%)}}{\text{Patient's HCT/Normal HCT*}}$$

$$*\text{Normal HCT} = 37.5\%$$

- **Feline viral screen:** The cat should be evaluated with an antigen test for FeLV and an antibody test for FIV. If the environmental history supports the need, a screen for feline coronavirus can be performed, recognizing the limitations of currently available tests.

Ancillary Diagnostics

- **Serum chemistry profile:** A serum chemistry profile can be helpful in looking for underlying disease, especially for nonregenerative anemia. Particular attention should be given to serum color, blood urea nitrogen (BUN), creatinine, alanine aminotransferase (ALT), alkaline phosphate (ALP), and total protein.

- **Bone marrow aspiration:** With unexplained nonregenerative anemias, bone marrow aspiration and cytology are usually indicated. Several sites are available for aspiration; the wing of the ilium is often used. A standard

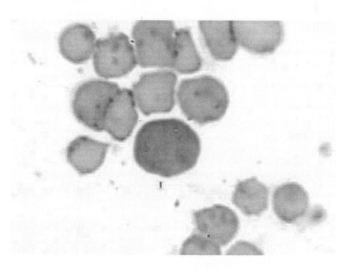

FIGURE 2.1. Anemia: The large dark cell is a macrocyte. It is a metarubricyte that has lost its nucleus. It is a reliable indicator of increased bone marrow activity and signals a regenerative anemia.

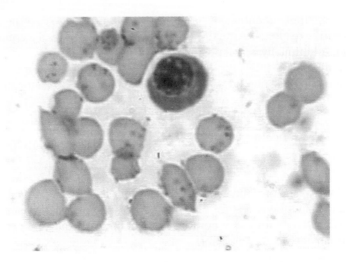

FIGURE 2.2. The large nucleated cell is a metarubricyte or nucleated red blood cell. It may or may not indicate bone marrow response.

internal medicine text may be consulted for details of the procedure. The bone marrow slides should be submitted to a veterinary pathologist, along with a tube of EDTA-anticoagulated blood drawn at the time of marrow aspiration.

- **Coombs' test:** A Coombs' test may be performed when an immune-mediated cause of anemia is suspected. An EDTA-anticoagulated tube of blood should be submitted to a veterinary diagnostic laboratory. It should be remembered that a positive test is *not* diagnostic of immune-mediated hemolysis; a variety of anemias may produce a positive Coombs' test. Feline Coombs' serum should be used for the test.
- **Radiography:** Thoracic and abdominal radiographs may be a useful component of the minimum database in cats with unexplained anemia.

Diagnostic Notes

- Mucous membrane color is a poor indicator of anemia in cats because the membranes are relatively pale compared with those in dogs.
- Nucleated red blood cells **do not** indicate a regenerative response unless also accompanied by an increase in reticulocytes.
- Regenerative anemias may take 5 to 6 days to respond to blood loss with an appropriate peripheral reticulocytosis. This time frame should be taken into consideration when the initial hemogram and reticulocyte count are consistent with *non*regenerative anemia but blood loss or hemolysis are likely.

- *Hemobartonella* organisms may detach from red blood cells after incubating in EDTA anticoagulant. A fresh blood smear should accompany the anticoagulated blood when hemobartonellosis is suspected.
- Increased numbers of Heinz bodies have been associated with hyperthyroidism, lymphoma, and diabetes mellitus.

T r e a t m e n t

Primary Therapeutics

- **Transfusion:** Blood transfusion may be indicated for acutely anemic cats and for some cases of chronic anemia. A standard reference should be consulted for details of managing the donor cat and for guidelines in transfusing the anemic cat.
- **Erythropoietin:** Human recombinant erythropoietin may be used in cases of nonregenerative anemia owing to renal failure. For other causes of anemia, this treatment is not indicated, because serum erythropoietin levels usually are already elevated.

Therapeutic Notes

- Emphasis should be placed on stabilizing the patient while aggressively pursuing the underlying disease process.
- For cats with anemia of chronic disease, specific treatment is rarely indicated. The practitioner should focus on identification and treatment of the underlying cause. If this treatment is successful, the anemia should resolve.

Prognosis

Prognosis for the anemic cat is totally dependent upon identification and successful management of the underlying cause. Generally, the prognosis is better for acute cases of anemia than for nonregenerative cases.

Suggested Readings

Cowell RL, Tyler RD. Diagnosis of anemia. In: August JR, ed. Consultations in feline internal medicine. Philadelphia: WB Saunders, 1991;335–342.

Rentko VT, Cotter SM. Feline anemia: the classifications, causes, and diagnostic procedures. *Vet Med* 1990;85:584–604.

Rentko VT, Cotter SM. The procedures for treating anemic cats. *Vet Med* 1990;85:605–612.

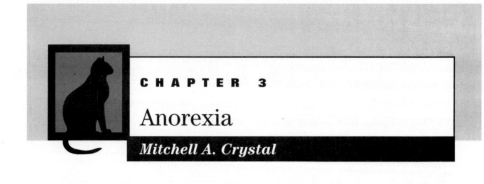

CHAPTER 3

Anorexia

Mitchell A. Crystal

Overview

Anorexia is the loss of appetite for food. Anorexia can result from numerous pathologic and nonpathologic conditions, including metabolic, gastrointestinal, or neurologic disorders, inflammatory/infectious diseases, reactions to drugs/toxins, neoplasia, fever, pain, environmental stress, and lack of diet palatability. Because so many conditions may lead to anorexia, other accompanying clinical signs are variable. Some cats will demonstrate anorexia or anorexia/lethargy/weight loss as the only presenting complaint of a disease process. Unlike many other animals, cats are obligate carnivores with special nutritional requirements. This is due to the cat's persistent use and loss of some nutrients and inadequate synthesis of others (Table 3.1). As a result, persistent or prolonged anorexia can lead to serious metabolic derangements, complicating an already present condition. An additional concern in prolonged anorexia in cats is the cat's potential to develop hepatic lipidosis. Therefore, anorexia in the cat warrants prompt diagnostic investigation and therapeutic intervention.

TABLE 3.1.

Special Nutrient Requirements of the Cat

Nutrient	Clinical Signs of Deficiency
Arginine	Ptyalism, hyperesthesia, vomiting, muscle tremors, ataxia; signs can develop within hours to days.
Taurine	Retinal degeneration, dilated cardiomyopathy, reproductive problems, decreased growth in kittens; signs develop over weeks to months.
Arachidonic acid	Dermatitis, dry hair coat, anemia, reproductive problems, decreased growth in kittens; signs develop over weeks to months.
Vitamin A	Retinal degeneration, weakness, dry/unkempt hair coat, decreased growth in kittens; signs develop over weeks to months.

Diagnosis

Primary Diagnostics

- **History:** Question the owner about the cat's environment (indoor versus outdoor and any recent moves, new pets, or members of the household), travel history (to areas endemic for infectious diseases), recent drug therapy, exposure to toxins, signs of other disease processes (e.g., polyuria/polydipsia, vomiting, diarrhea), or change in diet. Review the cat's vaccination history.

- **Physical examination:** Examine closely for wounds and abscesses, internal or external masses, lymphadenopathy, abnormal pulmonary auscultation, and pain. A complete oral examination is warranted to look for gingival or dental disease and to look under the tongue for a linear foreign body. A complete ophthalmologic examination (anterior chamber and retina) will sometimes disclose evidence of inflammatory/infectious diseases.

- **Database (CBC, chemistry profile, and urinalysis):** Abnormalities may suggest metabolic disorders, inflammatory/infectious diseases, or neoplasia.

- **FeLV/FIV test:** Positive results from either of these tests are not confirmatory for disease but are strong indicators of the source of anorexia.

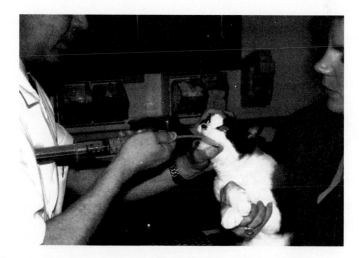

FIGURE 3.1. Anorexia: Orogastric tube feeding is an efficient way to administer blenderized food to a hospitalized cat.

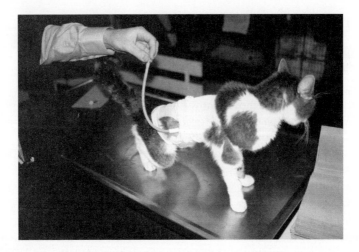

FIGURE 3.2. Gastrostomy tube feeding can be utilized when long-term feeding is required in a nonhospitalized patient.

Ancillary Diagnostics

- **Thoracic radiography and/or ultrasound:** Abnormalities may suggest inflammatory/infectious diseases, neoplasia, or cardiac disease.
- **Abdominal radiographs and/or ultrasound:** Abdominal imaging may reveal abnormalities in organ size and architecture, gastrointestinal obstruction, or neoplasia.

Diagnostic Notes

Dental disease is a rare cause of anorexia. A complete evaluation of any cat with anorexia is indicated prior to anesthesia and dental prophylaxis despite the presence of dental tartar. A complete evaluation will rule out the more common causes of anorexia and will confirm that anesthesia is not contraindicated.

 T r e a t m e n t

Primary Therapeutics

- **Treat underlying disease:** This is essential in restoring appetite.
- **Fluid support:** Fluids may be administered orally or parenterally if needed for dehydration.
- **Nutritional support:** Indications for nutritional support include weight loss of greater than 10% of body weight (greater than 5% in kittens),

anorexia longer than 3 to 5 days (longer than 1 to 2 days in kittens), hypo-albuminemia, lymphopenia, anemia, increased nutrient losses (vomiting, diarrhea, burns, large wounds, intestinal malassimilation, protein-losing nephropathies, peritonitis, pleuritis) and inability to eat because of a disease or therapy (e.g., oropharyngeal disease, chemotherapy). Each cat must be individually evaluated when deciding whether one or several of the above criteria should be present before initiating nutritional support. Nutrients may be provided via enteral (gastrostomy, esophagostomy, pharyngostomy, orogastric, jejunostomy or nasoesophageal tubes, or forced hand feeding) or parenteral routes.

Secondary Therapeutics

• **Appetite stimulants:** Appetite stimulants should only be used to help promote voluntary eating in cases in which a diagnosis has been achieved, specific therapy has been instituted, and immediate nutritional support is not feasible. Prior to using chemical agents, an attempt to stimulate eating should be made by offering a variety of foods of different flavors, odors, and textures, by warming foods, placing foods in a wide shallow bowl to prevent the sides of the bowl from contacting the cat's whiskers, and stroking and petting the cat at the time of feeding (or providing a quiet environment for the stressed cat such as a covered cage or a cardboard box). Chemical appetite stimulants reported effective in the cat include diazepam (0.2 mg/kg IV BID immediately prior to feeding), oxazepam (2.5 mg/cat PO BID 5 to 20 minutes prior to feeding) and cyproheptadine (2–4 mg/cat PO BID 5 to 20 minutes prior to feeding).

Therapeutic Notes

It is best to provide nutrition via the enteral route. This maintains gastrointestinal mucosal health, is less expensive, and provides a more natural means of nutrient absorption and utilization. If the gastrointestinal tract is unable to absorb and digest food, total or partial parenteral nutrition can be used.

Forced hand feeding is a less optimal means of enteral nutrition than tube feeding, because it significantly increases patient stress and generally cannot deliver the volumes necessary to meet the patient's nutritional requirements.

Intravenous fluids with 2.5 or 5% dextrose do not supply significant calories when delivered at rates at or moderately above maintenance; thus, they are only indicated in patients with hypoglycemia. Dextrose as a 5% solution contains 0.17 kcal per milliliter, which when delivered at maintenance for a 5 kg cat, provides only 51 kcal or about one-sixth of the daily caloric need.

If no significant response is seen after chemical appetite stimulants have been used for 24 hours, chemical appetite stimulants should be discontinued and nutritional support started.

P r o g n o s i s

The prognosis varies depending on the underlying disorder causing the anorexia.

S u g g e s t e d   R e a d i n g s

Case LP, Carey DP, Hirakawa DA. Canine and feline nutrition. A resource for companion animal professionals. St. Louis: CV Mosby, 1995;69–142.

Macy DW, Ralston SL. Cause and control of decreased appetite. In: Kirk RW, ed. Current veterinary therapy X. Small animal practice. Philadelphia: WB Saunders, 1989;18–24.

Wheeler SL, McGuire BH. Enteral nutritional support. In: Kirk RW, ed. Current veterinary therapy X. Small animal practice. Philadelphia: WB Saunders, 1989;30–37.

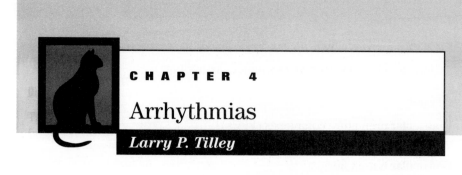

CHAPTER 4

Arrhythmias

Larry P. Tilley

Overview

The essentials of electrocardiography include the assessment of heart rate, heart rhythm, and the P-QRS-T wave forms. The ECG is needed to accurately diagnose cardiac arrhythmias, as it is extremely sensitive for this purpose. The ECG should be a standard part of the systemic disease workup, as well as part of the database in cats with suspected heart disease. An arrhythmia can be defined as (*a*) an abnormality in the rate, regularity, or site of origin of the cardiac impulse, or (*b*) a disturbance in conduction of the impulse such that the normal sequence of activation of atria and ventricles is altered. It is important to establish the causes of arrhythmias because such information affects prognosis and therapy. The possible sources of arrhythmias in dogs and cats can be divided into three basic categories: (*a*) autonomic nervous system; (*b*) cardiac sources; and (*c*) extracardiac sources. A classification of cardiac arrhythmias is as follows:

Sinus Rhythm

Normal sinus rhythm

Sinus tachycardia

Sinus bradycardia

Sinus arrhythmia

Wandering pacemaker

Abnormalities of Impulse Formation

Supraventricular

Sinus arrest

Atrial premature complexes (APCs)

Atrial tachycardia

Atrial flutter

Atrial fibrillation

Atrioventricular (AV) Junction

AV junctional escape rhythm (secondary arrhythmia)

Ventricular

Ventricular premature complexes (VPCs)

Ventricular tachycardia

Ventricular flutter, fibrillation

Ventricular asystole

Ventricular escape rhythm (secondary arrhythmia)

Abnormalities of Impulse Conduction

Sinoatrial (SA) block

Atrial standstill (hyperkalemia, sinoventricular conduction)

AV block

First degree

Second degree

Third degree (complete heart block)

Abnormalities of Both Impulse Formation and Impulse Conduction:

Pre-excitation (Wolff-Parkinson-White) syndrome, reciprocal rhythm (re-entry)

Parasystole

Other complex rhythms

 D i a g n o s i s

Differential Diagnoses

- **Autonomic nervous system:**
  Excitement, exercise, pain, or fever (sympathetic influence);
  Respiratory influences on vagal tone (not as pronounced in the cat);
  Organic brain disease causing sympathetic or vagal stimulation
- **Cardiac sources:**
  Hereditary (rare);
  Acquired damage to the conduction system, hypertrophic cardiomyopathy, neoplasia;
  Diseases of the atria and ventricles—arrhythmias occurring in neoplasia, hypertrophic cardiomyopathy, myocarditis (many causes)

- **Extracardiac sources:**

Hypoxia;

Disturbances of the acid-base balance;

Electrolyte imbalance;

Drugs;

Endocrine disease—hyperthyroidism, diabetes mellitus

Primary Diagnostics

- **Thoracic auscultation:** A markedly irregular cardiac rhythm on auscultation with an arterial pulse deficit may implicate arrhythmias such as ventricular premature complexes and atrial fibrillation but will require an ECG to differentiate among them.
- **Electrocardiography:** A systematic method for an accurate ECG analysis of a rhythm strip (usually lead II) should always include the following steps: (*a*) general inspection of the rhythm strip; (*b*) identification of P-waves; (*c*) recognition of QRS complexes; (*d*) relationship between P-waves and QRS complexes; and (*e*) summary of findings and final classification of the arrhythmia. Common examples of various feline arrhythmias are included in Figure 4.1.

Ancillary Diagnostics

- **Vagal stimulation:** This includes the mechanical application of pressure to receptors that cause a reflex increase in vagal tone (either by ocular pressure or carotid sinus massage). The effects of increasing vagal tone are mainly supraventricular, causing a slowing of the heart rate and a decrease in conduction through the AV junction.
- **Long-term ambulatory (Holter) recordings:** This technique monitors the ECG for extended periods of time. The long-term ECG recording technique is the most sensitive noninvasive test to demonstrate transient arrhythmias.
- **Echocardiography:** Arrhythmias can often be picked up as an incidental finding during the actual study or, in some cases, can affect the hemodynamics.

Diagnostic Notes

- A pronounced sinus arrhythmia, often normally auscultated in dogs, is rare in cats. Therefore, an irregular cardiac rhythm auscultated in the cat is generally an abnormal finding.
- It should be emphasized that severe, life-threatening arrhythmias, such as ventricular tachycardia or atrial tachycardia, may easily be missed on auscultation as the cardiac rhythm is often regular on auscultation. An ECG is the only way to accurately make this diagnosis.

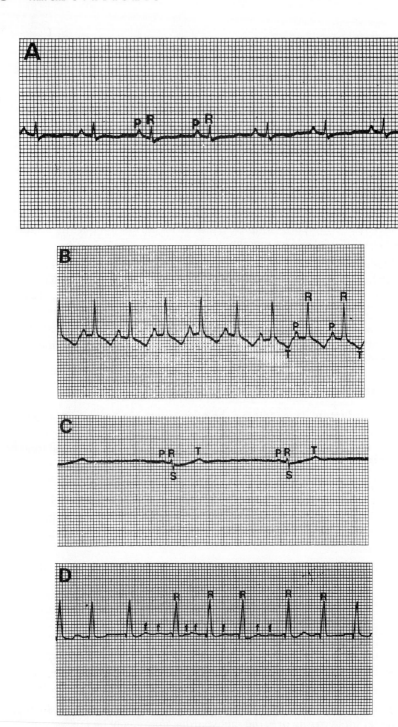

FIGURE 4.1. Examples of feline arrhythmias: *A*, normal sinus rhythm; *B*, sinus tachycardia; *C*, sinus bradycardia; *D*, atrial fibrillation; *E*, atrial tachycardia; *F*, complete AV block; *G*, ventricular premature complex.

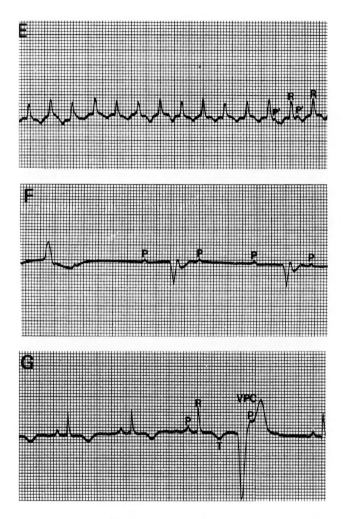

FIGURE 4.1. (*continued*)

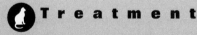 **T r e a t m e n t**

Primary Therapeutics

- **Antiarrhythmic drugs:** Beta-blockers (atenolol, propranolol), digoxin, and diltiazem are different drug groups used in the specific treatment of arrhythmias in the cat. Diltiazem and beta-blockers are currently the drugs of choice in cats because of their broad antiarrhythmic effects.

- **Digoxin:** Because of the recent use of enalapril in the cat, digoxin is used less often. Digoxin is used mainly to control the ventricular rate in atrial arrhythmias and for its inotropic effect in the improvement of cardiac performance in dilated cardiomyopathy.

Secondary Therapeutics

- **Treat the underlying disease:** Specific treatment for many of the arrhythmias present in cats often is not required. In the majority of cases, arrhythmias disappear when the underlying disease is brought under control. For example, the correction of hyperkalemia resulting from urethral obstruction by simply relieving the obstruction and restoring normal acid-base status and fluid volume may eliminate the associated arrhythmias.

Therapeutic Notes

Other antiarrhythmic drugs, including quinidine, procainamide, and lidocaine, have been shown to be dangerous in the cat. These drugs have not been used extensively in the cat because of their high risk of reactions and because ventricular arrhythmias are not common in the cat. Lidocaine could be used as an emergency ventricular antiarrhythmic drug in the cat, but very low doses should be used and only if the arrhythmia has not resolved by the treatment of the underlying cause.

Prognosis

The prognosis is variable depending upon the exact cause of the arrhythmia. In the majority of cases, arrhythmias disappear when the underlying disease is brought under control.

Suggested Reading

Tilley LP. Essentials of canine and feline electrocardiography, 3rd ed. Baltimore: Williams & Wilkins, 1992.

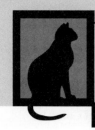

Ascites

John-Karl Goodwin

Overview

Ascites is the accumulation of fluid within the peritoneal cavity. Ascites is indicative of an underlying disease process (exception: overzealous fluid administration) and may be clinically significant if it restricts diaphragmatic excursions, impeding respiration.

 Diagnosis

Differential Diagnoses

The most common causes of ascites in the cat include:

- **Peritonitis**
  Feline infectious peritonitis
  Chylous peritonitis
  Bacterial peritonitis
- **Congestive heart failure**
  Dilated cardiomyopathy
  Hypertrophic cardiomyopathy
  Congenital cardiac anomaly (tricuspid dysplasia, cor triatriatum dexter)
  Pericardial effusion
- **Hypoalbuminemia**
  Chronic hepatic disease
  Urinary loss (glomerulonephritis)
  Protein-losing enteropathy
  Malnutrition (parasitic or dietary)
- **Abdominal neoplasia**
  Carcinomatosis

- **Hemorrhage**

  Warfarin toxicity

  Trauma

Primary Diagnostics

- **Mucous membrane color and CRT:** Pallor and delayed CRT may be present in cases of congestive heart failure or hemorrhage.
- **Thoracic auscultation:** In most cases of cardiomyopathy, a murmur and/or a gallop rhythm is present. Heart sounds are muffled when pericardial effusion is present.
- **Abdominal palpation:** This technique confirms the presence of ascites and grades severity. Organomegaly is suggestive of congestive heart failure or neoplasia.
- **Peritoneal fluid analysis:** Determine whether fluid is a transudate, exudate, hemorrhage, or chyle. Transudates are suggestive of congestive heart failure or hypoalbuminemia. Modified transudates are suggestive of feline infectious peritonitis and other infectious diseases or neoplasia.
- **CBC:** Evaluate for anemia.
- **Chemistry profile:** These tests may reveal hypoalbuminemia, elevation of liver enzymes, or low BUN (suggestive of hepatic insufficiency).
- **Radiography:** This is usually unrewarding when ascites is present other than to confirm the presence of ascites.

Ancillary Diagnostics

- **Bile acids:** Elevation of preprandial and postprandial bile acids are supportive of chronic liver disease.
- **Abdominal ultrasonography:** Ultrasound is indicated if abdominal disease is suspected.
- **Echocardiography:** An echocardiogram is indicated if cardiac disease is suspected.
- **Coronavirus test:** This should be performed when feline infectious peritonitis is suspected. See Chapter 54 for interpretation.

Diagnostic Notes

- The first condition to be ruled out when ascites is present in cats is feline infectious peritonitis.
- Analysis of peritoneal fluid should always be performed when ascites is present.
- Conditions that may mimic ascites include hepatomegaly, splenomegaly, obesity, large neoplasms, pyometra, hydrometra, pregnancy, and advanced obstipation.

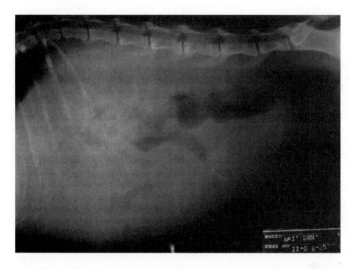

FIGURE 5.1. Ascites: Lateral radiography of ascites in a cat. The presence of fluid results in loss of distinction between abdominal organs. Scattered gas densities are seen within the intestinal tract.

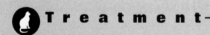

Treatment

Primary Therapeutics

- **Abdominocentesis:** This is essential when effusion is interfering with respiration. Approximately 50 to 75% of the ascites may be removed with minimal risk if a moderately sized (18 to 22 gauge) catheter is used.

Secondary Therapeutics

- **Furosemide:** This drug is indicated if ascites is secondary to congestive heart failure. A dose of 0.25–0.50 mg/kg SID is usually effective.
- **Address the underlying disease:** See specific chapters for guidelines.

Therapeutic Notes

Periodic abdominocentesis is better tolerated than long-term aggressive diuretic use.

Prognosis

The prognosis is variable depending upon the exact cause of the ascites. Most cats with respiratory distress can be stabilized with abdominocentesis.

Suggested Reading

Ettinger SJ. Ascites, peritonitis, and other causes of abdominal enlargement. In: Ettinger SJ, ed. Textbook of veterinary internal medicine, 3rd ed. Philadelphia: WB Saunders, 1993;131–138.

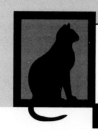

CHAPTER 6

Cardiopulmonary Arrest

John-Karl Goodwin

Overview

C ardiopulmonary arrest (CPA) is an immediately life-threatening condition that requires prompt recognition and appropriate intervention in order to restore circulatory function. In CPA, cessation of effective cardiac contractions and ventilation quickly leads to widespread hypoxia, with cerebral death occurring within 4 to 5 minutes.

CPA is usually a grave development, with survival rates of 2 to 5% reported even with optimal therapy. Considering this, the clinician should place a major emphasis on the recognition of impending CPA. Reversal of abnormalities placing the cat at risk of CPA are generally much more successful than cardiopulmonary resuscitation itself.

Signs of CPA include loss of consciousness, dilated pupils, agonal or absent respiration, absent heart sounds and arterial pulsations, cyanosis, and often opisthotonus. These signs may be abrupt and dramatic in a previously healthy cat or may occur rather inapparently in a moribund case.

D i a g n o s i s

Differential Diagnoses

Virtually any pathophysiologic state can deteriorate to the point at which CPA occurs. The most common clinical disorders predisposing cats to CPA are listed below.

Cardiopulmonary Disease

- Congestive heart failure (secondary to cardiomyopathy or other primary cardiac disease)
- Obstructive airway disease
- Heartworm disease

- Trauma (myocardial contusions, traumatic myocarditis)
- Pleural effusion
- Neoplasia
- Hemorrhage
- Trauma, surgical

Systemic Abnormalities

- Severe acid-base disturbances
- Severe electrolyte disturbances (e.g., hyperkalemia secondary to urethral obstruction)
- Overwhelming sepsis or endotoxemia

Other

- Drugs—particularly anesthetic agents
- Surges in parasympathetic tone (as may occur with tracheal intubation, manipulation of ocular, laryngeal, or pharyngeal areas) may precipitate CPA.

Primary Diagnostics

- Mucous membrane color and CRT: Look for pallor or cyanosis. CRT may be delayed.
- **Thoracic auscultation:** Look for absence of respiratory or heart sounds. In some cases, extreme bradycardia may be detected.
- **Electrocardiography:** Look for asystole (absence of complexes), slow ventricular escape rhythm, and idioventricular rhythm.

Ancillary Diagnostics

- Blood gas analysis: Look for severe hypoxemia, hypercapnia, and acidosis.

Diagnostic Notes

Intensive monitoring (vital signs, mucous membrane color, electrocardiograph) of cats with conditions predisposing them to CPA is essential.

 T r e a t m e n t

Prevention

- **Correct hypoxemia:** For anesthetized cats, discontinue anesthetic, increase oxygen flow, and confirm proper endotracheal tube placement. For cats with pulmonary edema, administer diuretics and supplemental oxygen.

- **Thoracocentesis:** This should be performed if significant pleural effusion is present.
- **Correct fluid deficits and electrolyte or acid-base disturbances**
- **Correct cardiac arrhythmias:** See Chapter 4.

Cardiopulmonary Resuscitation

- **ABCDs** of CPR:

  A = Airway: Clear the airway of any obstructive material. Endotracheal intubation should be performed, and tracheostomy should be considered if complete obstruction exists.

  B = Breathing: Provide respiratory support if spontaneous respiration is absent or insufficient. Provide 100% oxygen with an Ambu bag, through the reservoir bag of an anesthesia machine, or via a mechanical ventilator. Recent guidelines recommend rapid (2 to 3 per second) respirations, which should occur simultaneously with cardiac compressions.

  C = Circulation: External chest compression should occur at a rapid rate (2 to 3 per second). Displace the chest wall approximately 30% with each compression. Lateral recumbency is preferred for cats. Internal chest compressions are less likely in the cat to improve efficacy of CPR.

  D = Drugs: Administer atropine (0.02–0.05 mg/kg IV or 0.2–0.5 mg/kg intratracheally [IT]) if asystole or severe bradycardia is present. Give epinephrine (0.2 mg/kg [1 mL per 5 kg of the 1:1000 concentration] IV, or twice that if given IT). This may be repeated every 3 to 5 minutes. Give bicarbonate (0.5–1.0 mEq/kg IV) if acidosis or severe hyperkalemia present or if arrest duration has exceeded 10 minutes. Calcium is no longer recommended for routine CPR.

Therapeutic Notes

Intracardiac administration of emergency drugs is not recommended. If a central venous catheter is not available, administer drugs (atropine, epinephrine, lidocaine) intratracheally. Dilute the drugs with 5 to 10 mL of sterile saline and administer them through a catheter placed within the endotracheal (ET) tube. The tip of the catheter should be at the level of the carina. **The IT dose of emergency drugs is twice the IV dose.**

Defibrillation is rarely achieved with drugs. A defibrillator should be available for CPR, especially in critical care and emergency clinics.

A flowchart of ABCD steps should be placed in surgery and the intensive care area. Organization of efforts is essential. Prepare technicians with mock arrest situations. All technicians should be familiar with basic CPR. Establish a mobile "crash cart" of supplies and drugs needed for CPR.

Prognosis

The prognosis is best when CPA is unexpected (e.g., during elective anesthesia), not associated with significant underlying disease, and promptly detected. Otherwise, the prognosis is very poor.

Suggested   Reading

Beardow AW, Dhupa N. Cardiopulmonary arrest and resuscitation. In: Miller MS, Tilley LP, eds. Manual of canine and feline cardiology, 2nd ed. Philadelphia: WB Saunders, 1995;425–446.

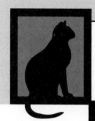

CHAPTER 7

Cervical Ventroflexion

Mitchell A. Crystal

Overview

Cervical ventroflexion is a syndrome characterized by muscle weakness or rigidity of the neck, causing an inability to raise the head. The neck may be so ventroflexed that the top of the head rests near or on the ground and the chin rests near the thoracic inlet. Other muscles of the body may also demonstrate weakness. The clinical signs are often acute in nature. The mechanism of cervical ventroflexion is variable depending on the etiology. It is uncertain why cervical muscles demonstrate greater weakness than other muscles in this syndrome. The differential diagnoses for cats with cervical ventroflexion are listed below. Hypokalemia is the most common cause of cervical ventroflexion. Organophosphate intoxication, thiamine-responsive disease, and hyperthyroidism are moderately common causes of this syndrome.

 Diagnosis

Differential Diagnoses

- Ammonium chloride toxicity (causes acidosis, which leads to intracellular potassium depletion)
- Polymyositis
- Diabetes mellitus
- Hypernatremia
- Hyperthyroidism
- Hypokalemia
- Idiopathic
- Myasthenia gravis
- Chronic organophosphate toxicity
- Portosystemic shunt
- Thiamine-responsive disease

Primary Diagnostics

- **History:** Investigate the possibility of exposure to ammonium chloride (such as urinary acidifiers) and organophosphates. Investigate the presence of other clinical signs that might suggest the etiology, such as polyuria and polydipsia (diabetes mellitus, hyperthyroidism, hypokalemia, portosystemic shunt), increased appetite with concurrent weight loss (diabetes mellitus, hyperthyroidism), neurologic signs (organophosphate toxicity, portosystemic shunt, thiamine-responsive disease), ptyalism (portosystemic shunt), and muscle pain or rigidity (hypokalemia, idiopathic polymyositis, thiamine deficiency).

- **Chemistry profile:** Evaluate for abnormalities in glucose (diabetes mellitus), sodium (hypernatremia), potassium (ammonium chloride toxicity, hypokalemia), liver enzymes (hyperthyroidism, portosystemic shunt), albumin (portosystemic shunt), creatine kinase (hypernatremia, hypokalemia, idiopathic polymyositis), and BUN and creatinine (hypokalemia secondary to renal disease).

- **Urinalysis:** Evaluate for glucosuria (diabetes mellitus) and decreased specific gravity (diabetes mellitus, hyperthyroidism, hypokalemia, portosystemic shunt).

- **Total T4:** This hormone is increased with hyperthyroidism.

Ancillary Diagnostics

- **Thoracic radiography:** Megaesophagus or thymic masses are occasionally seen in cats with myasthenia gravis.

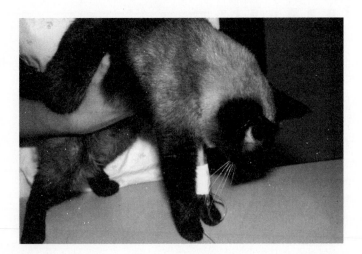

FIGURE 7.1. Cervical ventroflexion: Muscle weakness results in the cat's inability to lift its head.

- **Edrophonium chloride challenge:** 0.25 to 0.5 mg IV results in resolution of cervical ventroflexion and muscle weakness in most cats with myasthenia gravis.
- **Acetylcholine receptor antibody titer:** This is increased in most cases of acquired myasthenia gravis.
- **Serum cholinesterase activity:** This is reduced more than 50% in cats with organophosphate toxicity.
- **Fasting and postprandial serum bile acids:** These are increased in cats with portosystemic shunt.
- **Abdominal imaging:** Survey radiographs, ultrasound, per rectal ^{99m}Tc pertechnetate portal scintigraphy, and positive contrast portography often demonstrate abnormalities in cats with portosystemic shunts.
- **Electromyography/repetitive nerve stimulation:** Abnormalities are seen in cats with ammonium chloride toxicity, hypokalemia, idiopathic polymyositis, myasthenia gravis, and organophosphate toxicity.

Diagnostic Notes

Primary diagnostic tests should be performed in all cats with cervical ventroflexion along with a total T4 in cats over 7 years of age. Ancillary diagnostic tests should be performed if indicated by history, clinical signs, or chemistry abnormalities or if primary tests are nondiagnostic.

 T r e a t m e n t

Primary Therapeutics

Treat the primary disease process:

- **Thiamine (vitamin B$_1$ 25–50 mg/cat IM SID × 3 days).** All cats with cervical ventroflexion should receive thiamine because there is no diagnostic test available for thiamine deficiency, and cats on normal diets can occasionally develop thiamine-responsive cervical ventroflexion. Improvement is usually seen within 2 days.
- **Fluid support:** Administer fluid therapy if dehydration or renal disease is present or if prolonged lack of fluid intake is anticipated. If hypokalemia is present, potassium chloride should be added to the fluids at the rate of 40 to 60 mEq/L (for non–potassium-containing fluids).
- **Nutritional support:** Administer nutritional therapy if prolonged anorexia is anticipated.

Therapeutic Notes

Creatine kinase should be assessed prior to administration of any intramuscular (IM) medications.

P r o g n o s i s

The prognosis is excellent if the underlying disease can be identified and treated. Idiopathic polymyositis and myasthenia gravis carry less favorable prognoses as they are difficult to treat and may not respond to therapy.

S u g g e s t e d   R e a d i n g s

Joseph RJ, Carrillo JM, Lennon VA. Myasthenia gravis in the cat. *J Vet Int Med* 1988;2(2): 75–79.

Taboada J. Ventroflexion of the neck in cats. Proceedings of the Twelfth Annual Veterinary Medical Forum 1994;385–389.

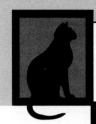

CHAPTER 8

Chronic Nasal Discharge

Gary D. Norsworthy

Overview

A nasal discharge that is present for over 30 days is considered to be chronic. There are at least eight types of disease that may be responsible, so a systematic diagnostic approach is important. The nature of the discharge is not indicative of the etiology; the presence of blood in the discharge does not correlate as strongly with neoplasia as it does in the dog. Affected cats usually have periodic episodes of severe sneezing. Most cats are not systemically affected, with the exception of cats with fungal infections or neoplasia.

 D i a g n o s i s

Differential Diagnoses

- **Viral infection**
  Feline herpesvirus, feline calicivirus
- **Bacterial infection**
  Pseudomonas aeruginosa, Proteus mirabilis, Staphylococcus aureus, others
- **Fungal infection**
  Cryptococcus neoformans, Histoplasma capsulatum
- **Neoplasia**
  Adenocarcinoma, lymphosarcoma, others
- **Inflammatory polyps**
- **Foreign body**
- **Food allergy**
- **Atopy**

Primary Diagnostics

- **Age of onset:** Cats with an age of onset of 6 years or less are more likely to have viral and bacterial infections. Cats with an age of onset of over 10 years are more likely to have neoplasia. The other diseases are not age-related.
- **Radiographs:** Lateral, open-mouth, and skyline views should be taken to localize the infection. It is important to know whether or not the frontal sinuses are involved.
- **Culture and cytology:** After the site of the lesion is identified by radiographs, a 20 or 22 gauge needle is drilled through the hard palate into the lesion. Material is aspirated for culture and cytology. If the site is chosen properly, a diagnostic-quality sample may be obtained. If this is not feasible or successful, a 3.5 Fr catheter is passed 1 to 2 cm into the nasal cavity and 10 mL of saline is flushed through the nasal cavity. The material is caught on a 2×2-inch gauze square in the pharynx. It is important that a cuffed endotracheal tube be in place. This method is not as likely to recover a diagnostic sample as is the aspiration technique.
- **Endoscopy:** A 2 to 3 mm rhinoscope can permit visualization of some aspects of the nasal cavity and recovery of material for histopathology.
- **Rhinotomy:** The nasal cavity can be explored surgically via an incision through the nasal bones. This procedure permits recovery of material for histopathology and the opportunity to remove foreign bodies.

Ancillary Diagnostics

- **Traumatic nasal flush:** This procedure is used to recover material for histopathology. The catheter should not be advanced past the medial canthus of the eye to prevent damaging the brain.
- **Viral culture:** This procedure is useful if it can be performed properly. Contact your laboratory for specific instructions.
- **Fungal serology:** False negatives are common, but high or increasing titers are indicative of fungal exposure (though not necessarily disease). Generally, titers for cryptococcosis are more reliable than those for other fungi.

Diagnostic Notes

- Radiographs are not sufficient to differentiate neoplasia from inflammatory polyps or infections. However, neoplasia tends to produce unilateral, aggressive lesions.
- Neoplasia often causes a distortion of the nasal planum or the entire nasal area.
- Inflammatory polyps often cause pressure necrosis of the nasal bone, resulting in draining tracts near the eye.

🐈 T r e a t m e n t

Primary Therapeutics

- **Antibiotics:** Antibiotics may offer temporary relief from most conditions because most are complicated with secondary bacterial infections. Enrofloxacin (4 mg/kg PO BID) is often effective, but others also may be effective on a short-term basis.
- **Hydration:** Fluid therapy, even when dehydration is not present, is helpful in thinning nasal secretions and making the cat more comfortable.

Therapeutic Notes

- Because there are so many differential diagnoses, it is imperative that a thorough workup be performed so that proper therapy may be instituted.
- See Chapters 90 and 91 for more specific therapy.

P r o g n o s i s

The prognosis depends upon the specific diagnosis. Many infections are treatable medically or surgically. Most tumors are adenocarcinoma or lymphosarcoma and have poor prognoses. Nasal polyps are difficult to remove completely, so they often recur. If the foreign body is removed, foreign body-induced nasal discharge is curable. Atopy and food allergies are often manageable.

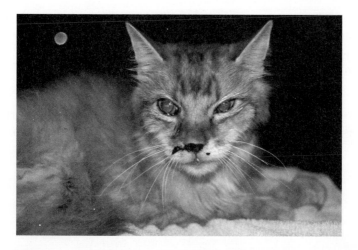

FIGURE 8.1. Chronic nasal discharge: The presence of blood in the nasal discharge does not correlate as highly with neoplasia in the cat as it does in the dog.

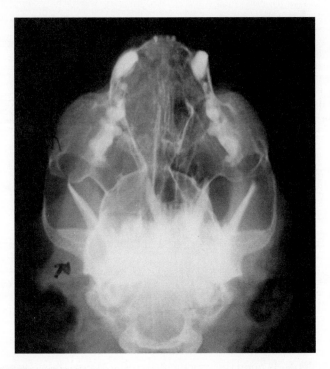

FIGURE 8.2. Radiographically, both nasal infection and neoplasia can result in increased density in the nasal cavity, as seen in this open-mouth view.

Suggested Readings

Cape L. Feline idiopathic chronic rhinosinusitis: a retrospective study of 30 cases. *J Am Anim Hosp Assoc* 1992;28:149–155.

Norsworthy GD. Chronic nasal discharge. In: Norsworthy GD, ed. Feline practice. Philadelphia: JB Lippincott, 1993;266–273.

Norsworthy GD. Finding the cause of chronic nasal discharge in cats. *Vet Med* 1995;90(11):1038–1047.

Norsworthy GD. Treating chronic nasal discharge in cats. *Vet Med* 1995;90(11):1048–1054.

O'Brien RT, Evans SM, Wortman JA, Hendrick MJ. Radiographic findings in cats with intranasal neoplasia or chronic rhinitis: 29 cases (1982–1988). *J Am Vet Med Assoc* 1996;208(3):385–389.

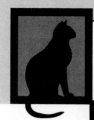

CHAPTER 9

Coughing

Gary D. Norsworthy

Overview

Coughing is not a common occurrence in the cat. Although it is closely related to cardiac disease in the dog, cats in heart failure typically do not cough.

Diagnosis

Differential Diagnoses

- Bronchial asthma
- Heartworm disease
- Chylothorax
- Pulmonary larval migration
- Lungworm disease
- Tracheal disease

Primary Diagnostics

- **Thoracic radiograph:** This is the test that should be done first to determine the presence of bronchial asthma, pleural effusion (including chylothorax), heartworm disease, and tracheal disease.

Ancillary Diagnostics

- **CBC:** Many cats with bronchial asthma and some cats with heartworm disease and lungworms have a peripheral eosinophilia.
- **Bronchoalveolar lavage:** This can be a meaningful way to collect samples for cytologic examination.

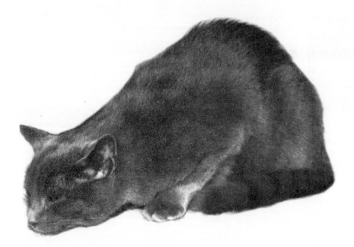

FIGURE 9.1. Coughing: This is the characteristic coughing position assumed by most allergic cats. The cat sits in a crouched position with its neck extended.

- **Lung aspiration:** The finding of large numbers of eosinophils is strongly suggestive of bronchial asthma. Heartworm disease also produces a transient pulmonary eosinophilia.
- **Thoracic fluid analysis:** When pleural effusion is present, this an important test.
- **Fecal flotation:** This will detect the presence of ascarid ova; however, one negative sample does not rule out their presence.
- **Baermann fecal examination:** This is important for cats from lungworm-endemic areas.
- **Heartworm antibody and antigen tests:** These tests should be performed when the thoracic radiographs reveal enlarged or tortuous pulmonary arteries.
- **Tracheal endoscopy:** This procedure will evaluate the trachea for the presence of abnormal secretions, stricture, or collapse. The use of a brush can provide meaningful cytologic samples.

T r e a t m e n t

Therapeutic Notes

Typically, coughing in cats is not life threatening or debilitating, although it may be a sign of serious disease. It is not necessary to suppress the cough. One's efforts should be directed at determining and treating the underlying cause.

Prognosis

The prognosis is variable depending upon the underlying disease.

Suggested Readings

Levy JK, Ford RB. Diseases of the upper respiratory tract. In: Sherding RG, ed. The cat: diseases and clinical management, 2nd ed. New York: Churchill Livingstone, 1994;947–978.

Norsworthy GD. Dyspnea. In: Norsworthy GD, ed. Feline practice. Philadelphia: JB Lippincott, 1993;172–190.

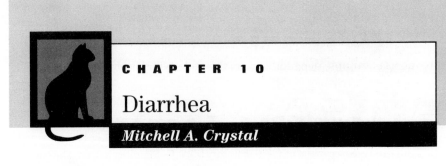

CHAPTER 10

Diarrhea

Mitchell A. Crystal

Overview

Diarrhea results from excessive fecal water. There are four pathophysiologic types of diarrhea: osmotic, secretory, altered permeability (exudative), and altered motility. Osmotic diarrhea is caused by an increase in unabsorbed solutes within the gastrointestinal lumen, which leads to an increase in fecal water. An increase in unabsorbed solutes may result from dietary overload, maldigestion/malabsorption (e.g., exocrine pancreatic insufficiency [EPI], lymphangiectasia), and small intestinal mucosal disease (e.g., inflammatory bowel disease [IBD]). Secretory diarrhea is caused by excessive secretion of fluid into the gastrointestinal lumen. An increase in gastrointestinal fluid secretion may result from bacterial enterotoxins, cholinergic agonists, deconjugated bile acids, and hydroxy fatty acids. Altered permeability is caused by disease processes that damage or destroy the gastrointestinal mucosa, leading to maldigestion, malabsorption, and leakage of fluid, electrolytes, and large particles into the gastrointestinal tract and, subsequently, diarrhea. Altered permeability may be caused by ulcers/erosions (e.g., nonsteroidal anti-inflammatory drugs, liver disease), mucosal inflammation (e.g., viral enteritis, IBD), and mucosal infiltration (e.g., lymphoma). Altered motility leads to diarrhea as a result of decreased fluid absorption owing to decreased contact time between the intestinal absorptive epithelium and the luminal contents (decreased gastrointestinal transit time). The cause is most often a decrease in rhythmic segmentation and much less commonly an increase in peristalsis. Altered motility may contribute to other mechanisms of diarrhea and is uncommonly the primary disorder causing diarrhea, such as irritable bowel syndrome and dysautonomia. Determining the pathophysiologic mechanism causing the diarrhea helps to determine the best initial supportive care for the patient.

Classifying diarrhea based on chronicity, severity, and anatomical site is clinically helpful in determining the etiologic/specific cause of the problem. This helps direct the best initial diagnostic approach and is also helpful in selecting the initial therapeutic management. Diarrhea should be categorized as acute versus chronic, serious versus nonserious, and small bowel versus large bowel. Acute diarrhea is

TABLE 10.1.

Differentiating Features of Small and Large Bowel Diarrhea

Characteristic	Small Bowel Diarrhea	Large Bowel Diarrhea
Frequency	2–3 times normal	>5 times normal
Volume	Increased	Normal to decreased
Type of blood if present	Melena	Frank
Presence of mucus	Absent	± Present
Dyschezia	Absent	Present
Urgency	Normal to mildly increased	Increased

less than and chronic diarrhea greater than 2 to 3 weeks in duration. Parameters indicating serious diarrhea include loss of 10% or more of body weight, dehydration of 3 to 5% or more, evidence of significant mucosal compromise (hemorrhagic diarrhea), severe electrolyte disturbances, and pyrexia greater than 104°F. Features of small and large bowel diarrhea are listed in Table 10.1.

The remainder of the assessment of the diarrhea patient includes listing specific diseases considered likely based on the above criteria. Both gastrointestinal and extragastrointestinal diseases should be included, as many metabolic, neoplastic, and infectious/inflammatory diseases may manifest gastrointestinal signs despite lacking primary gastrointestinal involvement. Differential diagnoses for diarrhea are listed below under diagnosis.

 D i a g n o s i s

Differential Diagnoses

- **Extragastrointestinal**
  Hyperthyroidism
  Renal failure
  Exocrine pancreatic insufficiency
  Hepatic disease
  Extragastrointestinal neoplasia
  FeLV/FIV-related diseases
- **Gastrointestinal**
  Nonspecific enterocolitis
  Food intolerance

Food allergy

Toxins

Infectious diseases (*Salmonella, Campylobacter*)

Parasites (nematodes, *Giardia, Cryptosporidium*)

Inflammatory bowel diseases

Neoplasia (lymphoma, carcinoma, and others)

Primary Diagnostics

- **Database (CBC, chemistry profile, and urinalysis):** A data base should be submitted to evaluate for liver disease (hyperbilirubinemia, decreased BUN, increased ALT, ALP, and GGT, bilirubinuria), renal disease (elevated BUN and creatinine with a decreased urine specific gravity), signs of hyperthyroidism (increased ALT or ALP, a mild increase in PCV, low urine specific gravity), and signs of lymphoma (occasional cats demonstrate circulating lymphoblasts and anemia). Protein-losing enteropathy from a variety of causes is an uncommon finding in cats with diarrhea (hypoalbuminemia, hypoglobulinemia).
- **Fecal:** A zinc sulfate flotation should be performed to evaluate for nematodes and *Giardia.*
- **Total T4:** This test should be performed on all cats over 10 years of age with diarrhea to evaluate for hyperthyroidism.
- **FeLV/FIV Test:** These tests are not confirmatory for specific disease but are good indicators that other diseases are likely to be present.

Ancillary Diagnostics

- **Feline-specific trypsin-like immunoreactivity (TLI):** A 12-hour fasting serum sample can be submitted to evaluate for EPI.
- **Fecal culture for *Salmonella* and *Campylobacter:*** Fecal samples can be submitted for *Salmonella* and *Campylobacter* culture and sensitivity. Samples are best submitted in special media (selenite or tetrathionate media for *Salmonella; Campylobacter* media for *Campylobacter*), as high numbers of normal enteric bacteria present in feces tend to overgrow and mask *Salmonella* and *Campylobacter* growth. A positive culture without evidence of other disease processes supports a diagnosis. A negative culture does not necessarily eliminate the possibility of infection (see Chapter 109).
- **Fecal evaluation for *Cryptosporidium*:** Feces and fecal smears can be submitted for concentration techniques and special staining. Fecal ELISA and IFA assays are also available at many laboratories.
- **Intestinal biopsy/histopathology:** This procedure should be performed in cases of chronic diarrhea to investigate for primary intestinal diseases after other noninvasive procedures have been completed. Biopsies may be

collected via endoscopy, exploratory laparotomy, or, in the case of diffuse or focal intestinal thickening greater than 2 to 3 cm, by ultrasound guidance. Histopathology may reveal IBD, alimentary lymphoma, and/or *Cryptosporidium.*

Diagnostic Notes

A complete diagnostic workup is indicated in cats with chronic diarrhea and acute, serious diarrhea. Cats with acute, nonserious diarrhea can be treated with supportive care without an extensive workup if fecal and quick assessment tests (PCV, total protein, glucose test strip, BUN strip, urine dipstick, and specific gravity) are unremarkable.

 T r e a t m e n t

Primary Therapeutics

- **Treat underlying disease:** This is the key to long-term cure.

- **Deworm:** Anthelminthics are indicated in indoor/outdoor cats even if a negative fecal is obtained. Fenbendazole at 25 mg/kg PO SID for 3 days, repeating in 2 to 3 weeks, is the drug of choice because it is effective against nematodes and *Giardia.*

- **Water only for 24–48 hours:** Osmotic diarrhea will resolve and altered permeability will improve. Removing food will not affect secretory diarrheas.

- **Oral isotonic glucose, amino acid, and electrolyte solutions:** These solutions will improve secretory diarrheas and may help with other types of diarrhea.

Secondary Therapeutics

- **Motility modifiers:** Diarrhea with a significant functional component may improve with opioid motility modifiers such as loperamide at 0.08–0.16 mg/kg PO BID, diphenoxylate at 0.05–0.1 mg/kg PO BID, or paregoric-containing solutions at 0.05–0.06 mg/kg PO BID.

- **Fluid and electrolytes:** Fluid and electrolyte therapy IV, SQ, or PO should be administered based on the degree of dehydration and the amount of fluid loss in the feces.

- **Omega-3 fatty acids:** These fatty acids have been shown to have anti-inflammatory effects on the gastrointestinal tract and may prove helpful in the management of IBD. Omega-3 fatty acid supplementation can be found as part of some balanced commercial cat foods (see Appendix E).

Therapeutic Notes

Fructo-oligosaccharides are fibers that are digested by intestinal bacteria. These nutrients are believed to increase beneficial and decrease pathogenic populations of intestinal bacteria. In doing this, they may help promote intestinal mucosal health by enhancing short-chain fatty acid production (which intestinal epithelial cells use for a majority of their energy), improving intestinal water absorption, reducing putrefactive substances, and suppressing toxin release. These nutrients are currently used in some human and canine foods and in the future may prove to be beneficial in feline intestinal health.

P r o g n o s i s

The prognosis varies depending on the cause of the diarrhea.

S u g g e s t e d   R e a d i n g s

Burrows CF, Batt RM, Sherding RG. Diseases of the small intestine. In: Ettinger SJ, Feldman EC, eds. Textbook of veterinary internal medicine, 4th ed. Philadelphia: WB Saunders, 1995;1169–1232.

Guilford WG, Strombeck DR. Classification, pathophysiology, and symptomatic treatment of diarrheal diseases. In: Strombeck's small animal gastroenterology, 3rd ed. Philadelphia: WB Saunders, 1996;351–366.

Lieb MS, Matz ME. Diseases of the large intestine. In: Ettinger SJ, Feldman EC, eds. Textbook of veterinary internal medicine, 4th ed. Philadelphia: WB Saunders, 1995;1232–1260.

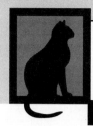

CHAPTER 11

Draining Tracts and Nodules

Gary D. Norsworthy

Overview

T here are numerous common and rare diseases that cause either the formation of a draining tract or the occurrence of one or more nodules. Few can be diagnosed on clinical appearance alone, so an aggressive diagnostic approach is indicated. Some of these diseases are limited to specific geographic regions in the United States.

 Differential Diagnoses

Relatively Common Diseases

- **Systemic mycoses**
  Cryptococcosis
  Histoplasmosis
  Coccidioidomycosis
- **Neoplasia**
  Squamous cell carcinoma
  Basal cell carcinoma
  Cutaneous lymphosarcoma
  Others
- **Cuterebriasis**

Relatively Uncommon Diseases

  Blastomycosis
  Pemphigus foliaceus/erythematosus
  Botryomycosis
  Actinomycosis

Nocardiosis

Tuberculosis

Feline leprosy

Atypical mycobacteriosis

Phaeohyphomycosis

Mycetoma

Sporotrichosis

Xanthomatosis

 D i a g n o s i s

Primary Diagnostics

- **Biopsy and histopathology:** This is the test of choice for most of the diseases in this category.
- **Aspiration cytology:** This test can be diagnostic in many of these diseases; therefore, it is good practice to perform it prior to biopsy because of its minimally invasive nature.

Ancillary Diagnostics

- **Culture:** Culturing of systemic fungi is not a common practice because of the public health aspects related to growing the organisms. Most of these

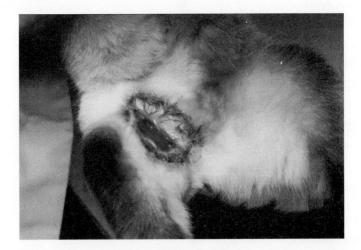

FIGURE 11.1. Draining tracts and nodules: This draining tract in the axillary space in not characteristic of any specific disease. It is important that diagnostics be performed to narrow the differential list.

organisms are fastidious or require very specific media or growing conditions. Culturing is unrewarding in most cases.

Diagnostic Notes

The lesions caused by many of these diseases are clinically indistinguishable from common fight wound abscesses, so they are generally treated accordingly with antibiotics. Any wound that does not promptly respond to therapy should be biopsied.

 T r e a t m e n t

Primary Therapeutics

There is no symptomatic treatment that is likely to be effective in many of these diseases. Few of them respond to antibiotics. Therefore, obtaining a confirmed diagnosis is imperative.

P r o g n o s i s

The prognosis is dependent on the diagnosis.

S u g g e s t e d   R e a d i n g s

Merchant SR. The skin: fungal diseases. In: Norsworthy GD, ed. Feline practice. Philadelphia: JB Lippincott, 1993;504–510.

Moriello KA. Diseases of the skin. In: Sherding RG, ed. The cat: diseases and clinical management, 2nd ed. Philadelphia: WB Saunders, 1994;1907–1968.

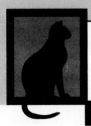

CHAPTER 12

Dyspnea

Gary D. Norsworthy

Overview

Dyspnea is defined as difficulty breathing. The term is frequently used to describe polypnea or tachypnea, two terms that mean rapid breathing, which is more common than true dyspnea in cats. Although the cat's normal respiratory rate is 20 to 60 breaths per minute, a rate over 50 is suspicious for disease. The causes of dyspnea are numerous; they may be divided into categories according to the part of the respiratory system that is involved in their pathogenesis. Because many dyspneic cats are fragile patients, initial care and assessment must be handled quickly and judiciously.

 Diagnosis

Differential Diagnoses

The diseases that cause dyspnea have been classified in the following manner:

- **Oxygen deprivation**

  Anemia

  Methemoglobinemia

- **Upper airway**

  Rhinitis

  Nasopharyngeal masses

  Tracheal collapse or compression

- **Pulmonary/lung**

  Pulmonary edema (cardiac or pulmonary disease)

  Pneumonia (viral, bacterial, fungal, foreign body, parasitic)

  Pulmonary trauma (contusion, torsion, cysts)

Heartworm disease

Bronchial asthma

Emphysema

Pulmonary neoplasia (primary or metastatic)

- **Pleural space**

Chylothorax (primary or secondary)

Pyothorax

Hemothorax (trauma, coagulopathy, bleeding disorder, torsion),

Pneumothorax (trauma, parasitic, iatrogenic)

Diaphragmatic hernia (trauma, congenital)

Neoplasia (lymphosarcoma, mesothelioma, thymoma, pulmonary neoplasia)

Hydrothorax (cardiogenic, pericardial disease, mediastinal mass, feline infectious peritonitis, diaphragmatic hernia, lung lobe torsion)

Primary Diagnostics

- **Mucous membrane and tongue color:** The presence of cyanosis indicates that a respiratory crisis is present and dictates that emergency therapeutic measures be taken before further diagnostics.
- **Auscultation:** Lung and heart sounds should be assessed initially.
- **Radiographs:** The most meaningful diagnostic test is a set of well-exposed radiographs of the chest, cervical area, and/or skull. The presence of pleural effusion must be determined because it is frequently present in dyspneic cats.
- **Thoracentesis:** Aspiration of the pleural space can determine the presence of air or fluid.
- **Pleural fluid analysis:** If fluid is recovered from the pleural space, the following tests should be performed: (*a*) Total protein content and/or specific gravity; (*b*) white blood cell count; and (*c*) cytology.

Ancillary Diagnostics

- **Pleural fluid analysis:** If bacteria are found on cytology, aerobic and anaerobic cultures should be performed. If the fluid is milky white in color, serum and fluid triglyceride levels should be compared.
- **Celiogram:** If diaphragmatic hernia is suspected, but the chest radiographs are inconclusive, this study should be performed.
- **FeLV antigen test:** If the cytology is suggestive of lymphosarcoma, this test should be done. It will not rule this disease in or out, but it will document a contagious state.

- **CBC:** If bronchial asthma is suspected, the diagnosis is supported by the presence of eosinophilia.
- **Tracheal wash:** This can be helpful in determining the presence of asthma and certain pneumonias.
- **Echocardiography:** This should be performed when cardiomyopathy is suspected.
- **Coronavirus test:** This should be performed when feline infectious peritonitis is suspected. See Chapter 54 for interpretation.

Diagnostic Notes

- If a radiograph is not feasible (because of the critical condition of the cat or as a result of financial limitations), thoracentesis that removes fluid or air can stabilize the patient; if fluid is recovered, it can be analyzed as part of the diagnostic workup.
- In a 4-kg cat, a minimum of 50 mL of pleural effusion must be present for it to be radiographically discernible.

 T r e a t m e n t

Primary Therapeutics

- **Oxygen:** Placing the cat in an oxygen cage or oxygen tent can be life saving.
- **Cage confinement:** Even if an oxygen cage is not available, placing the cat in a cage away from the sight or sound of dogs or other cats can help to

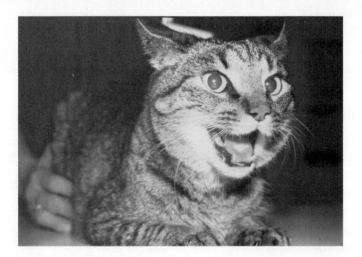

FIGURE 12.1. Dyspnea: Open-mouth breathing is a sign of serious airway obstruction and demands immediate diagnostics and therapy.

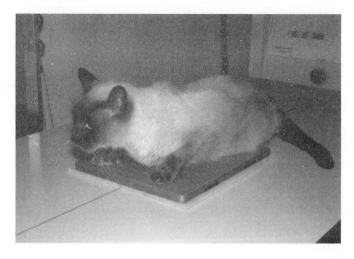

FIGURE 12.2. The safest position for radiographing a dyspneic cat is the ventrodorsal view. Many cats will lie unrestrained for the radiograph to be made.

stabilize the cat. This confinement may be necessary between various diagnostic procedures.

- **Thoracentesis:** The removal of 60+ mL of air or fluid can stabilize the cat.

Secondary Therapeutics

- **Furosemide:** One 25-mg IV dose can be life saving to cats with pulmonary edema. Its only contraindication is dehydration.

- **Corticosteroids:** One dose of a short-acting steroid (5 mg of dexamethasone sodium phosphate) can be very helpful to a cat with severe bronchial asthma. Because these cats are likely to have secondary bacterial pneumonia, steroids should not be repeated until antibiotics are started.

Therapeutic Notes

The administration of IV fluids should be done very cautiously or not at all. Catheter placement can be stressful, and fluid overload can be fatal to cats with pulmonary edema or other serious lung disease.

Prognosis

The prognosis is variable depending on the condition at the time of presentation, the response to emergency treatment, and the primary disease.

S u g g e s t e d   R e a d i n g s

Henik RA, Yeager AE. Bronchopulmonary diseases. In: Sherding RG, ed. The cat: diseases and clinical management, 2nd ed. New York: Churchill Livingstone, 1994;979–1052.

Norsworthy GD. Dyspnea. In: Norsworthy GD, ed. Feline practice. Philadelphia: JB Lippincott, 1993;172–190.

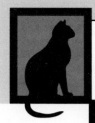

CHAPTER 13

Dystocia

Gary D. Norsworthy

Overview

D ystocia is difficulty during parturition. Causes can generally be classified into one of two categories: maternal or fetal.

 D i a g n o s i s

Differential Diagnoses

- **Maternal**
  Geriatrics
  Obesity
  Narrowed birth canal
  Uterine contraction disorders (primary and exhaustive)
  Uterine torsion
  Uterine rupture
  Ectopic pregnancy
- **Fetal**
  Excessive fetal size (often seen with litters of one or two kittens)
  Excessive fetal head size (often seen in brachycephalic breeds)
  Fetal death
  Fetal morphologic abnormalities
  Fetal malposition

Primary Diagnostics

- **Clinical signs:** Dystocia should be suspected when any one of these occur: (*a*) 20 minutes of intense labor without birth; (*b*) 10 minutes of intense labor without birth of a kitten in the birth canal; (*c*) acute depression (usually associated with uterine rupture); (*d*) fever; or (*e*) fresh vaginal bleeding of more than 10 minutes' duration.

- **Palpation:** This is the least accurate test, but it can permit one to make some determination of fetal size.
- **Radiology:** Fetal size, number, and position can be assessed. In some cases, fetal death can be determined by the presence of intrauterine gas or the collapsing of fetal cranial bones. The size and shape of the birth canal can be assessed.

Ancillary Diagnostics

- **Ultrasound:** Fetal viability can be determined most accurately by observance of fetal movement and cardiac contraction.

Diagnostic Notes

The use of radiographs frequently causes one to underestimate litter size.

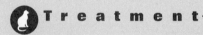 T r e a t m e n t

Primary Therapeutics

- **Oxytocin:** This drug is given at 2–4 U IM every 20 to 30 minutes for two or three injections. Additional doses are not recommended.
- **Calcium:** When combined with oxytocin, calcium gluconate (1–2 mL of a 10% solution given slowly IV) can be even more effective than oxytocin alone.

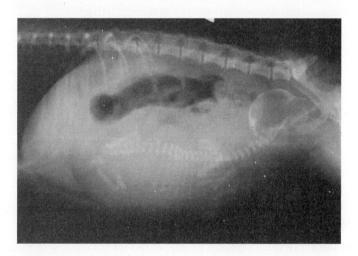

FIGURE 13.1. Dystocia: A large kitten's head may be too large to traverse the pelvic canal. This is most common in brachycephalic breeds.

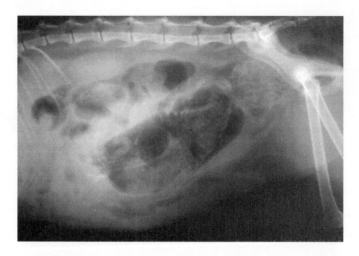

FIGURE 13.2. The presence of gas within the uterus is a sign of fetal death.

- **Cesarean section:** Surgical removal of the kittens is recommended when oxytocin and calcium are not effective, if uterine disease is present (inertia, torsion, rupture), or if the pelvic:fetal ratio prohibits fetal passage.

Therapeutic Notes

- The queen can voluntarily control parturition, so environmental stress can prolong it or delay its onset.
- Cesarean section can be a lifesaving procedure for both the queen and kittens. It should not be delayed unnecessarily.

Prognosis

The prognosis is excellent for the queen and kittens if medical or surgical intervention occurs quickly.

Suggested Readings

Eilts BE, Paccamonti DL, Causey R. In: Norsworthy GD, ed. Feline practice. Philadelphia: JB Lippincott, 1993;458–476.

Johnson CA. Female reproduction and disorders of the female reproductive tract. In: Sherding RG, ed. The cat: diseases and clinical management, 2nd ed. Philadelphia: WB Saunders, 1994;1855–1876.

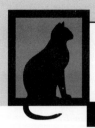

CHAPTER 14

Fever

Mitchell A. Crystal

Overview

Fever is an elevation of body temperature in response to a disease process or drug. Fever (or pyrexia) should be differentiated from hyperthermia, as causes and therapies differ. Fever describes elevations in body temperature owing to endogenous heat formation secondary to an elevation of the hypothalamic thermoregulatory set point. Hyperthermia describes elevations in body temperature with the thermoregulatory set point at its normal setting, such as those resulting from an external heat source or excessive activity. Fevers result from disease processes or drugs that either directly or indirectly (via release of pyrogenic substances, which cause cytokine production from leukocytes) elevate the thermoregulatory set point. Disease processes that cause fevers include infectious/inflammatory, neoplastic, and immune-mediated diseases. Common drugs that can cause fever in the cat include cephalosporins, griseofulvin, methimazole, penicillins, propylthiouracil, sulfa or trimethoprim/sulfa drugs, tetracyclines, and thiacetarsamide; of these, the tetracyclines are most likely to cause fever. Clinical signs of fever in the cat include lethargy, anorexia, and atypical behavior such as hiding or irritability. Other clinical signs of the underlying disease causing the fever may also be present.

The term fever of unknown origin (FUO) is often used to describe cats that have been febrile for 1 to 2 weeks, have no obvious cause of fever, and have no abnormalities on routine diagnostic evaluation. This syndrome is common in cats.

Diagnosis

Primary Diagnostics

- **History:** Question the owner about the cat's environment (indoor or outdoor), travel history (to areas endemic for infectious diseases), and drug therapy. Review vaccination history.

- **Physical examination:** Examine closely for wounds and abscesses, internal or external masses, lymphadenopathy, joint effusion, abnormal pulmonary auscultation, and pain. A complete ophthalmologic examination (anterior chamber and retina) will sometimes disclose evidence of infectious diseases.
- **Database (CBC, chemistry profile, urinalysis, FeLV antigen, FIV antibody):** Abnormalities may suggest neoplastic, inflammatory or infectious diseases, or organ dysfunction.
- **Thoracic radiography:** Abnormalities may suggest neoplastic or infectious diseases.

Ancillary Diagnostics

- **Abdominal radiographs or ultrasound:** Abnormalities may suggest neoplastic or infectious diseases.
- **Blood and urine culture and sensitivity:** These may be helpful but are often nondiagnostic and expensive.

Diagnostic Notes

Because less body fat decreases the diagnostic quality of radiographs, abdominal ultrasound is often more helpful than abdominal radiographs in normal-to-thin cats with fever. Abdominal palpation approaches the usefulness of abdominal radiography in these cases.

FeLV/FIV tests should be repeated 1 to 2 months following an initial positive or negative test in indoor/outdoor cats with FUO.

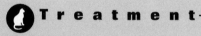

Treatment

Primary Therapeutics

Treat the underlying disorder: This is the key to long-term care.
- **Fluid support:** This should be provided if needed for dehydration.
- **Antibiotics:** Because bacterial infections are a common cause of fever, a short course of therapy with a bactericidal, broad-spectrum antibiotic is indicated for cats with FUO.

Secondary Therapeutics

- **Nutritional support:** This may be needed if prolonged anorexia has occurred.
- **Antipyretics:** Use only when fever exceeds 106°F. Aspirin (10 mg/kg QOD PO) or dipyrone (25 mg/kg SID or BID IM, SQ, or IV) as needed to control fever.

Therapeutic Notes

Antipyretic agents should not be administered unless fever is greater than 106°F. Antipyretics will interfere with both the ability to follow the course of the disease as well as the effectiveness of and response to therapy. Fevers below 106°F will not lead to brain or organ damage or dysfunction.

Nonsteroidal anti-inflammatory drugs have prolonged elimination times in cats and should be used with caution to prevent toxicity.

Emphasize to the owner the importance of not administering acetaminophen.

Prognosis

The prognosis is variable depending on the underlying disorder. With appropriate support, most cats with FUO recover uneventfully.

Suggested Readings

Allen DG. Fever of unknown origin. In: Allen DG, ed. Small animal medicine. Philadelphia: JB Lippincott, 1991;53–60.

Greene CE. Fever. In: Green CE, ed. Infectious diseases of the dog and cat. Philadelphia: WB Saunders, 1990;64–71.

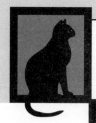

CHAPTER 15

Icterus

Sharon K. Fooshee

Overview

I cterus, a common clinical disorder in cats, occurs when excess bilirubin is deposited in tissues. Clinically apparent tissue icterus generally does not occur until serum levels of bilirubin exceed 2.0 mg/dL, whereas the serum is visually icteric at about 1.5 mg/dL. Therefore, the total bilirubin may exceed the normal range before serum and tissue icterus is present. Although the workup for an icteric cat can be complicated, it is often simplified if the causes are broken down into three main categories: prehepatic, hepatic, and posthepatic. Prehepatic icterus is associated with disorders leading to red blood cell destruction (hemolysis). Hepatic causes are related to diseases primarily or secondarily involving the liver. Posthepatic causes are associated with obstructive processes in the liver or extrahepatic biliary tree. The distinctions are not always clear cut, and some causes may overlap between categories. Clinical findings are referable to the underlying disease but usually include anorexia and lethargy. Tissue icterus is first seen in the mucosa of the hard palate.

D i a g n o s i s

Differential Diagnoses

- **Prehepatic causes (hemolytic)**

  Cytauxzoonosis

  Babesiosis

  Hemobartonellosis*

  Immune-mediated disease

- **Hepatic causes**

  Endotoxemia/bacteremia

  Hepatic necrosis: toxins, drugs, plants (pine oil, arsenicals, tetracyclines, acetaminophen, griseofulvin, ketoconazole)

Cholangitis/cholangiohepatitis complex ($\pm$ sludged bile)*

Infectious disease: Feline infectious peritonitis (FIP)*, feline leukemia virus-related disorders*, less commonly, panleukopenia, Calicivirus, fungal diseases, toxoplasmosis

Hepatic lipidosis*

Liver flukes

Primary or metastatic neoplasia (especially lymphoma)

- **Posthepatic causes**

Neoplasia

Sludged bile

Pancreatitis

Abscess/granuloma

Cholelithiasis

Liver flukes

Primary Diagnostics

- **History:** The history is often vague, as general symptoms (anorexia, lethargy, vomiting, etc.) are present. More specifically, the history of a previously obese cat that has undergone a period of anorexia may point to hepatic lipidosis. Cats that have traveled or lived in the southeast or Hawaii may have liver flukes.

- **Clinical signs:** Lethargy, weakness, and pale mucous membranes may be evident with hemolytic disease (see Chapter 2). The spleen and liver may be enlarged, although the liver may also be palpably enlarged with primary liver disease. Abdominal pain is most suggestive of an obstructive process. Neurologic signs and ptyalism may indicate hepatic encephalopathy. A complete ophthalmologic examination is essential to aid in identifying multisystemic disease (lymphosarcoma, FIP).

- **CBC:** With prehepatic causes of icterus, the hematocrit and reticulocyte count may indicate a regenerative anemia. The smear should be examined for red blood cell parasites. A nonregenerative anemia is more suggestive of primary hepatic disease. Microcytosis (decreased mean corpuscular volume [MCV]) may point to portosystemic shunting. The leukogram is nonspecifically affected.

- **Chemistry profile:** Liver enzymes may be increased with hepatic and posthepatic causes of icterus; in most cases, they are normal or only marginally increased with prehepatic causes. Hemolysis in serum is usually caused by collection and handling problems; massive hemolysis is

*Common causes.

necessary to cause serum discoloration. With primary liver disease, the level of albumin does not usually fall until the liver is functioning at less than 80% capacity.

- **Urinalysis:** The presence of bilirubin in feline urine is *never* normal and warrants immediate investigation. Isosthenuria may result from the medullary washout associated with chronic liver disease.

- **Viral screen:** Icteric cats should be tested for FeLV, FIV, and FIP. The limitations of FIP serology (relative to specificity) should be recognized.

Ancillary Diagnostics

- **Abdominal radiography and ultrasound:** The size and architecture of the liver, the patency of the biliary system, and the structure of the gall-bladder may be evaluated with these diagnostic imaging techniques. Ultrasound is usually more specific than radiology.

- **Liver aspirate:** Aspiration of the liver with a 25-gauge needle is a relatively noninvasive means of screening for many liver disorders and does not usually require sedation or anesthesia. It is useful for establishing the presence of excess fat in the liver, many neoplasias, fungal diseases, etc. Aspiration cytology does not provide information as to liver architecture, so biopsy may still be needed.

- **Liver biopsy:** Clotting profiles should be determined prior to liver biopsy, regardless of whether the procedure involves an ultrasound-guided biopsy or laparotomy. Core biopsy and fine-needle techniques are utilized.

- **Coagulation profile:** The liver must be severely and diffusely affected to cause coagulopathy. An activated clotting time (ACT) may be performed in-house; prothrombin time (PT) and activated partial thromboplastin time (APTT) must usually be sent to a diagnostic laboratory.

- **Coombs' test:** A feline Coombs' test may be indicated if evidence of immune-mediated hemolytic anemia is present (a prehepatic cause).

Diagnostic Notes

- It may be easier to palpate the cat's liver if the forequarters are held up, allowing the viscera to fall farther down into the abdominal cavity. In general, cats with liver disease (including cirrhosis) do not have small livers. One exception to this is liver disease owing to a portosystemic shunt.

- Normal liver enzymes do not eliminate the possibility that primary liver disease is present.

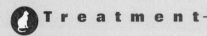**T r e a t m e n t**

Primary Therapeutics

- **Specific therapy:** No therapy is indicated for icterus, but for the underlying disease.
- **Treatment of primary disease:** Therapy should be based upon a diagnosis of the underlying disease.

Secondary Therapeutics

- **Ursodeoxycholic acid:** Some cats with cholestasis may benefit from ursodeoxycholic acid at 10–15 mg/kg PO q 24 hr until cholestasis subsides. Ursodeoxycholic acid should not be used when extrahepatic bile duct obstruction is suspected.
- **Vitamin K$_1$:** This vitamin may need to be supplemented in cholestatic disorders. Dosage is 5 mg/kg once or twice daily until coagulation tests are normalized.
- **Fluids and electrolytes:** Appropriate attention should be given to fluid and electrolyte balance in icteric cats. Fluids may need to be supplemented with potassium.

Therapeutic Notes

- Generally, tetracyclines *should be avoided in cats with liver disease.* Metronidazole or penicillins (e.g., amoxicillin) are useful to treat anaerobic

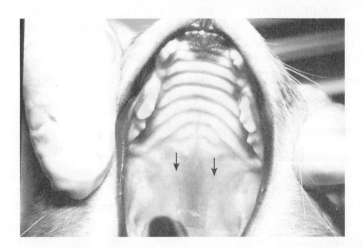

FIGURE 15.1. Icterus: The first place that icterus can be detected is usually the mucosa of the hard palate (arrows). Special attention should be paid to this area during the physical examination of any sick cat.

bacteria, while enrofloxacin or gentamicin are of value for suspected gram-negative bacteria.

- Methionine is *contraindicated* in the management of cats with liver disease, as it may exacerbate hepatic encephalopathy.

Prognosis

The prognosis will depend upon the underlying cause of icterus.

Suggested Readings

Center SA. Feline liver disorders and their management. *Compend Contin Educ* 1986; 8:889–902.

Day DG. Diseases of the liver. In: Sherding RG, ed. The cat: diseases and clinical management. Philadelphia, WB Saunders, 1994;1297–1340.

Rogers KS, Cornelius LM. Feline icterus. *Compend Contin Educ* 1985;7:391–402.

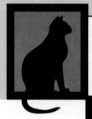

CHAPTER 16

Kidneys: Abnormal Size

Gary D. Norsworthy

Overview

T he size of the feline kidney can be determined by palpation, radiographs, or ultrasound. It should be approximately two and one-half times the length of the body of the second lumbar vertebrae. A significant change in size signals a pathologic state.

Differential Diagnosis

Abnormally Small

- Congenital renal hypoplasia
- Chronic tubulointerstitial nephritis
- Other chronic nephritis

Abnormally Large

- Polycystic renal disease
- Feline infectious peritonitis (FIP)
- Lymphosarcoma
- Hydronephrosis
- Other neoplasia
- Perinephric pseudocyst
- Nephrotoxins, especially ethylene glycol

Treatment

Primary Therapeutics

- **Renal failure therapy:** This is the state that causes clinical signs and must be treated aggressively. See Chapter 37.

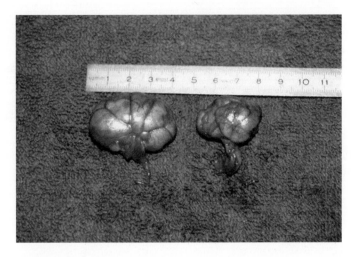

FIGURE 16.1. Kidney: abnormal size: The kidney on the left is normal in size; the kidney on the right is abnormally small.

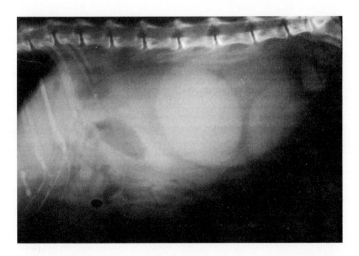

FIGURE 16.2. Radiographs can be used to identify changes in size of kidneys. These kidneys are enlarged.

- **Relief of the underlying disease:** Sometimes this is possible for hydronephrosis, pyelonephritis, glomerulonephritis, benign tumors, and perinephric pseudocysts.
- **Nephrectomy:** This can be curative for unilateral hydronephrosis and unilateral tumors. It is important to establish functionality of the contralateral kidney with an excretory urogram prior to surgery.

Prognosis

The prognosis will depend upon the underlying disease; however, most cats in severe renal failure with either large or small kidneys have a poor prognosis.

Suggested Reading

DiBartola SP, Rutgers HC. Diseases of the kidneys. In: Sherding RG, ed. The cat: diseases and clinical management, 2nd ed. Philadelphia: WB Saunders, 1994;1711–1767.

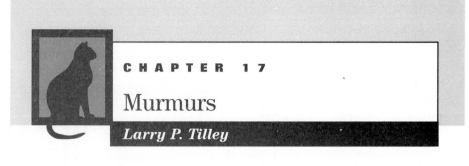

CHAPTER 17

Murmurs

Larry P. Tilley

Overview

Murmurs are defined as vibrations caused by disturbed blood flow associated with high flow through normal or abnormal valves or with structures vibrating in the blood flow. A murmur can include flow disturbances associated with outflow obstruction or forward flow through stenosed valves or into a dilated great vessel. Murmurs can also indicate flow disturbances associated with regurgitant flow through an incompetent valve, septal defect, or patent ductus arteriosus.

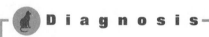**Diagnosis**

Differential Diagnosis

- Other abnormal heart sounds (e.g., split sounds, ejections sounds, gallop rhythms, and clicks)
- Abnormal lung sounds and pleural rubs
- Anemia (usually a pale mucous membrane is present)
- Location and radiation of a murmur and timing during the cardiac cycle can help determine the cause of the murmur. See the algorithm in Figure 17.1.

Primary Diagnostics

- **Grading of murmurs:** Grade I: barely audible; Grade II: soft, but easily ausculted; Grade III: intermediate loudness (most hemodynamically important murmurs are at least grade III); Grade IV: loud, with palpable thrill; Grade V: very loud and audible with stethoscope barely touching the chest, with palpable thrill; Grade VI: very loud and audible without the stethoscope touching the chest, with palpable thrill.

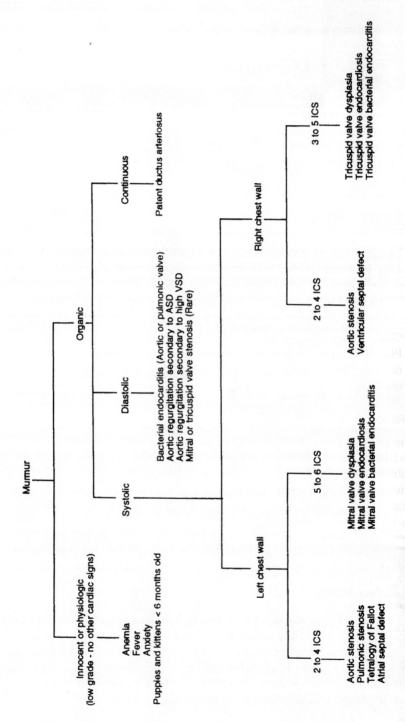

FIGURE 17.1. Murmurs: Differential diagnosis of cardiac disease based on the timing and location of murmurs. (Adapted from Allen DG. Murmurs and abnormal heart sounds. In: Allen DG, Kruth SA, eds. Small animal cardiopulmonary medicine. Philadelphia: BC Decker, 1988;13.)

- **Configuration of murmur:** Plateau murmurs have uniform loudness and are typical of regurgitant murmurs such as mitral and tricuspid insufficiency and ventricular septal defect. Crescendo-decrescendo murmurs get louder and then softer and are typical of ejection murmurs such as pulmonic and aortic stenosis and atrial septal defect. Decrescendo murmurs start loud and then get softer and are typical of diastolic murmurs such as aortic or pulmonic insufficiency.

- **Location of murmur:** Mitral area: left fifth to sixth intercostal space one-quarter the ventrodorsal distance from sternum; Aortic area: left second to third intercostal space just above the pulmonic area; Pulmonic area: left second to third intercostal space one-third to one-half the ventrodorsal distance from sternum; Tricuspid area: right fourth to fifth intercostal space one-quarter the ventrodorsal distance from sternum.

Ancillary Diagnostics

- **Thoracic radiographs:** These are useful for evaluating heart size and pulmonary vasculature in hopes of determining the cause and significance of the murmur.

- **Echocardiography:** This is recommended when a cardiac cause is suspected and the nature of the defect is unknown.

- **CBC-differential:** Anemia is found in animals with anemic murmurs. Polycythemia is present in animals with right-to-left shunting congenital defects. Leukocytosis is expected with a left shift in animals with endocarditis.

Diagnostic Notes

The causes of systolic murmurs include mitral and tricuspid valve endocardiosis, cardiomyopathy, anemia, valve dysplasia, septal defects, pulmonic stenosis, aortic stenosis, thyroid disease, and heartworm disease. The causes of continuous murmur include patent ductus arteriosus. The causes of diastolic murmurs include mitral and tricuspid valve stenosis and aortic and pulmonic valve endocarditis.

T r e a t m e n t

Primary Therapeutics

Most cats are treated as outpatients unless heart failure is evident. Treatment decisions are based on the cause of the murmur and associated clinical signs. No treatment is indicated for a murmur alone.

Secondary Therapeutics

- **Drugs and fluids:** Their use depends on the cause of the murmur and associated clinical signs.

- **Heart failure treatment:** If the murmur is associated with structural heart disease, signs of congestive heart failure (e.g., dyspnea) may develop. Treatment for heart failure can include diuretics, ACE inhibitors, and cage rest.

Therapeutic Notes

- Murmurs present since birth are generally associated with congenital defects or physiologic flow murmurs.
- Acquired murmurs in geriatric cats are usually associated with cardiomyopathy, hyperthyroidism, or hypertension.

Prognosis

The prognosis is variable depending upon the exact cause of the murmur.

Suggested Reading

Smith FWK Jr, Tilley LP. Rapid interpretation of heart sounds, murmurs, and arrhythmias: a guide to cardiac auscultation in dogs and cats. Baltimore: Williams & Wilkins, 1992.

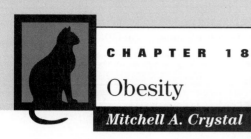

C H A P T E R   1 8

Obesity

Mitchell A. Crystal

Overview

O besity is the excess of body fat that occurs as a result of increased energy intake (increased food intake and/or increased energy-dense food) or decreased energy use (decreased activity and/or, very uncommonly, decreased thyroid function). The most common cause of obesity in cats is overeating, usually owing to free-choice feeding. Obesity can complicate several medical conditions, such as dyspnea, cardiovascular disease, hypertension, diabetes mellitus, and musculoskeletal problems. It can also create an increased risk for anesthesia and surgery, decrease reproductive performance, predispose the cat to hepatic lipidosis, create heat intolerance, and possibly lower resistance to infectious diseases.

Diagnosis

Primary Diagnostics

- **History:** The owner should be questioned about the cat's diet, method of feeding (free-choice versus scheduled feedings), treats or other foods given outside of normal diet, and activity level.
- **Physical examination:** Subjective findings of obesity include lack of ability to see or feel the ribs and excessive intra-abdominal or inguinal fat depots.

Ancillary Diagnostics

- **Abdominal radiographs:** In cases of marked abdominal distention, abdominal radiographs may be needed to differentiate obesity from organomegaly or intra-abdominal neoplasia.

Diagnostic Notes

Hypothyroidism is extremely rare in the cat and should not be diagnosed unless other obvious signs of hypothyroidism are present (truncal alopecia, bradycardia, low body temperature, hypercholesterolemia on a fasted serum chemistry profile, low-grade nonregenerative anemia on CBC).

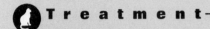 **T r e a t m e n t**

Primary Therapeutics

- **Diet:** Calorie restriction. This can be accomplished by feeding less food or by changing to a calorie-restricted diet (see Appendix E). Caloric need should be calculated based on the formula:

$$\text{kcal to feed} = [\text{body weight in kg} \times 30] + 70$$

This is an appropriate maintenance diet for the cat with low to moderate activity. Obese cats should be fed 66% of the calculated maintenance kilocalories until an optimum body weight is reached. Cats should be fed their recommended caloric intake in two to three divided meals, although continual feeding is acceptable as long as the total daily energy requirements are not exceeded.

- **Avoid foods other than diet:** No treats or table food should be fed to the cat unless they are figured into the daily caloric intake.

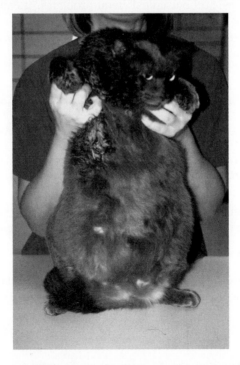

FIGURE 18.1. Obesity: This 28-pound cat is in serious need of weight reduction. Cats of this size often have respiratory and musculoskeletal problems.

> • **Exercise:** Increase activity by increasing play or acquiring another pet.
>
> **Therapeutic Notes**
>
> An effective way to facilitate weight loss is to set a specific weight goal and establish an in-hospital weight-check program in which the client brings the cat in every 1 to 2 weeks to be weighed on the same hospital scale.

Prognosis

The prognosis for obesity is excellent if a weight reduction program is selected and followed. Obesity, if not corrected, may increase the morbidity and mortality of cats with illness and cats needing anesthesia and surgery.

Suggested Reading

MacEwen EG. Obesity. In: Kirk RW, Bonagura JD, eds. Current veterinary therapy XI. Small animal practice. Philadelphia: WB Saunders, 1992;313–318.

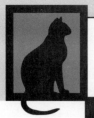

CHAPTER 19

Pleural Effusion

Gary D. Norsworthy

Overview

F luid flow through the pleural space is a continuous process. Its source is the high-pressure parietal circulation. As it forms, it is removed via the low-pressure visceral circulation so that constant movement occurs. An abnormal collection of fluid in the pleural space constitutes a pleural effusion. Although the pleural space is a negligible space in the healthy cat, the presence of fluid causes pulmonary compression, enlarging the pleural space so that 200 mL or more of fluid may be present.

There are five mechanisms responsible for the formation of pleural effusion. They are:

- Increased venous or capillary hydrostatic pressure.
- Decreased capillary oncotic pressure due to hypoalbuminemia.
- Increased capillary membrane permeability.
- Lymphatic obstruction or spillage.
- Hemorrhage (hemothorax is disputably included as a form of pleural effusion).

Cats of any age, breed, or sex may be affected. Most of these cats are reported to have an acute onset of dyspnea or tachypnea. However, most causes of pleural effusion are not peracute. The cat's ability to hide disease until the crisis stage is reached prevents many owners from detecting disease in the early stage. Many cats with pleural effusion will have a history of lethargy and anorexia of one day's duration to several days'. Some will also have weight loss.

The physical examination may reveal tachypnea, open-mouth breathing, cyanosis, fever, and dehydration. The notable sign in advanced disease is dyspnea; however, diseases of slower onset may cause systemic changes (lethargy, anorexia) that may cause the owner to seek veterinary care. Some of these cats will only be experiencing tachypnea that may not be perceptible to the owner. The cat's respiratory pattern should be observed carefully while it is on the examination table.

D i a g n o s i s

Primary Tests

- **Thoracic radiograph:** Dorsoventral (DV) and lateral views are desirable, but the amount of dyspnea present may prevent radiography altogether, or it may permit only a DV view, which is the least stressful.

- **Fluid analysis:** Initial tests should include gross observation, protein determination, specific gravity, cell count, and cytologic examination of sediment. This permits the fluid to be categorized as a transudate, modified transudate, nonseptic exudate, septic exudate, chylous, or hemorrhagic effusion. See Table 19.1 for categorizing and interpreting the fluid analysis.

Secondary Tests

- **Fluid analysis:** Secondary tests are based on the findings from the primary tests. These include anaerobic and aerobic culture and triglyceride and cholesterol determinations.

- **CBC, chemistry profile, feline viral screen:** These tests are to determine the presence of systemic diseases that are known to cause pleural effusion. The viral screen should include tests for feline leukemia virus antigen and coronavirus antibody.

- **Thoracic ultrasonography:** This procedure is most effective if it is utilized when fluid is still present. It allows visualization of small masses and adhesions present in the effusion that may not be visualized radiographically.

Diagnostic Notes

Pleural effusion causes dyspnea; sometimes it is severe enough to be life threatening. It is imperative that diagnostics not be so aggressive that respiratory failure results. Thoracentesis may be necessary before diagnostics can be employed.

T r e a t m e n t

Primary Therapeutics

- **Oxygen administration:** Oxygen may relieve dyspnea and cyanosis. However, it should be administered in a nonstressful manner. Many cats will fight a face mask so that the beneficial effects of oxygen are negated. An oxygen cage is most desirable. An oxygen tent, made from a clear plastic bag, can be very effective.

| TABLE 19.1. |

Interpretation of Pleural Fluid Analysis

	T	MT	NSE	SE	CE	HE
Color	Colorless to pale yellow	Yellow	Yellow or pink	Yellow or pink brown	Milky to red	Red
Turbidity	Clear	Clear to cloudy	Clear to cloudy	Cloudy to opaque; flocculent	Opaque	Opaque
Protein (g/dL)	<1.5	2.5–5.0	3.0–6.0 (FIP: 3.5–8.5)	3.0–7.0	2.5–6.0	>3.0
Fibrin	Absent	Absent	Present	Present	Variable	Present
Trigly-ceride	Absent	Absent	Absent	Absent	Present	Absent
Bacteria	Absent	Absent	Absent	Present	Absent	Absent
Nucleated cells/μL	<1,000	1,000–7,000 LSA: up to 100,000	5,000–20,000 LSA: up to 100,000	5,000–300,000	1,000–20,000	Like peripheral blood
Cytology	Mesothelial cells	Macrophages; mesothelial cells; nondegenerate PMN; neoplastic cells	Nondegen PMN; macrophages	Degenerate PMN; some macrophages neoplastic cells	Small lymphocytes; some macrophages	Erythrocytes; some macrophages engulfing erythrocytes
Diseases	Hypoalbuminemia; early CHF	Chronic CHF; neoplasia diaphragmatic hernia	FIP; neoplasia; diaphragmatic hernia; lung lobe torsion; pancreatitis	Pyothorax	Chylothorax (obstructed or ruptured thoracic duct; HW; neoplasia; CHF)	Hemothorax (trauma; coagulopathies, lung lobe torsion; neoplasia)

Abbreviations: T: Transudate; MT: Modified transudate; NSE: Nonseptic exudate; SE: Septic exudate; CE: Chylous effusion; HE: Hemorrhagic effusion; FIP: Feline infectious peritonitis; LSA: Lymphosarcoma; CHF: Congestive heart failure; PMN: Polymorphonuclear leukocytes or neutrophils; HW: Heartworms.

Adapted from Sherding RG. Diseases of the pleural cavity. In: Sherding RG, ed. The cat: diseases and clinical management, 2nd ed. New York: Churchill Livingstone, 1994;1053–1091.

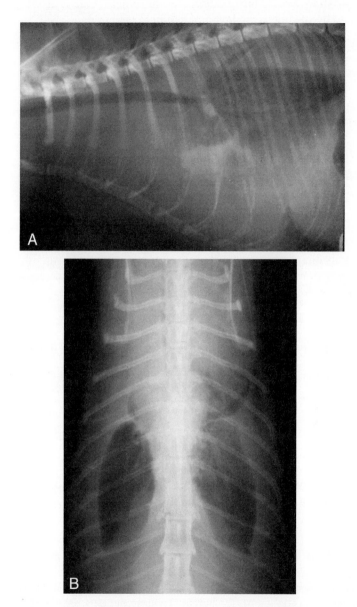

FIGURE 19.1. Pleural effusions: The radiographic signs of pleural effusion include fissure lines between lung lobes, rounding of lung borders (*A, B*), mediastinal widening (*B*), ventral scalloping of lung borders (*A*), obscure cardiac and/or diaphragmatic silhouettes (*A, B*), and separation of lung margins from the thoracic wall (*B*).

- **Cage confinement:** This can be life saving even if oxygen administration is not possible. Do not hurry. Allow the cat time to recover from the stress produced by getting to the hospital and being examined.
- **Thoracentesis:** Ideally, removal of large amounts of fluid is desirable to restore normal respiration. The use of 10 mg of ketamine intravenously will produce enough sedation in the average 4-kg cat that thoracentesis can be performed safely. However, the owner should be told that sedation of a severely dyspneic cat can be fatal. The fluid should be saved for analysis.

Secondary Therapeutics

- **Specific therapy:** This is only possible after a diagnosis has been made. Refer to the chapters concerning these diseases for recommendations on specific therapy.
- **Thoracostomy tube:** Certain conditions producing pleural effusion are treatable and curable; however, the course of therapy may require daily or twice-daily chest drainage for up to 2 weeks. A thoracostomy tube permits drainage with minimal stress and discomfort to the patient. Its use should be limited to treatable diseases.

Therapeutic Notes

Pleural effusion is not a disease. It is a symptom of a serious underlying disease that should be diagnosed before involved therapy begins, especially because many of the diseases are not treatable.

P r o g n o s i s

The prognosis depends on the success of relieving the dyspneic crisis and the diagnosis. Pleural effusion signals the need for aggressive diagnostics and therapy, but the outcome for many cats is very good.

S u g g e s t e d   R e a d i n g

Sherding RG. Diseases of the pleural cavity. In: Sherding RG, ed. The cat: diseases and clinical management, 2nd ed. New York: Churchill Livingstone, 1994;1053–1091.

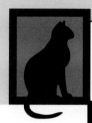

CHAPTER 20

Polyphagic Weight Loss

Mitchell A. Crystal

Overview

Polyphagic weight loss describes the condition of progressive decrease in body weight in the presence of an increased appetite. The two most common diseases that result in this condition are hyperthyroidism and diabetes mellitus. Hyperthyroidism leads to polyphagic weight loss by causing an increase in metabolic rate and a decrease in intestinal transit time. Hyperthyroidism can also cause loss of nutrients as a result of intermittent vomiting. Diabetes mellitus leads to polyphagic weight loss as a result of decreased utilization of glucose, loss of glucose through the urine, and decreased detection of circulating calories by the satiety center in the brain. Less common diseases that can cause polyphagic weight loss include exocrine pancreatic insufficiency (EPI) (usually resulting from chronic interstitial pancreatitis) and intestinal lymphangiectasia. These disorders result in maldigestion (EPI) and malabsorption (lymphangiectasia). Inflammatory bowel disease (IBD), alimentary lymphoma, and some neoplastic diseases are common diseases that present for weight loss, usually in association with normal or decreased appetite, but may rarely present with polyphagic weight loss. These disorders result in malabsorption (IBD, alimentary lymphoma) or increased metabolism (neoplasia). In kittens, and rarely in adult cats, intestinal parasitism can lead to polyphagic weight loss via decreased intestinal absorption.

Because hyperthyroidism and diabetes mellitus most commonly result in this condition, most cats with polyphagic weight loss are older than 10 years of age and often present with polyuria/polydipsia. Cats with polyphagic weight loss due to intestinal diseases or EPI often demonstrate diarrhea with or without vomiting.

Diagnosis

Differential Diagnoses

- Hyperthyroidism
- Diabetes mellitus

- Exocrine pancreatic insufficiency
- Intestinal lymphangiectasia
- Inflammatory bowel disease
- Alimentary lymphoma
- Intestinal parasitism

Primary Diagnostics

- **Cervical palpation for thyroid enlargement:** See Chapter 73 for technique.
- **Chemistry profile:** Around 90% of hyperthyroid cats have an elevation of either ALT or ALP. Hyperglycemia will be present in cats with diabetes mellitus. Hypoalbuminemia and hypoglobulinemia (panhypoproteinemia) may be present in cats with diseases causing intestinal malabsorption.
- **Urinalysis:** Poorly or nonconcentrated urine may be present as a result of hyperthyroidism and/or diabetes mellitus. Glucosuria, and possibly ketonuria, will be present in cats with diabetes mellitus.
- **Fecal examination:** A fecal flotation should be performed to evaluate for parasites.
- **Total T_4 (TT_4):** This test should be performed on all cats over 10 years of age with polyphagic weight loss. The serum TT_4 is elevated in 90–98% of hyperthyroid cats. Some cats have normal TT_4 levels as a result of either fluctuation of TT_4 levels in and out of the normal range or suppression of elevated TT_4 levels into the normal range secondary to concurrent nonthyroidal illness.

Ancillary Diagnostics

- **CBC:** A CBC may demonstrate a mildly elevated PCV in cases of hyperthyroidism and may rarely reveal abnormalities in leukocytes in cases of eosinophilic gastroenteritis and lymphoma.
- **T_3 suppression test:** This test should be performed if there is evidence of hyperthyroidism (palpable thyroid, clinical signs) and a normal TT_4. (See Chapter 73.)
- **FeLV/FIV test:** Retrovirus infection may predispose cats to some causes of intestinal malabsorption.
- **Feline-specific trypsin-like immunoreactivity (TLI):** This test is diagnostic for EPI and should be performed after hyperthyroidism and diabetes mellitus have been ruled out. A 12-hour fasting serum sample is submitted. Decreased pancreatic function leads to decreased leakage of trypsinogen into the vascular space, resulting in a subnormal value of TLI.
- **Intestinal biopsy/histopathology:** This procedure should be performed after hyperthyroidism and diabetes mellitus have been ruled out to investigate for primary intestinal diseases. Biopsies may be collected via

endoscopy, exploratory laparotomy, or, in the case of diffuse or focal intestinal thickening greater than 2 to 3 cm, by ultrasound guidance.

- **Thoracic radiographs:** Thoracic radiography may reveal metastatic disease in the case of polyphagic weight loss due to neoplasia.

Diagnostic Notes

Cats with alimentary lymphoma are usually FeLV negative (see Chapter 82).

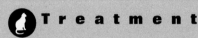 **Treatment**

Primary Therapeutics

- **Treat the underlying disease:** See Chapters 45, 51, 73, and 77.

Prognosis

The prognosis varies depending on the underlying disorder causing the polyphagic weight loss. With appropriate therapy, hyperthyroidism (treated with radioactive iodine or surgery) and intestinal parasitism carry an excellent prognosis for cure. With lifelong appropriate therapy, hyperthyroidism (treated medically), diabetes mellitus, and EPI carry a very good prognosis for controlling the disease, although occasional clinical problems may arise. Lymphocytic-plasmacytic IBD is often controllable with intermittent therapy. Other forms of IBD and intestinal lymphangiectasia do not usually respond to therapy. The prognosis with alimentary lymphoma varies (see Chapter 82). The prognosis for other types of neoplasia vary depending on the tumor type.

Suggested Readings

Hawkins EC. Diagnostic approach to polyphagia and weight loss. In: August JR, ed. Consultations in feline internal medicine. Philadelphia: WB Saunders, 1991;237–242.

Steiner JM, Williams DA. Feline trypsin-like immunoreactivity as a diagnostic tool for diseases of the exocrine pancreas in the cat. *Vet Previews* 1995;2(2):7–9.

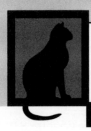
Polyuria/Polydipsia

Mitchell A. Crystal

Overview

Polyuria and polydipsia (PU/PD) are defined as excessive urination (greater than 50 mL/kg/day) and fluid intake (greater than 100 mL/kg/day), respectively. PU/PD results from alterations in the normal homeostatic mechanisms that control thirst and urine formation. These alterations may result from osmotic diuresis, lack of sufficient vasopressin activity, lack of responsiveness to vasopressin, altered hypothalamic/pituitary/adrenal axis, decreased renal tubular function, and decreased renal medullary interstitial concentration gradient. PU/PD should be differentiated from pollakiuria (frequent urination), which commonly results from lower urinary tract diseases. (See Chapter 56.)

PU/PD is a common complaint and may result from a variety of disease processes. Clinical signs aside from excessive thirst and urination vary depending on the underlying disease causing the PU/PD.

Diagnosis

Differential Diagnoses

- **Common causes**
  Chronic renal failure
  Diabetes mellitus
  Hyperthyroidism
  Pyometra
- **Less common causes**
  Liver disease
  Diabetes insipidus
  Psychogenic polydipsia
  Chronic pyelonephritis

Hypokalemia

Acute renal failure

Hypercalcemia (most commonly caused by lymphoma)

Acromegaly (presents for insulin-resistant diabetes mellitus)

Hyperadrenocorticism (usually presents for insulin-resistant diabetes mellitus and dramatic dermatologic signs)

Primary Diagnostics

- **Database (CBC, chemistry profile, and urinalysis):** These should be submitted to evaluate for diabetes mellitus, acromegaly, and hyperadrenocorticism (hyperglycemia, glucosuria, low urine specific gravity, ketonuria), liver disease (hyperbilirubinemia; decreased BUN; increased ALT, ALP, and gamma-glutamyltransferase [GGT]; bilirubinuria), renal disease (elevated BUN and creatinine with a decreased urine specific gravity, hyperphosphatemia), hyperthyroidism (increased ALT and/or ALP, mild increase in packed cell volume [PCV], low urine specific gravity) and electrolyte derangements (hypokalemia, hypercalcemia).

- **Total T$_4$:** This test should be performed on all cats over 10 years of age with PU/PD to evaluate for hyperthyroidism.

Ancillary Diagnostics

- **Abdominal imaging:** Abdominal radiographs or ultrasound will help identify pyometra, renal disease, and liver disease.

- **Thoracic radiographs:** These are indicated if hypercalcemia is documented as the cause of PU/PD to look for lymphoma (mediastinal masses).

- **Pituitary/adrenal screening tests:** Dexamethasone suppression, ACTH stimulation, and/or urinary cortisol:creatinine ratio testing is indicated in the rare case of insulin-resistant diabetes mellitus and dramatic dermatologic signs consistent with hyperadrenocorticism.

- **Water deprivation test:** This test is indicated after common causes of PU/PD have been excluded to evaluate for diabetes insipidus and psychogenic polydipsia.

Diagnostic Notes

- A urine specific gravity will help confirm if PU/PD is present. A specific gravity less than 1.025 supports PU/PD.

- There is currently no reliable test for confirming acromegaly aside from demonstrating a pituitary mass on MRI or CT scan of the head.

- Water deprivation testing is contraindicated in cats with renal insufficiency.

ⓒTreatment————————————————

Primary Therapeutics

- **Treat underlying disease:** This is essential in obtaining a cure.
- **Water:** Adequate quantities of water should be available at all times to prevent dehydration.

Secondary Therapeutics

- **Fluid support:** Fluid therapy is indicated in cats with PU/PD that are dehydrated.

P r o g n o s i s

The prognosis varies depending on the cause of the PU/PD.

S u g g e s t e d   R e a d i n g s

Feldman EC, Nelson RW. Hyperadrenocorticism in cats. In: Canine and feline endocrinology and reproduction, 2nd ed. Philadelphia: WB Saunders, 1996;256–261.

Feldman EC, Nelson RW. Water metabolism and diabetes insipidus. In: Canine and feline endocrinology and reproduction, 2nd ed. Philadelphia: WB Saunders, 1996;2–37.

Meric SM. Polyuria and polydipsia. In: Ettinger SJ, Feldman EC, eds. Textbook of veterinary internal medicine, 4th ed. Philadelphia: WB Saunders, 1995;159–163.

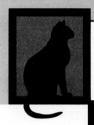

CHAPTER 22

Seizures

Sharon K. Fooshee

Overview

Seizures are defined as clinically apparent disturbances in the electrical activity of the brain. They do not represent a disease entity per se, but rather indicate the presence of another underlying disorder. The clinical appearance of the seizure may vary depending on the location and severity of the hypersynchronous electrical activity. A seizure is generally divided into three stages: pre-ictus, ictus, and post-ictus. An effort should be made to follow a thorough, appropriate evaluation of the patient. Although epilepsy is poorly understood in cats, it is a diagnosis of exclusion and should not be considered without an attempt to investigate other possible causes. The most common causes of seizures in cats involve a structural disorder within the nervous system; functional disturbances are relatively less common.

D i a g n o s i s

Differential Diagnoses

- **Anomaly/congenital**
  Epilepsy: primary or secondary
  Hydrocephalus
  Metabolic storage disease (rare)
  Cerebellar hypoplasia
- **Metabolic**
  Thiamine deficiency
  Hypoglycemia
  Hypocalcemia
  Portosystemic shunt
  Hyperthyroidism

Epilepsy

Primary

Secondary (meningitis, encephalitis, etc.)

- **Infectious/inflammatory**

Nonsuppurative meningoencephalitis

Bacterial disease

Viral disease: FIP, FIV, rabies, pseudorabies

Fungal disease: Cryptococcosis (less common: histoplasmosis, blastomycosis, coccidioidomycosis)

Protozoal disease: Toxoplasmosis, cytauxzoonosis

- **Neoplastic**

Lymphoma

Meningioma

Metastatic tumor

- **Toxic**

Ethylene glycol

Lead

Organophosphates

Metronidazole

- **Trauma**
- **Vascular disturbances**

Feline ischemic encephalopathy

Primary Diagnostics

- **General history:** Details should be sought that relate to the health of the queen during pregnancy, signs of illness in the affected cat or kitten, history of trauma, exposure to toxins, type of diet and relationship of the seizure to eating, travel history, source from which the cat was obtained (i.e., cattery, shelter, etc.), exposure to other animals (swine, wildlife), and recent administration of medications (e.g., insulin, metronidazole). A valid rabies vaccination history *must* be established—(in most cases, the vaccination is not considered valid unless it has been administered by a licensed veterinarian. State laws vary with requirement for frequency of rabies vaccination.

- **History related to seizure activity:** The practitioner should be sure that the owner is describing seizure activity, not signs referable to cardiac or vestibular disease. The description should include loss of consciousness and involuntary movement of the legs, head, etc. Urination, defecation, and salivation are frequently noted. Additional information should include frequency of seizure activity, time of day/night for seizure occurrence, length of the seizure, and possible precipitating events. Characteristics of the pre-ictal and post-ictal period may be important.

- **Physical examination:** A complete neurologic examination should be performed. Cranial nerve deficits, proprioceptive deficits, lateralizing signs, and vision disturbances are just a few of the abnormalities that may help pinpoint the underlying cause. The head should be evaluated for the presence of a "dome" shape or open fontanelle; these may point to hydrocephalus. A thorough ophthalmologic examination is essential to identify inflammatory retinal lesions.

- **Minimum database:** Any seizure investigation should start with a CBC, chemistry profile, and urinalysis. These will help to assess the general health of the patient and may provide clues as to the under-lying cause.

Ancillary Diagnostics

- **Radiography:** In general, skull radiographs do not provide meaningful information except with trauma and some cases of hydrocephalus.

- **Serum bile acids:** Fasting *and* postprandial serum bile acids are useful in identifying portosystemic shunts. Determination of bile acids may be especially appropriate for kittens and young adult cats.

- **Ultrasonography:** For many cats, the brain can be imaged by placing the transducer over the temporal bone cranial to the base of the pinna.

- **Cerebrospinal fluid (CSF) analysis:** Standard texts may be consulted for details of performing the CSF tap. Because the fluid must be analyzed within 20–30 minutes and because the procedure poses some risk for the patient, it often is appropriate to refer the patient to a specialist or a university hospital. Complete analysis includes measurement of protein content, cytologic analysis, and occasionally culture or serologic testing (e.g., *Cryptococcus*, bacterial disease). The CSF tap *should not* be performed if there is suspicion for increased intracranial pressure.

- **Serology:** Appropriate serologic testing should be submitted if there is suspicion of infectious disease. In-clinic testing often includes FIV and FeLV. Local diagnostic laboratories may perform toxoplasmosis serology. If coronavirus (FIP) serology is obtained, results should be interpreted with recognition of test limitations (i.e., specificity for FIP virus).

- **Serum protein electrophoresis:** Serum electrophoresis may be helpful, especially when FIP is a suspected cause. See Chapter 54 for details on interpretation.

- **Computed tomography (CT) and magnetic resonance imaging (MRI):** Specialized imaging techniques are very helpful in identifying focal brain lesions. If not locally available, most veterinary teaching hospitals have a CT and/or an MRI unit.

Diagnostic Notes

- When the cat presents for a first-time seizure, it is rarely necessary to embark upon a complicated diagnostic evaluation. At most, diagnostics may need to include only a history, physical examination, and perhaps a minimum database (especially glucose and calcium).

- If seizure activity becomes frequent, it may be helpful for the owner to keep a notebook that records pertinent comments related to the seizures (see "History" above). In some cases, clues as to the underlying cause may become apparent.

- If a cat with historical seizure activity requires sedation, ketamine should be avoided because it increases intracranial pressure. Phenothiazines (acepromazine) are always contraindicated because of their effect on lowering the seizure threshold.

- Whenever a cat with unexplained neurologic signs bites a human, appropriate public health officials should be notified. Usually, local animal control officers can assist with this. It is always advisable to submit the cat for necropsy should it die. If the owner is reluctant, the cat's cerebellum may be retrieved and submitted for rabies examination. *DO NOT FREEZE THE TISSUE!*

 T r e a t m e n t ───────────────────────

Primary Therapeutics

- *Status epilepticus:* Diazepam (5 mg/mL) may be administered intravenously to effect at 0.5 to 1.0 mg/kg every 10 to 15 minutes for a total of three doses. Cats are slow to eliminate this drug, so repeated treatments should be given with caution. If more sustained anticonvulsant control is needed in-hospital, phenobarbital may be given, although it may be 15 to 20 minutes before it crosses the blood-brain barrier. Calcium and glucose should be administered, if appropriate. Although thiamine deficiency is uncommon, it is reasonable to administer injectable vitamin B_1 or B-complex. Body temperature should be carefully monitored. Oxygen may be required.

- **Maintenance anticonvulsant therapy:** Phenobarbital and diazepam are used as maintenance anticonvulsants in cats. Phenobarbital is dosed at 1.5 to 2 mg/kg BID; serum levels can be monitored, as for dogs, although recommendations for appropriate concentrations of the drug in cats are still being determined. The maximum dose is 10 mg/kg BID. Diazepam is dosed at 0.25 to 0.5 mg/kg BID or TID; on average, this translates to 2 to 5 mg per cat TID. Other anticonvulsants (including primidone) are currently under investigation.

- **Corticosteroids:** Glucocorticoids may be administered for cases of suspected cerebral edema or granulomatous meningitis. Trauma and brain tumors may require the anti-inflammatory effects of steroids.

- **Antimicrobials:** When antimicrobial therapy is required, consideration must be given to distribution limitations posed by the blood-brain barrier. Generally, sulfas and chloramphenicol more readily penetrate the barrier, although others may cross over, especially when inflammation is present.

- **Bathing:** Any suspicious odor or appearance to the haircoat may suggest dermal exposure to toxins; the cat should be immediately bathed.

- **Surgery:** Meningiomas can often be removed after the exact location is established through examination and specialized imaging techniques. This procedure should only be performed by those with specialized training in cranial surgery.

Therapeutic Notes

- Nonsuppurative meningoencephalitis is a fairly common cause of seizures in cats. It is only diagnosed with histopathology. Therefore, a therapeutic trial of corticosteroids is indicated in cats with seizures whose workup is nondiagnostic.

- Injectable diazepam should not be combined with lactated Ringer's solution. It is incompatible with a number of other drugs so is best injected alone.

- Once a cat is placed on long-term anticonvulsant therapy, the medication should never be abruptly terminated; this may precipitate uncontrolled seizure activity.

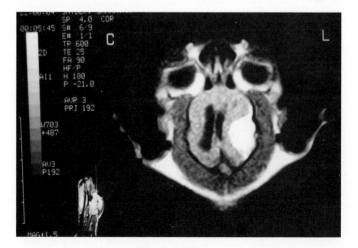

FIGURE 22.1. Seizures: Seizures can be caused by many diseases, including brain tumors. This cat has a large meningioma compressing the left cerebrum and the ventricles.

- A changing seizure pattern may reflect inappropriate seizure control rather than progressive neurologic disease.
- Serious side effects, including death, have recently been reported with oral diazepam in cats.

P r o g n o s i s

Prognosis is entirely dependent upon the identification and resolution of the underlying cause of the seizures along with appropriate seizure control.

S u g g e s t e d   R e a d i n g s

Center SA, Elston TH, Rowland PH, et al. Fulminant hepatic failure associated with oral administration of diazepam in 11 cats. *J Am Vet Med Assoc* 1996;209(3);618–625.

Dyer KR, Shell LG. Managing patients with status epilepticus. *Vet Med* 1993;88:654–659.

Fenner WR. Diseases of the brain, spinal cord, and peripheral nerves. In: Sherding RG, ed. The cat: diseases and clinical management. Philadelphia: WB Saunders, 1994;1507–1568.

Quesnel AD, Parent JM, McDonell W, Percy D, Lumsden JH. Diagnostic evaluation of cats with seizure disorders: 30 cases (1991–1993). *J Am Vet Med Assoc* 1997;210(1):65–71.

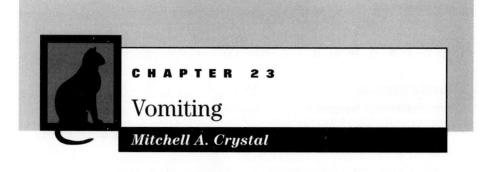

CHAPTER 23

Vomiting

Mitchell A. Crystal

Overview

Vomiting is the forceful, reflexive ejection of gastric contents from the stomach through the mouth. Vomiting is mediated via two higher centers within the brain, the chemoreceptor trigger zone and the vomiting center. The vomiting center is thought to be the final center that mediates/initiates vomiting. These areas are important in the pharmacologic control of vomiting. Prior to beginning diagnostic evaluation and therapeutic management, vomiting must be differentiated from regurgitation (the passive, retrograde expulsion of food from the esophagus). Characteristics of vomiting include the presence of nausea (ptyalism, swallowing, retching, depression, restlessness, licking of lips); abdominal muscle contraction; and bile or digested blood or food in the vomitus. Characteristics of regurgitation include lack of nausea, lack of abdominal contractions and/or bile in the vomitus; and the presence of nondigested food in a tubular shape.

Once vomiting is assessed as acute or chronic and serious or nonserious, potential causes can be considered and initial diagnostic or therapeutic management begun. Chronic/serious, chronic/nonserious, and acute/serious vomiting warrants a complete diagnostic evaluation, whereas acute/nonserious vomiting can initially be supported without an in-depth investigation. If the problem recurs or persists, then additional, more complete evaluation is necessary. In some cases, chronic intermittent vomiting may result from trichobezoars (hairballs). This may be normal or may indicate underlying disease. In either case, the vomiting may require evaluation and management (see Chapter 120).

Vomiting may be caused by gastrointestinal or extragastrointestinal disease. When performing a diagnostic workup of the vomiting cat, the veterinarian should evaluate common causes of extragastrointestinal disease prior to performing diagnostics to investigate for primary gastrointestinal disease. Once common extragastrointestinal diseases that cause vomiting have been excluded, causes of vomiting from primary gastrointestinal disease can be considered.

D i a g n o s i s

Differential Diagnoses
Extragastrointestinal Diseases

- **Metabolic diseases:** renal failure, urinary tract obstruction, hepatobiliary disease, electrolyte and acid/base disorders
- **Endocrinopathies:** hyperthyroidism, complicated diabetes mellitus
- **Less common diseases:** neurologic, cardiovascular, pancreatic, heartworm, FeLV/FIV-associated diseases, and behavior disorders

Gastrointestinal Diseases

- Obstruction: foreign body, neoplasia, intussusception, stricture
- Nonspecific gastroenteritis
- Toxicity
- Dietary intolerance
- Parasitism
- Inflammatory bowel disease
- Lymphoma and other GI neoplasia
- *Helicobacter* gastritis
- Obstipation
- Functional gastrointestinal disorders

Primary Diagnostics

- **History:** The owner should be questioned about the cat's exposure to toxins, access to foreign bodies, or changes in diet.
- **Oral examination:** It is important to look closely under the tongue for a linear foreign body.
- **Database (CBC, chemistry profile, and urinalysis):** A database should be submitted to evaluate for diabetes mellitus (hyperglycemia, glucosuria, ketonuria, low urine specific gravity), liver disease (hyperbilirubinemia, decreased BUN, increased ALT, ALP, and GGT, bilirubinuria), renal disease (elevated BUN and creatinine with a decreased urine specific gravity), signs of hyperthyroidism (increased ALT and/or ALP, a mild increase in PCV, low urine specific gravity), electrolyte and acid/base derangements (changes in sodium, potassium, chloride, calcium, and total carbon dioxide [TCO_2]), and signs of lymphoma (occasional cats demonstrate circulating lymphoblasts and anemia).
- **Fecal:** A fecal flotation should be performed to evaluate for parasites.

- **Total T$_4$:** This test should be performed on all vomiting cats over 10 years of age to evaluate for hyperthyroidism.
- **FeLV/FIV Test:** These tests are not confirmatory of disease but allow one to more specifically direct investigation.

Ancillary Diagnostics

- **Abdominal radiographs and/or ultrasound:** Abdominal imaging may reveal abnormalities in organ size and/or architecture, gastrointestinal obstruction, or neoplasia.
- **Feline-specific trypsin-like immunoreactivity (TLI):** A 12-hour fasting serum sample can be submitted to evaluate for pancreatitis. Some cases of pancreatitis have elevations in TLI, although many are normal. (See Chapter 96.)
- **Heartworm testing:** Heartworm serology is indicated in cats with chronic vomiting who live in endemic areas when other more common causes have been excluded. Heartworm serology should be performed in conjunction with other diagnostic tests to screen for heartworm disease (i.e., CBC, thoracic radiographs, transtracheal wash). (See Chapter 64.)
- **Intestinal biopsy/histopathology:** This procedure should be performed to investigate for primary intestinal diseases in cases of chronic vomiting after other noninvasive procedures have been completed. Biopsies may be collected via endoscopy, exploratory laparotomy, or, in the case of diffuse or focal intestinal thickening greater than 2 to 3 cm, by ultrasound guidance. Histopathology may reveal IBD, lymphoma, or other gastrointestinal neoplasia and/or *Helicobacter* gastritis.
- **Urea test (CLOtest*) on gastric biopsies:** This test can be performed to evaluate for indirect evidence of *Helicobacter*. (See Chapter 65.)

Diagnostic Notes

The presence of a hypochloremic metabolic alkalosis on a chemistry profile is suggestive of a pyloric outflow obstruction and is most commonly seen with gastroduodenal foreign bodies.

 T r e a t m e n t

Primary Therapeutics

- **Treat underlying disease:** This is essential for long-term cure.
- **Gut rest:** Keep the cat NPO (nothing by mouth) for 24–48 hours.

*Campylobacter-like organism test.

- **Correct fluid, electrolyte, and/or acid base derangements:** Intravenous or subcutaneously administered fluids are recommended.
- **Diet:** Feed a low-fat, easily digestible diet (see Appendix E).

Secondary Therapeutics

- **Antiemetic therapy:** Antiemetics are useful when vomiting compromises hydration/acid base/electrolyte status, is frequent enough to cause significant stress or discomfort, and/or is present in animals at risk for aspiration pneumonia. Table 23.1 lists antiemetics commonly used in the vomiting cat.

Therapeutic Notes

Antiemetics are contraindicated in cases of gastrointestinal obstruction.

TABLE 23.1.

Antiemetics Commonly Used in the Vomiting Cat

Drug	Location of Action*	Dose (mg/kg unless noted)	Side Effects
Metoclopramide	CRTZ, GIS	0.2–0.4 PO, SQ, IM TID-QID or 1–2 mg/kg/day constant rate IV infusion	Diarrhea, disorientation, extra-pyramidal signs**
Cisapride	GIS	2.5–7.5 mg/cat PO BID-TID	
Chlorpromazine	VC, CRTZ	0.2–0.4 SQ, IM TID-QID	Hypotension, sedation
Prochlorperazine	VC, CRTZ	0.2–0.4 SQ, IM TID-QID	Hypotension, sedation

*VC, vomiting center; CRTZ, chemoreceptor trigger zone; GIS, gastrointestinal smooth muscle

**involuntary limb movements, torticollis, stiffness, tremors, loss of righting reflex

P r o g n o s i s

The prognosis varies depending on the cause of the vomiting.

S u g g e s t e d   R e a d i n g s

Guilford WG. Approach to clinical problems in gastroenterology. In: Strombeck's small animal gastroenterology, 3rd ed. Philadelphia: WB Saunders, 1996;50–62.

Strombeck DR, Guilford WG. Vomiting: pathophysiology and pharmacologic control. In: Strombeck's small animal gastroenterology, 3rd ed. Philadelphia: WB Saunders, 1996;256–260.

Washabau RJ, Elie MS. Antiemetic therapy. In: Bonagura JD, ed. Kirk's current veterinary therapy XII. Small animal practice. Philadelphia: WB Saunders, 1995;679–684.

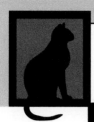

CHAPTER 24

Weight Loss

Mitchell A. Crystal

Overview

Weight loss occurs with decreased hydration and/or negative energy balance, i.e., energy needs exceed intake. Weight loss **from dehydration** occurs rapidly (within hours to days) and is considered significant when it exceeds 3–5% of normal body weight or sooner in animals that cannot normally conserve fluids (e.g., animals with renal failure, causes of PU/PD, burns/wounds). Other signs of dehydration include dry, tacky mucous membranes, pallor, poor skin turgor, and sunken eyes. Dehydration can be associated with a great number of disease processes and thus may demonstrate a wide variety of additional clinical signs. Diagnostic evaluation is based on significant clinical signs. Therapy involves replacing the fluid deficit, meeting maintenance fluid requirements, and providing additional fluids for continuing losses.

Weight loss due to **negative energy balance** occurs slowly, i.e., days/weeks to months. Negative energy balance can result from **decreased energy intake** (anorexia, decreased access to food, decreased quality of food) or **increased energy use/loss** (increased activity, pregnancy, lactation, growth, disease states). Weight loss becomes significant when it exceeds 10% of normal body weight (5% in kittens). Anorexia, polyphagic weight loss, and other conditions leading to a decreased body weight must be investigated when significant weight loss occurs. (See Chapters 3 and 20.) Usually, other clinical signs resulting from the underlying disease process will be present, suggesting the appropriate diagnostic approach.

D i a g n o s i s

Differential Diagnoses

- **Dehydration**
- **Metabolic diseases**
  Renal failure

Hepatobiliary disease

Pancreatic diseases

- **Endocrinopathies**

Hyperthyroidism

Diabetes mellitus

- **Gastrointestinal (GI) diseases**

Stomatitis

Parasites

Inflammatory bowel disease

Alimentary lymphoma and other GI neoplasia

Helicobacter gastritis

Esophagitis

Gastritis

Oral disease, including jaw fractures

- **Cardiovascular disease**

Hypertrophic cardiomyopathy

- **Infectious diseases**

Fungal disease

Protozoal disease

Viral disease

- **Neoplasia of other organs**

Primary Diagnostics

- **History:** The client should be questioned about the cat's access to food and water, diet, diet changes, appetite, thirst and urination, reproductive status, and whether any other clinical signs are present.
- **Oral examination:** The oral cavity should be examined for abnormalities that might inhibit eating.
- **Abdominal palpation:** The cat's abdomen should be palpated organ by organ to look for abnormalities in size and shape and to determine if abdominal masses are present.
- **Fundic examination:** Infectious diseases and lymphoma may demonstrate uveitis and/or chorioretinitis.
- **Database (CBC, chemistry profile, and urinalysis):** A data base should be submitted to evaluate for signs of metabolic diseases, endocrinopathies, gastrointestinal diseases, infectious diseases, and neoplasia.
- **Fecal:** A fecal flotation should be performed to evaluate for parasites.
- **Total T$_4$:** This test should be performed on all cats over 10 years of age that are demonstrating weight loss to evaluate for hyperthyroidism.

- **FeLV/FIV test:** These tests may signal the presence of other diseases.

Ancillary Diagnostics

- **Thoracic radiographs:** Thoracic radiographs should be submitted to evaluate for signs of cardiovascular diseases, infectious diseases, and neoplasia.
- **Abdominal radiographs and/or ultrasound:** Abdominal imaging should be performed to investigate organs (size, location, contour, and architecture) and to look for masses.
- **Electrocardiogram (ECG):** An ECG should be performed to evaluate for signs of cardiovascular disease.

Diagnostic Notes

Additional diagnostics should be based on specific clinical signs and initial test results.

 T r e a t m e n t

Primary Therapeutics

- **Treat underlying disease:** This is the cornerstone of successful treatment.

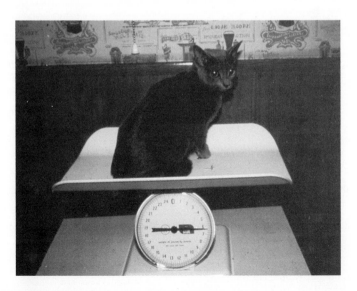

FIGURE 24.1. Weight loss: Owners should be encouraged to weigh their cats on the same scale each time to determine if weight changes are occurring. This is especially important for geriatric cats.

- **Correct fluid and electrolyte disturbances:** This should be done within the first 24 hours.

Secondary Therapeutics

- **Nutritional Support:** See Chapter 3.

Therapeutic Notes

Daily changes in weight are a good indicator of hydration status.

P r o g n o s i s

The prognosis varies depending on the cause of the weight loss.

S u g g e s t e d   R e a d i n g

Greco DS. Changes in body weight. In: Ettinger SJ, Feldman EC, eds. Textbook of veterinary internal medicine, 4th ed. Philadelphia: WB Saunders, 1995;2–5.

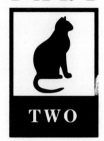
DISEASES

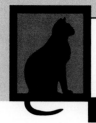

CHAPTER 25

Acetaminophen Toxicosis

Sharon K. Fooshee

Overview

Acetaminophen toxicosis usually occurs when well-intentioned owners, unaware of the significant toxicity of this drug in cats, administer this drug for a variety of reasons. Ingestion of 50–60 mg/kg of acetaminophen may be fatal for cats. This amounts to one regular-strength tablet for a 4–5 kg cat. Acetaminophen preys on several of the cat's metabolic peculiarities and leads to development of life-threatening methemoglobinemia and Heinz-body hemolytic anemia. Acetaminophen ingestion leads to depletion of cellular stores of glutathione, the compound that normally binds with toxic metabolites and leads to their excretion as nontoxic conjugates. Whereas the methemoglobinemia is reversible, Heinz-body formation (and damage to the red blood cell [RBC] membrane) is not. Earliest signs include vomiting and salivation. The appearance of cyanotic or brown-colored mucous membranes (usually within a few hours) heralds the onset of methemoglobinemia. Edema of the face and paws is common. As Heinz-body hemolytic anemia ensues, the mucous membranes become pale and sometimes jaundiced.

Diagnosis

Primary Diagnostics

- **History:** Because the clinical signs are not distinctive, a history of acetaminophen administration is critical to a confirmed diagnosis.
- **Clinical signs:** The appearance of cyanotic or brown-colored mucous membranes and facial edema is noteworthy.
- **CBC:** Typical findings include decreased hematocrit and formation of Heinz bodies on the red cell membrane. Reticulocytes may appear several days later.

Diagnostic Notes

Attendant methemoglobinemia is usually the cause of death and occurs within 18–36 hours.

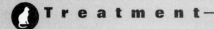

Treatment

Primary Therapeutics

- **Removal of the toxin:** If ingestion has occurred very recently, vomiting should be induced and followed by activated charcoal and a saline cathartic.
- **Acetylcysteine (Mucomyst):** This drug in a 5% solution is recommended as a specific antidote. An initial oral or intravenous dose of 130–140 mg/kg should be followed by 70 mg/kg every 4–6 hours (PO or IV); treatment may need to be continued for 2 to 3 days. The available solutions are in 10% and 20% concentrations and should be appropriately diluted.

Secondary Therapeutics

- **Ascorbic acid (vitamin C):** 30 mg/kg PO should be given every 6 hours. It may help reduce the amount of unbound toxic metabolite while glutathione stores are being replenished. It should not be substituted for acetylcysteine therapy. It has not been conclusively proven to be of value.
- **Transfusion:** Administration of whole blood may be useful in cats with severe hemolytic anemia.
- **Cimetidine:** This drug has been advocated by some for potential inhibition of toxic metabolite formation. Its usefulness has not been proven, and it should not be the sole therapy for acetaminophen toxicosis.
- **Supportive therapy:** This includes intravenous fluids and electrolytes, oxygen, and limited handling of the patient.

Therapeutic Notes

Signs of recovery within 48 hours indicate a positive response to treatment.

Prognosis

A grave prognosis is indicated when the methemoglobinemia and Heinz-body hemolytic anemia are severe and unresponsive to appropriate therapy. For cats that recover, no long-term effects have been reported.

Suggested Reading

Groff RM, Miller JM, Stair EL, Hall JO, et al. Toxicoses and toxins. In: Norsworthy GD, ed. Feline practice. Philadelphia: JB Lippincott, 1993;559–560.

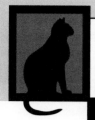

CHAPTER 26

Acne

Gary D. Norsworthy

Overview

Feline acne typically occurs in mature or geriatric cats instead of in young cats. It begins with the formation of comedones or blackheads. If infection occurs, it can progress to furunculosis or folliculitis, at which time the chin becomes swollen. It is associated with a lack of proper grooming but can be secondary to demodicidosis, dermatophytosis, or *Malassezia* infections.

Diagnosis

Primary Diagnostics

- **Clinical appearance:** This is diagnostic.
- **Cytologic preparation, bacterial and fungus culture:** These are appropriate to determine the presence of an underlying disease.

Treatment

Primary Therapeutics

- **Clipping of hair:** This is important to permit application of medications.
- **Cleansing of the chin:** This is best accomplished by hot packing the chin for a few minutes to open the pores, then gently scrubbing with 2.5% benzoyl peroxide.
- **Antibiotic:** The drug of choice is erythromycin (Cleocin-T). It is applied topically one or two times per day.

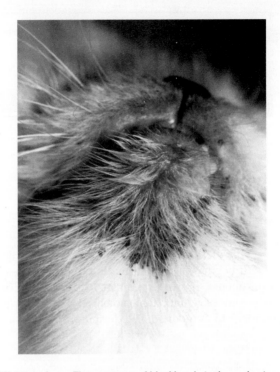

FIGURE 26.1. Acne: The presence of blackheads is the early sign of acne.

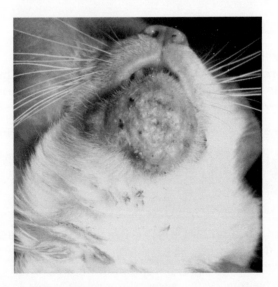

FIGURE 26.2. When infection occurs, the chin becomes swollen and alopecic.

Secondary Therapeutics

- **Anti-inflammatories:** The author has found that many cats with severe acne respond faster if megestrol acetate is administered (5 mg/cat SID for 5 days ONLY).

Therapeutic Notes

Megestrol acetate can cause significant side effects. Owners should be informed of this and their permission secured before using this drug.

Prognosis

The prognosis is good, but recurrence is common.

Suggested Readings

Merchant SR. The skin: diseases of unknown or multiple etiology. In: Norsworthy GD, ed. Feline practice. Philadelphia: JB Lippincott, 1993;532–539.

Moriello KA. Diseases of the skin. In: Sherding RG, ed. The cat: diseases and clinical management, 2nd ed. New York: Churchill Livingstone. 1994;1907–1968.

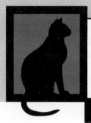

CHAPTER 27
Anal Sac Impaction and Infection

Gary D. Norsworthy

Overview

The anal sacs secrete a foul-smelling substance that is part of the cat's defense system. Many household cats, especially geriatric cats, live a stress-free lifestyle that never calls for natural anal sac expression. Consequently, the anal sac excretion desiccates and thickens. At this stage, the anal sacs are said to be impacted; the cat exhibits pain when defecating and may experience tenesmus. The cat responds to that by licking or biting at the tailhead region. If infection occurs within the sacs, pain will increase. The skin over the anal sac may rupture, expelling purulent material.

Diagnosis

Primary Diagnostics

- **Clinical signs:** The signs of tenesmus, licking at the perineal region, and a draining tract are characteristic of anal sac disease.

Diagnostic Notes

- Anal sac disease of dogs usually produces scooting. This is not a common finding in cats with anal sac disease.
- Some cats with anal sacculitis may lick the perineal area and the caudal thighs, producing a symmetrical pattern of alopecia.

Treatment

Primary Therapeutics

- **Manual expression:** This procedure should permit removal of thickened secretions.

- **Irrigation:** An antiseptic solution is used to flush remaining dried debris from the anal sacs. Sedation of the cat generally is required.
- **Antibiotic instillation:** Local treatment with antibiotics is indicated.
- **Systemic antibiotics:** Systemic antibiotics speed recovery.

Secondary Therapeutics

- **Surgical drainage:** Anal sac abscesses that have not ripened and drained will heal faster if surgical drainage is performed.
- **Anal Sacculectomy:** This procedure should be considered in recurrent cases.

Therapeutic Notes

This disease is uncommon in the cat.

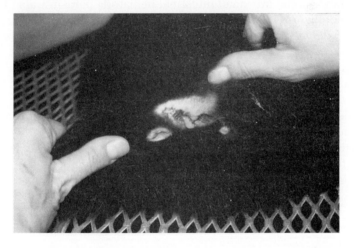

FIGURE 27.1. Anal sacculitis: When anal sacs become infected, they may rupture and drain purulent material lateral to the anus.

Prognosis

The prognosis is good. However, aggressive therapy as outlined should occur.

Suggested Reading

RM Bright, MS Bauer. Surgery of the digestive system. In: Sherding RG, ed. The cat: diseases and clinical management, 2nd ed. New York: Churchill Livingstone, 1994;1353–1401.

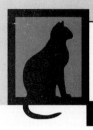

CHAPTER 28

Ancylostoma Infection

Mitchell A. Crystal

Overview

Ancylostoma are small intestinal nematode parasites also known as hookworms. Three types of hookworms are found in the cat: *Ancylostoma tubaeforme* (most common), *Ancylostoma braziliense*, and *Uncinaria stenocephala*. *A. tubaeforme* is a moderately bloodsucking parasite, whereas *A. braziliense* and *U. stenocephala* are minimally bloodsucking parasites. Hookworms are acquired via ingestion of infected feces and have a 2-week to 3-week life cycle without extra-intestinal migration, although infection is occasionally acquired via skin penetration; transplacental and transmammary infection does not occur. Clinical signs are more severe in kittens than in adult cats and include diarrhea, dark stools, vomiting, weight loss or failure to gain weight (kittens), and weakness or lethargy due to anemia (kittens). Infection may also be asymptomatic. Physical examination may be normal, reveal evidence of weight loss (kittens) or diarrhea, or demonstrate pallor (kittens).

D i a g n o s i s

Primary Diagnostics

- **Fecal flotation:** Eggs are seen on microscopic examination.

Ancillary Diagnostics

- **Direct saline smear:** Eggs are sometimes seen on microscopic examination.

Diagnostic Notes

Clinical signs may develop in kittens before eggs are detected in the feces.

Treatment

Primary Therapeutics

- **Pyrantel pamoate:** Give 20 mg/kg PO, repeating in 2 to 3 weeks.
- **Praziquantel/pyrantel pamoate (Drontal):** Give per label instructions, repeating in 2 to 3 weeks.

Secondary Therapeutics

- **Fenbendazole:** Give 25 mg/kg PO for 3 days, repeating in 2 to 3 weeks.
- **Ivermectin:** Give 200 mg/kg PO, repeating in 2 to 3 weeks.
- **Dichlorvos:** Give 11 mg/kg PO, repeating in 2 to 3 weeks.
- **Disophenol:** Give 10 mg/kg SQ, repeating in 2 to 3 weeks.

Therapeutic Notes

Treat kittens routinely or if hookworm infection is suspected, even if fecal floatation is negative.

A second treatment is needed 2 to 3 weeks following initial therapy to kill new adults arising from eggs and larva that were initially resistant to therapy.

Disophenol may be useful in cats that vomit oral anthelminthics but causes death at doses greater than 35 mg/kg.

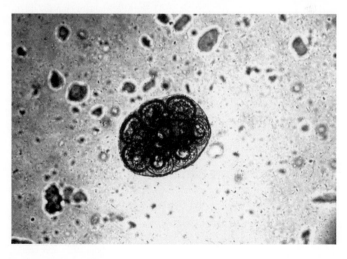

FIGURE 28.1. Ancylostoma: The egg of *Ancylostoma tubaeforme* may be found on a fecal flotation.

Prognosis

The prognosis is excellent for cure, although hookworms often persist in the environment and lead to reinfection. This may be a problem in outdoor cats. Sodium borate may be applied to the environment at a rate of 5 kg/100 square feet to kill hookworm larvae.

Suggested Readings

Burrows CF, Batt RM, Sherding RG. Diseases of the small intestine. In: Ettinger SJ, Feldman EC, eds. Textbook of veterinary internal medicine, 4th ed. Philadelphia: WB Saunders, 1995;1196–1198.

Reinemeyer CR. Feline gastrointestinal parasites. In: Kirk RW, Bonagura JD, eds. Kirk's current veterinary therapy XI. Small animal practice. Philadelphia: WB Saunders, 1992;626–630.

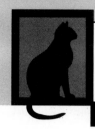

CHAPTER 29

Aortic Stenosis

John-Karl Goodwin

Overview

Congenital narrowing of the left ventricular outflow tract, aortic valves, or supravalvular aorta has been reported in the feline. Although there are several acquired abnormalities that cause left ventricular outflow obstruction (i.e., hypertrophic cardiomyopathy), congenital aortic stenosis in the cat is rare. Of the different types of aortic stenosis noted in the cat, supravalvular stenosis appears to be most commonly encountered lesion. Aortic stenosis may be seen concurrently with other congenital defects such as mitral valve dysplasia.

Left ventricular concentric hypertrophy occurs when significant outflow obstruction is present. The elevated left ventricular pressures may eventually result in left-sided congestive heart failure in severely affected cats.

Physical examination reveals a left basilar systolic ejection-type murmur and potentially late-rising femoral pulses, which are difficult to note at high heart rates.

 Diagnosis

Primary Tests

- **Echocardiography:** Left ventricular concentric hypertrophy, left atrial enlargement, high-velocity turbulent systolic flow in the left ventricular outflow tract as demonstrated by spectral or color-flow Doppler echocardiography, systolic anterior movement of the anterior mitral valve leaflet, mitral regurgitation, aortic regurgitation, and premature closure of the aortic valves may be present.
- Cardiac catheterization and selective angiocardiography may be used for definitive diagnosis but often is unnecessary.

Ancillary Diagnostics

- **Electrocardiography:** Increased R-wave amplitude, suggestive of left ventricular enlargement; wide P-waves, suggestive of left atrial enlargement; and atrial and ventricular tachyarrhythmias may be present.
- **Thoracic radiography:** Left atrial and ventricular enlargement, dilation of the ascending aorta, and signs consistent with left-sided congestive heart failure, such as pulmonary edema, may be present.
- **Angiocardiography:** Contrast studies of the heart may demonstrate the lesion.

Diagnostic Notes

This congenital abnormality is rare in the cat.

 T r e a t m e n t

Primary Therapeutics

Medical management of left-sided congestive heart failure consists of the use of diuretics, vasodilators such as ACE inhibitors, digoxin, and moderate dietary salt restriction.

Surgical intervention or balloon valvuloplasty of the stenotic lesion is difficult in cats.

Secondary Therapeutics

Atenolol (Tenormin=AE) 6.25–12.5 mg PO SID may be effective in reducing ventricular and supraventricular arrhythmias.

Therapeutic Notes

Medical management of this abnormality often is unrewarding, especially if significant aortic regurgitation is present.

Prophylactic antibiotic therapy is indicated at times of potential bacteremia (i.e., dental procedures), as these patients (even those with mild stenosis) are predisposed to valvular endocarditis.

P r o g n o s i s

The prognosis of aortic stenosis is directly related to the severity of the outflow obstruction. Patients with significant pressure gradients across their outflow tract (i.e., >100 mm Hg) have a guarded-to-poor prognosis. As with other causes of ventricular concentric hypertrophy, there is an increased risk of sudden cardiac death.

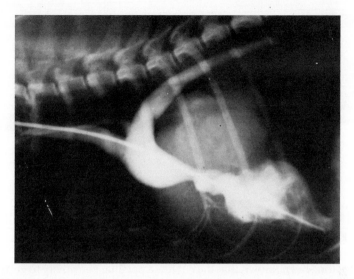

FIGURE 29.1. Aortic stenosis: An angiocardiogram showing supravalvular aortic stenosis.

Considering the genetic potential, breeding of affected cats should be discouraged.

S u g g e s t e d   R e a d i n g

Fox PR. Congenital feline heart disease. In: Fox PR, ed. Canine and feline cardiology. New York: Churchill Livingstone, 1988;391–408.

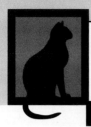

CHAPTER 30

Aspirin Toxicosis

Sharon K. Fooshee

Overview

I t has long been known that the cat has a peculiar sensitivity to certain drugs. One of the primary reasons for this is the cat's relative deficiency of hepatic glucuronyl transferase, an enzyme important in drug conjugation and excretion. Deficiency of this enzyme greatly prolongs the effective half-life of many therapeutic agents. Aspirin, one such drug, may be safely given to cats as long as the dosing interval is increased appropriately. Aspirin may be safely administered to cats at a dose of 20 mg/kg every 48 hours. Nonspecific signs such as anorexia, vomiting, tachypnea, fever, and depression may be seen first. If a history of aspirin ingestion is unrecognized, it is difficult to make a specific diagnosis at this time. The likelihood of respiratory or gastrointestinal hemorrhage (with potential perforation) is increased with repeated dosing of the drug. Drug-induced hepatitis may lead to icterus. Muscular weakness, ataxia, seizures, coma, and death may follow within days.

 D i a g n o s i s

Primary Diagnostics

- **History:** Because the clinical signs are nonspecific, it is important to query the owner about the administration of aspirin.
- **CBC:** Anemia due to bone marrow suppression and the presence of Heinz bodies are occasionally noted on the CBC. Thrombocytopenia and leukocytosis with a left shift also are reported.
- **Acid-base evaluation:** An initial respiratory alkalosis with subsequent high anion gap metabolic acidosis may be noted.

Ancillary Diagnostics

Larger commercial laboratories may be equipped to measure serum salicylate levels.

Diagnostic Notes

- The presence of a condition requiring analgesic or antithrombotic medication may prompt the clinician to suspect aspirin toxicosis in the patient.
- Ethylene glycol toxicity is an important differential diagnosis.

 T r e a t m e n t

Primary Therapeutics

- **Removal:** If early intervention is possible, emesis may be induced or gastric contents removed by lavage. Activated charcoal should be given orally at 2 g/kg.
- **GI:** Gastrointestinal ulceration should be treated with appropriate protectants (sucralfate).

Secondary Therapeutics

- **Supportive care:** This should include fluid therapy, as needed, and attention to the patient's body temperature.
- **Acid-base:** The patient should be monitored and treated for ongoing acid-base disturbances. Sodium bicarbonate therapy may combat metabolic acidosis and hasten elimination of the drug.

P r o g n o s i s

The prognosis should be favorable with early intervention and the cessation of aspirin administration.

S u g g e s t e d   R e a d i n g s

Groff RM, Miller JM, Stair EL, et al. Toxicoses and toxins. In: Norsworthy GD, ed. Feline practice. Philadelphia: JB Lippincott, 1993;560.

Rumbeiha WK, Oehme FW, Reid FM. Toxicoses. In: Sherding RG, ed. The cat: diseases and clinical management. Philadelphia: WB Saunders, 1994;215–249.

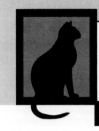

CHAPTER 31

Asthma

Gary D. Norsworthy

Overview

Feline asthma is also known as chronic bronchitis, bronchial asthma, and allergic bronchitis. Serotonin is the primary mediator in feline mast cells that contributes to airway smooth muscle contraction. Inhaled antigens within airways cause acute mast cell degranulation and thus a release of serotonin. This results in a sudden contraction of the airway smooth muscle. The disease is often progressive, resulting in bronchiectasis and emphysema. The antigens that initiate serotonin release are usually undiagnosed, but the common suspects are grass and tree pollens, smoke (cigarette or fireplace), sprays (hair sprays, flea sprays, household deodorizers), dusty cat litter, and flea powders; food allergy is also a consideration. Cigarette smoke is becoming a greater suspect in smokers' households because the pollutants gravitate to the floor or carpet. The cat's respiratory intake is on or near this level. The most common clinical sign is coughing. Asthmatic cats usually assume a characteristic crouched position. Cats with severe cases exhibit expiratory dyspnea, wheezing, open-mouth breathing, and cyanosis.

Diagnosis

Primary Diagnostics

- **Clinical signs:** Asthma should always be suspected in a coughing cat, especially if the cat assumes the characteristic crouched position.
- **Radiographs:** The most common pattern is interstitial, but patchy alveolar densities may occur. The right middle lung lobe may collapse in some cats. Right heart enlargement and lung overinflation, aerophagia, or emphysema may occur.
- **CBC:** A peripheral eosinophilia has been reported 20 to 75% of the time.

Ancillary Diagnostics

- **Bronchial wash or BAL:** An increase in eosinophils is expected, but eosinophils are commonly found in the respiratory tract of normal cats.
- **Heartworm Antibody and Antigen Tests:** Heartworms are an important cause of coughing.

Diagnostic Notes

- Coughing is an uncommon sign in cats; the most common cause of coughing is asthma.

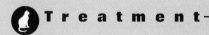 **T r e a t m e n t**

Primary Therapeutics: Respiratory Crisis

- **Oxygen therapy:** Oxygen can be administered via face mask, nasal catheter, tent (made from a plastic bag), or oxygen cage. The first two are usually too stressful for a cat in a crisis.
- **Corticosteroids:** Intravenously administered, rapidly acting steroids should be administered. Dexamethasone (0.2–2.2 mg/kg) or prednisolone sodium succinate (30 mg/kg) is recommended.
- **Bronchodilators:** Aminophylline (5 mg/kg IV) or terbutaline (0.01 mg/kg SC or IV) can be given. Owners can be taught to give terbutaline subutaneously for asthmatic crises. It can be repeated in 15–30 minutes if response does not occur.

Secondary Therapeutics: Respiratory Crisis

- **Adrenergics:** Epinephrine (0.1 mL of a 1:10,000 solution SC) or isoproterenol (0.1–0.2 mL of a 1:5,000 solution SC) can be given if there is no response to the primary therapeutics.
- **Anticholinergics:** Atropine (0.04 mg/kg SC or IM) can be given if there is no response to the adrenergics.
- **Airway suctioning:** A life-threatening collection of mucus in the airway can be removed with suction through an 8-Fr feeding tube. However, this procedure requires anesthetic, which may be dangerous in this situation.

Primary Therapeutics: Mild Signs

- **Corticosteroids:** Oral or reposital injectable steroids are effective on a short-term and a long-term basis. Prednisolone is given at 1 mg/kg BID for 10–14 days, then tapered over 1–2 months to a maintenance dose of 5–10

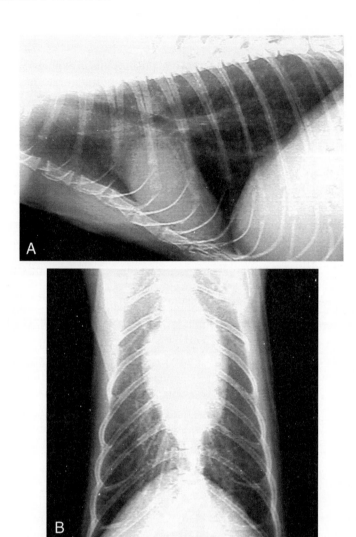

FIGURE 31.1. Asthma: Radiographic signs of asthma include increased pulmonary radiolucency (*A,B*) and bronchial thickening (*A,B*).

mg every other evening. If administration is a problem, a long-acting repository steroid is used.

- **Bronchodilators:** The preferred drug is time-release theophylline (Theo-Dur). The usual dose is 10 mg/kg every evening. It should not be used without corticosteroids. Terbutaline (0.625 mg/kg BID) is also effective.

- **Antibiotics:** Many asthmatic cats have bacterial or *Mycoplasma* infections. If culture and sensitivity are not available, the preferred drugs are enrofloxacin (2.2 mg/kg BID PO) or doxycycline (5 mg/kg BID PO).

Secondary Therapeutics

- **Weight reduction:** If indicated, this can be very helpful.

- **Avoidance of allergens:** Restricting the cat's access to the items listed in the overview section, especially dusty kitty litter and cigarette smoke, should be tried.

- **Food trial:** A 4–8 week food elimination trial should be considered, although the success rate is low.

- **Cyproheptadine:** This is a serotonin-receptor blocker that should be considered for cats intolerant of prolonged oral terbutaline. A 4–5-kg cat is dosed at 2 mg BID PO.

- **Cyclosporin A:** This drug blocks interleukin-2 synthesis and can be very effective at 10 mg/kg BID PO. It has adverse side effects in many cats, so it should be used only as a drug of last resort.

Prognosis

The prognosis is good in the short term; however, some chronically affected cats develop pulmonary fibrosis and emphysema.

Suggested Readings

Henik RA, Yeager AE. In:Sherding RG, ed. The cat: diseases and clinical management, 2nd ed. New York: Churchill Livingstone, 1994;979–1052.

Norsworthy GD. Asthma. In: Norsworthy GD, ed. Feline practice. Philadelphia: JB Lippincott, 1993;231–235.

Padrid, P. New strategies to treat feline asthma. *Vet Forum* 1996;13(10):46–50.

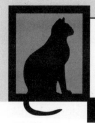

CHAPTER 32

Atopy

Gary D. Norsworthy

Overview

Atopy is a type I hypersensitivity reaction common in cats. It does not appear to have the genetic influence that is so strong in dogs. The clinical signs are more variable than in dogs; the most common sign is truncal alopecia with or without miliary dermatitis. Diseases of the eosinophilic granuloma complex are thought to be allergic manifestations. Head and neck pruritus is common. Less common manifestations include self-mutilation, foot chewing, and recurrent otitis externa. Because of excessive licking, cats may have an increase in vomition of hairballs or constipation caused by hair ingestion.

 D i a g n o s i s

Primary Diagnostics

- **Clinical signs:** Truncal alopecia, with or without obvious pruritus, should raise suspicion of atopy. Lesions typical of the eosinophilic granuloma complex diseases and miliary dermatitis also indicate that atopy is likely.
- **Intradermal skin testing:** This is the gold standard for confirming atopy.

Ancillary Diagnostics

- **In vitro testing:** The radioallergosorbent test (RAST) and enzyme-linked immunosorbent assay (ELISA) have been used in cats, but most authorities question their specificity for use in feline patients.
- **Response to corticosteroids:** Most atopic cats respond dramatically to oral or injectable steroids. However, this is not specific for atopy.
- **Trichogram:** This is a microscopic examination of the distal ends of hair. Blunt, broken hairs indicate licking, scratching, or chewing and are consistent with atopy. For details on technique, see Appendix F.

Diagnostic Notes

The technique used for skin testing cats is somewhat different from the technique used with dogs. Positive reactions are often not as pronounced and may take 4 to 6 hours to occur.

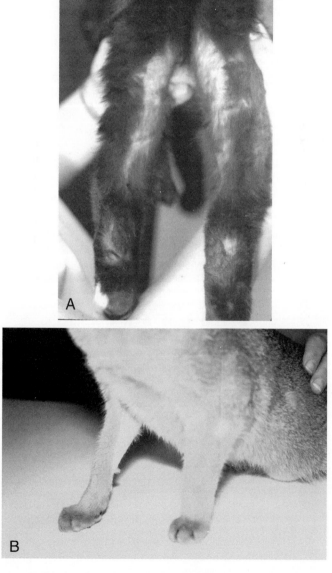

FIGURE 32.1. Atopy: Atopic cats usually are pruritic. They often lick hair from the caudal aspects of the rear legs (*A*) and in focal areas anywhere on the skin, including the front legs (*B*).

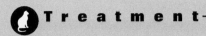

Treatment

Primary Therapeutics

- **Avoidance of exposure:** This is the ideal method of treatment but is usually not possible because of an inability to identify the allergen(s) or an inability to halt exposure.
- **Hyposensitization:** This is the method of choice. One study reported a success rate of 73%.
- **Corticosteroids:** This is a commonly used approach because of its effectiveness and its lack of side effects in cats. Oral prednisolone is preferable at 0.5 to 2.2 mg/kg every other evening. Methylprednisolone (Depo-Medrol) is generally effective at 20 to 40 mg/cat IM or SC every 4 weeks.

Secondary Therapeutics

- **Chlorpheniramine:** This antihistamine has been reported to be effective in relieving pruritus due to atopy at a dose of 2 mg/cat PO BID/TID. It may take 6 to 10 weeks for response, which makes client compliance problematic.
- **Essential fatty acid supplements:** Derm Caps™ (DVM) have been reported to also relieve pruritus at two to four times the labeled dose. It, too, may take 6 to 10 weeks for response.

Prognosis

The prognosis is excellent if there is good response to hyposensitization. Corticosteroids, antihistamines, or essential fatty acids also are good options for successful therapy.

Suggested Reading

Moriello KA. Diseases of the skin. In: Sherding RG, ed. The cat: diseases and clinical management, 2nd ed. Philadelphia: WB Saunders, 1994;1907–1968.

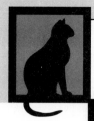

Basal Cell Tumor

Mitchell A. Crystal

Overview

B asal cell tumors are common, making up 11–30% of feline skin tumors. Basal cell tumors occur in adult cats (usually older than 7 years of age) and may be benign (benign basal cell tumor, basal cell epithelioma, basaloid tumor, basaloma) or malignant (basal cell carcinoma), although most behave in a benign manner. Tumors arise from epidermal basal cells and usually appear as well-circumscribed, solitary, 0.5–2.0 cm raised, ulcerated, melanotic, occasionally cystic intradermal masses on the head, neck, and thorax (and occasionally on the nasal planum and eyelids). Tumors appear in all breeds, although Siamese (carcinoma) and Himalayan and Persian (benign basal cell tumor) breeds may be predisposed to their development. Basal cell tumors have no known etiology, although a strong correlation exists in humans between ultraviolet light exposure and tumor formation. Clinical signs are limited to the presence of the mass. Differential diagnoses include squamous cell carcinoma, melanoma, mast cell tumor, cutaneous hemangioma or hemangiosarcoma, hair follicle tumors, and sebaceous gland tumors.

 D i a g n o s i s

Primary Diagnostics

- **Surgical removal and histopathology:** This is the most accurate means of diagnosis.

Ancillary Diagnostics

- **Fine-needle aspiration/cytology:** This may reveal the diagnosis prior to surgery.

Diagnostic Notes

Tumors usually behave in a benign manner even if assessed as a carcinoma by histopathology.

Treatment ——————————————————————

Primary Therapeutics

- **Surgical excision:** Complete removal of the tumors is curative in most cases.

Secondary Therapeutics

- **Laser ablation, cryotherapy, electrosurgery:** These methods have been successful.
- **Observation without treatment:** Some tumors cease growing.

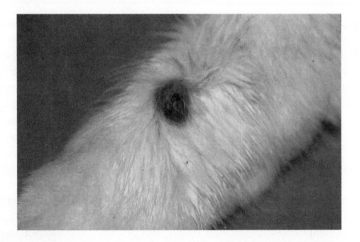

FIGURE 33.1. Basal cell tumor: Basal cell tumors often occur as small masses on the skin.

Prognosis

The prognosis for cure is excellent with complete surgical excision in nearly all cases.

Suggested Readings

Elmslie RE. Basal cell tumor. In: Smith FWK, Tilley LP, eds. The 5-minute veterinary consult. Baltimore: Williams & Wilkins, 1996;386–387.

Scott DW, Miller WH, Griffin CE. Miller & Kirk's small animal dermatology, 5th ed. Philadelphia: WB Saunders, 1995;1007–1008.

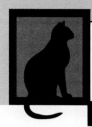

C H A P T E R   3 4

Bartonellosis

Mitchell A. Crystal

Overview

*B*artonella spp. (previously named *Rochalimaea* spp.) are fastidious, intra- or epi-erythrocytic gram-negative bacteria that cause the human ailment cat-scratch disease (CSD), as well as bacillary angiomatosis, bacillary peliosis hepatitis, endocarditis, granulomatous hepatosplenic syndrome, retinitis and optic nerve swelling, osteolytic lesions, and pulmonary granulomas. The most common species of *Bartonella* associated with CSD is *B. henselae*. The mode of transmission of *Bartonella* spp. in both humans and cats has not been determined, although contact with cats (scratches, bites) and insect vectors (fleas, ticks, lice) are considered as possibilities. The role of *Bartonella* spp. as a disease-causing organism in cats is uncertain. Up to 41% of healthy cats have been documented to have *Bartonella* spp. bacteremia. Experimental infections in cats have resulted in self-limiting febrile episodes of 48–72 hours duration, and intracellular *Bartonella*-like organisms have been demonstrated in some cats with idiopathic peripheral lymphadenopathy. Clinical signs of CSD in humans include lymphadenopathy, fever, malaise, myalgia, and headache. *Bartonella* spp. is considered of zoonotic importance in both immunocompetent and immunocompromised individuals. Any person demonstrating clinical signs consistent with CSD or other *Bartonella*-induced diseases should be referred to a physician for confirmation. If *Bartonella* spp. is confirmed, discontinuation of exposure to and contact with the affected animal should be recommended.

Diagnosis

Primary Diagnostics

- **Indirect fluorescent antibody (IFA) or enzyme-linked immunosorbent assay (ELISA) for antibodies to *Bartonella* spp.:** These are the tests of choice. They are available from the Centers for Disease Control for determination of *Bartonella* spp. antibodies in human patients.

Ancillary Diagnostics

- **Culture and sensitivity:** Cultures are performed using blood agar media in a 5% carbon dioxide and high humidity environment and may require up to 56 days to grow visible colonies.
- **PCR:** Amplification of *Bartonella* spp. DNA from tissue samples via polymerase chain reaction (PCR) has been described but it is not currently commercially available for feline patients.

Diagnostic Notes

IFA or ELISA for antibodies to *Bartonella* spp. may be useful in acutely infected cats, but antibody kinetics for chronically infected cats have not been established.

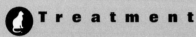 **T r e a t m e n t**

Primary Therapeutics

- **Antibiotics:** Doxycycline, erythromycin, rifampin, penicillin, ceftriaxone, and ciprofloxacin have all been reported to have some efficacy in humans.

Therapeutic Notes

The treatment of choice in humans remains controversial as a result of limited clinical studies.

No definitive treatment recommendations can be made for cats as the significance of *Bartonella* as a pathogen and antimicrobial efficacy has not been established in cats.

P r o g n o s i s

Cats with *Bartonella* spp. usually have inapparent infections and thus have an excellent prognosis of not developing any serious illness. CSD in humans is usually self-limiting or responds well to antibiotic therapy, although relapses requiring prolonged treatment may occur in immunocompromised individuals.

S u g g e s t e d   R e a d i n g s

Breitschwerdt EB. Bartonellosis and culture negative endocarditis. Proceedings of the Thirteenth Annual Veterinary Medical Forum 1995;311–313.

Kordick DL, Lappin MR, Breitschwerdt EB. Feline Rickettsial diseases. In: Ettinger SJ, Feldman EC, eds. Textbook of veterinary internal medicine, 4th ed. Philadelphia: WB Saunders, 1995:289.

Groves MG, Harrington KS. *Rochalimaea henselae* infections: newly recognized zoonoses transmitted by domestic cats. *J Am Vet Med Assoc* 1994;204(2):267–271.

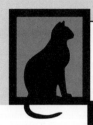

CHAPTER 35

Blastomycosis

Sharon K. Fooshee

Overview

*B*lastomyces dermatitidis, the etiologic agent of feline blastomycosis, is a dimorphic, saprophytic organism. The disease is rare in the cat; only a limited number of cases have been reported. Inhalation of infective spores is the primary mechanism for establishment of infection. Once in the lung, the mycelial phase transforms to a thick-walled yeast phase, with dissemination by hematogenous and possibly lymphatic routes. Reproduction occurs by budding from the parent organism. The organism is worldwide in distribution; in the United States, it is endemic in the Mississippi, Ohio, and Missouri River valleys. Attempts to isolate the organism from soil have met with only limited success. The infected cat must have a competent cell-mediated immune response to overcome the disease. The yeast phase is not considered contagious to humans, although caution should be exercised with open draining tracts. Public health risk is derived from a shared environmental exposure.

Disseminated disease is common in the few feline cases reported. Vague signs such as anorexia, fever, weight loss, and depression are expected. Pulmonary disease and related signs (dyspnea, tachypnea, increased lung sounds) represent the most common organ-specific involvement. Inflammatory ocular lesions, lymphadenopathy, draining tracts, osteomyelitis, and central nervous system (CNS) signs have been reported.

 D i a g n o s i s

Primary Diagnostics

- **Clinical signs:** Respiratory signs and signs of systemic disease in cats in the endemic area should raise one's index of suspicion.
- **Cytology:** The organism is usually easily recognized in exudative lesions and infected organs. It has a characteristic thick, refractile wall.

Budding organisms are attached to the parent organism by a broad base. The associated inflammatory response is usually pyogranulomatous.

Ancillary Diagnostics

- **Radiography:** The most common radiographic finding is a diffuse miliary nodular pattern in the lung parenchyma; this is very suggestive of fungal pneumonia. Pleural and peritoneal effusions have been reported.
- **CBC:** Nonregenerative anemia is common.
- **Serologic and intradermal skin testing:** These *are not* reliable indicators of infection. *Identification of the organism is essential for confirmation of a diagnosis.*

Diagnostic Notes

- The broad-based attachment that is present during reproduction is helpful in distinguishing *Blastomyces* from *Cryptococcus neoformans.*
- *Blastomyces* may not stain reliably with routine histopathologic stains. If blastomycosis is suspected, the pathologist should be advised so that other stains may be used. Cytology may be the preferred method for demonstrating the organism, as it stains well with modified Wright's stains.
- A travel history should always be obtained for any sick cat. Cats housed exclusively indoors are still at risk for infection.

 T r e a t m e n t

Primary Therapeutics

- Itraconazole is the antifungal drug of choice. It should be dosed at 5 mg/kg PO BID and given with a meal; an acid environment in the stomach enhances absorption of the drug. The capsule may be opened and the contents divided into plain gelatin capsules or mixed into canned food.

Therapeutic Notes

Itraconazole is better tolerated than ketoconazole by most cats. However, it is still recommended to periodically check serum chemistries. For cats with *clinical* evidence of hepatotoxicity (anorexia, jaundice), the drug should be discontinued, at least temporarily. Asymptomatic cats with increased liver enzymes (alanine aminotransferase [ALT]) do not necessarily need cessation of therapy but should be closely monitored.

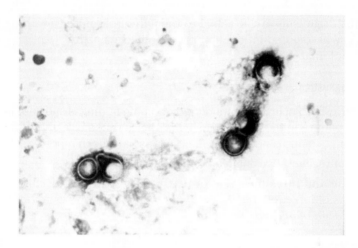

FIGURE 35.1. Blastomycosis: *Blastomyces dermatitidis* can be recovered from body fluids or aspirates. They are 6–20 micrometers (μm) in diameter and have a double wall.

Prognosis

In general, the prognosis for infected cats has improved with the introduction of itraconazole. However, severely debilitated cats with advanced systemic disease still have a guarded prognosis.

Suggested Readings

Breider MA, Walker TL, Legendre AM, VanEe RT. Blastomycosis in cats: five cases (1979–1986). *J Am Vet Med Assoc* 1988;193:570–572.

Fooshee SK, Woody BW. Systemic fungal diseases. In: Norsworthy GD, ed. Feline practice. Philadelphia: JB Lippincott, 1993;540–550.

Taboada J, Merchant SR. Treatment of fungal diseases. In: Proceedings of the American College of Veterinary Internal Medicine, Thirteenth Annual Meeting. 1995;800.

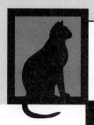

CHAPTER 36

Cholangiohepatitis Complex

Gary D. Norsworthy

Overview

Cholangitis and cholangiohepatitis (CHT) are inflammatory and/or infectious diseases affecting the intrahepatic biliary system and the biliary system and hepatic parenchyma, respectively. This complex includes three diseases in a continuum of occurrence. **Acute** or **suppurative** CHT is caused by Eschenchia bacteria that generally ascend the bile duct into the intrahepatic biliary system. *Escherichia coli* is the most commonly recovered organism, but gram-positive anaerobes have also been found. Liver aspirations or biopsies of this form reveal inflammatory cells that are primarily neutrophils and macrophages. **Chronic** or **lymphocytic** CHT causes a sterile inflammatory process that is usually a sequela to acute CHT and may be perpetuated by an abnormal immune response. The predominant infiltrating cells are lymphocytes and plasma cells, which suggest immune disease. **Cirrhosis** is the end-stage of the spectrum, resulting in terminal liver failure. It is the least common form because many cats die before the chronic form progresses to cirrhosis. The clinical signs of each of the diseases in this complex are similar. Icterus, lethargy, anorexia, and vomiting can occur with each disease. Fever is common in the acute form but uncommon in the others. Ascites occasionally occurs during cirrhosis. Cats with the chronic form have recurrent episodes of clinical signs interspersed with weeks or months of normalcy. Extrahepatic biliary obstruction due to inspissated bile can occur with the acute or chronic forms.

Diagnosis

Primary Diagnostics

- **Clinical signs:** Cats with systemic signs that have acute or recurrent icterus should be suspected of one of these diseases. Ascites is an uncommon finding in cats and should raise one's index of suspicion for cirrhosis.

- **Chemistry profile:** The ALT, AST, ALP, and total bilirubin are elevated; however, these elevations are not specific for this disease. Mild anemia, hyperglobulinemia, and hypoalbuminemia are common in the chronic form.
- **Liver cytology or histopathology:** Histopathology is diagnostic and is the preferred test. Cytology can identify the characteristic infiltrating cells, but it usually cannot differentiate CHT from other infectious or inflammatory liver diseases, including feline infectious peritonitis.

Ancillary Diagnostics

- **Ultrasound:** The increased echogenicity commonly found is not specific for acute or chronic CHT, and the study may appear normal. Cirrhotic livers are usually hyperechoic. Ultrasound is very useful in determining the presence of extrahepatic biliary obstruction.
- **Radiography:** Radiographs of cats with the acute and chronic forms are usually normal, although the liver may be enlarged. It is usually enlarged when cirrhosis is present.
- **Culture:** If a liver biopsy is performed, aerobic and anaerobic cultures should be performed on the liver parenchyma and the bile.

Diagnostic Notes

Many of these cats have clotting disorders. Percutaneous liver biopsies can result in significant bleeding. The safest biopsy is via laparotomy so hemorrhage can be controlled adequately.

 T r e a t m e n t

Primary Therapeutics

- **All forms:** Supportive care in the form of IV or SC fluids and enteral nutritional support are important in stabilizing these cats. Famotidine (0.2 mg/kg SID PO) is the author's choice for controlling vomiting induced by liver disease.
- **Acute form:** Antibiotics are the basis of treatment. Drugs or combinations that are effective on aerobes and anaerobes are indicated. Enrofloxacin (2.2 mg/kg BID PO) and amoxicillin (11 mg/kg BID PO) or amoxicillin and metronidazole (12.5 mg/kg BID PO) are good choices when culture and sensitivity results are not available. Corticosteroids (prednisolone: 2–3 mg/kg SID PO) are also helpful in many cats. Antibiotics should be given for 3–4 weeks and longer if indicated.
- **Chronic form:** Antibiotics are indicated, but corticosteroids (prednisolone: 2.2 to 4.4 mg/kg SID PO) are the basis of treatment.

Because this is a chronic disease, continuous use of corticosteroids is needed in many cats.

- **Cirrhosis:** There is no known treatment to reverse cirrhosis. Ascites should be controlled with low-salt diets and loop diuretics (furosemide: 2.5–5.0 mg/kg q24 to 48h PO). Angiotensin-converting enzymes inhibitors (enalapril: 0.125–0.25 mg/kg SID PO) may be helpful in refractory cases.

Secondary Therapeutics

- **Surgery:** Extrahepatic biliary obstruction should be relieved with cholecystoduodenostomy or with cholecystotomy and bile duct flushing or cannulization.

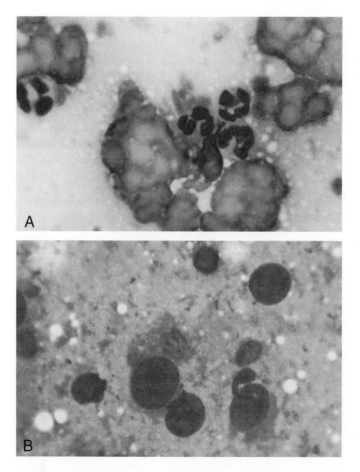

FIGURE 36.1. Cholangiohepatitis complex: The predominant cell in the acute (suppurative) form is the neutrophil (*A*); the predominant cell in the chronic form is the lymphocyte (*B*).

- **Ursodeoxycholic acid (urosdiol, Actigall):** This drug has choleretic properties. It has been very helpful in some cats to relieve intrahepatic cholestasis when dosed at 10 mg/kg SID PO.

Therapeutic Notes

- Because the acute form may progress to the chronic form, it is important to extend antibiotic therapy for at least 3 weeks. Antibiotic selection should be based on culture and sensitivity if at all possible.
- Enrofloxacin has little effect on anaerobes. It should not be used alone.
- Tetracycline and diazepam are contraindicated in hepatic disease.

Prognosis

The prognosis varies with the form of the disease. Most cats with the acute form recover clinically in a few days. The chronic form requires continuous therapy in many cats. Those that respond well have a good prognosis, but those that progress to cirrhosis have a poor prognosis. Cirrhosis is the least common of the forms because many cats with the chronic form die or are euthanized.

Suggested Reading

Day DG. Diseases of the liver. In: Sherding RG, ed. The cat: diseases and clinical management, 2nd ed. New York: Churchill Livingstone. 1994;1297–1340.

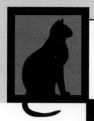

C H A P T E R   3 7
Chronic Tubulointerstitial Nephritis

Gary D. Norsworthy

Overview

T he most common renal disease in cats is chronic tubulointerstitial nephritis, formerly called chronic interstitial nephritis. It may be the result of any chronic renal disease, including glomerulonephritis, pyelonephritis, or amyloidosis, but the cause of most cases is unknown. Because most affected cats are geriatric, it is likely, in part, to be the result of the normal aging process. The most common clinical signs are weight loss, anorexia, lethargy, polyuria, and polydipsia. Vomiting may occur, but much later in the disease than in dogs. Many cats with advanced disease are dehydrated and emaciated and have pale mucous membranes. The cat's kidneys are smaller than normal; this may be documented by palpation, radiography, or ultrasonography.

 D i a g n o s i s

Primary Diagnostics

- **Clinical signs:** Geriatric cats that are anorectic, polydipsic, and polyuric and have experienced significant weight loss should be suspected of having chronic renal disease.
- **Laboratory findings:** The common laboratory findings include nonregenerative anemia, azotemia, hyperphosphatemia, metabolic acidosis, and low urine specific gravity.

Diagnostic Notes

- The serum creatinine level is less influenced by nonrenal factors than is the serum urea nitrogen, so it is a more specific and preferred test.
- Many cats in renal failure are hypertensive; therefore, blood pressure determination is desirable. Restoration of renal function often makes the cat normotensive, so long-term treatment with hypotensive agents may not

be necessary unless signs of retinal hemorrhage or detachment are present. However, there is evidence in dogs that renal failure and hypertension may aggravate each other.

 T r e a t m e n t

Primary Therapeutics: Initial Treatment Phase

- **Rehydration and diuresis:** This is best accomplished by placement of an intravenous catheter and administration of an isotonic, balanced fluid such as lactated Ringer's solution.
- **Tube feeding:** Anorexia is a consistent finding, and vomiting is not; therefore, feeding of a balanced diet via orogastric or nasogastric tube is very desirable. The cat's hydration status and general well-being improve rapidly when adequate nutrition is supplied.
- **Potassium:** Hypokalemia is a consistent result of anorexia and further reduces renal function. Intravenous fluid administration aggravates hypokalemia. Forty to 60 mEq of potassium chloride should be added to each liter of intravenous fluids, or 4–8 mEq of potassium gluconate (Tumil-K, Daniels Pharmaceuticals) should be given orally each day. (IMPORTANT: see Therapeutic Notes.)
- **Phosphate binder:** The use of calcium acetate (PhosLo, 1/4 tablet BID with food) helps reduce phosphate absorption from the digestive tract. Amphujel is also effective.
- **B-vitamins:** The loss of water-soluble B complex vitamins likely is due to polyuria.

Secondary Therapeutics: Initial Treatment Phase

- **Blood transfusion:** This measure is unlikely to be needed but should be considered when the hematocrit is below 15%.
- **Antiemetic:** Famotidine (0.5 mg SID PO) should be used to control vomiting. This is important to facilitate enteral feeding. There is some evidence that gastric hyperacidity causes nausea and results in anorexia; thus, famotidine may be helpful in any anorectic cat in renal failure.

Primary Therapeutics: Maintenance Phase

- **Special diet:** A low-protein diet will reduce phosphate intake and nitrogenous waste production. Both result in the cat's feeling and eating better. These diets are also non-acidifying, which is desirable.
- **Potassium:** Oral potassium should be continued long-term at a dose of 2–4 mEq per cat per day. Potassium gluconate (Tumil-K, Daniels Pharmaceuticals) is recommended.

- **Phosphate binder:** PhosLo or Amphojel should be continued long-term at 1/4 tablet BID with food if needed to control hyperphosphatemia.
- **Fluids:** Subcutaneously administered fluids (lactated Ringer's solution or normal saline solution) should be given one to seven times per week based on the cat's clinical response and serial creatinine levels. The average dose is 150 mL/cat.

Secondary Therapeutics: Maintenance Phase

- **Calcitriol:** The use of this active form of vitamin D is controversial. Calcitriol's proponents feel that it may enhance gastrointestinal absorption of calcium and reduce parathyroid hormone secretion. These processes help to control renal secondary hyperparathyroidism.
- **Erythropoietin:** Persistent, severe anemia may be correctable with injections of this exogenous hormone. It is dosed initially at 100 u/kg SC three times per week until clinical response occurs; the dose then is tapered.
- **Hypotensive agent:** Because hypertension may be corrected with improvement of renal function, these drugs may not be needed long-term; however, blood pressure monitoring is highly recommended. The drugs of choice are amlodipine (0.625 mg/cat SID PO) and benazepril (1.25 mg/cat SID or BID PO).
- **Sodium bicarbonate:** Persistent acidosis (serum bicarbonate less than 16 mEq/L) may resolve with the oral administration of this drug.
- **Anabolic steroids:** The use of these products is controversial; they are intended to increase the cat's hematocrit. The preferred drugs are nandrolone decanoate (1 mg/kg q7d SC or IM) and stanozolol (1–2 mg/cat BID PO).

Therapeutic Notes

- Nondehydrated cats that are presented with mild elevations in serum creatinine levels may not require intravenous fluids. Their stress level can be reduced by administering fluids subcutaneously and, in select cases, by treating the cats as outpatients.
- An economical and practical solution of famotidine can be made by crushing three 10-mg tablets and adding them to 1 ounce of a palatable, liquid vitamin solution. This yields a concentration of 1 mg/mL. The suspension should be well shaken before use.
- Overdosing with intravenous potassium can be fatal. Care should be taken not to administer IV potassium too rapidly. Do not exceed 0.5 mEq/kg/hr. However, it is difficult to create hyperkalemia with orally administered potassium.
- Some potassium supplements for human use contain phosphates. These should be avoided.

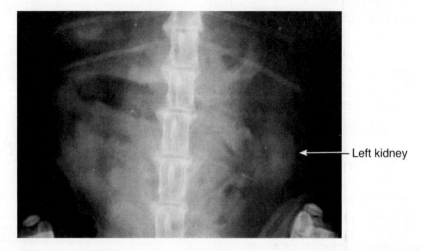

Left kidney

FIGURE 37.1. Chronic tubulointerstitial nephritis: One of the typical findings in chronic tubulointerstitial nephritis is kidneys of reduced size. The left kidney of this cat is considerably shorter than two to two-and-one-half times the length of the body of L2.

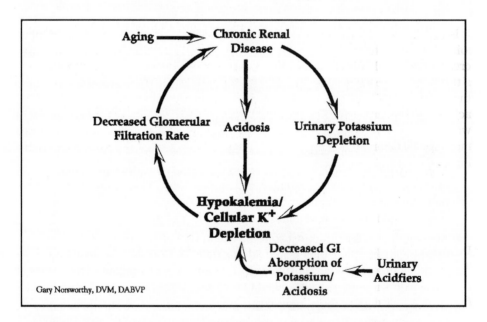

FIGURE 37.2. The interaction of potassium and renal failure is depicted in this diagram in which a vicious cycle of potassium loss and reduced renal function begins a self-perpetuating set of events that is complicated by acidosis and urinary acidifiers.

- Calcitriol should not be used if the product of the serum calcium and phosphorus levels is greater than 60. This avoids the potential for intracellular calcification. An elevated parathyroid hormone (PTH) level should be documented before calcitriol is administered.

- Erythropoietin is expensive, and about one-third of cats receiving it will develop antibodies that will destroy both exogenous and endogenous erythropoietin, making the cat transfusion-dependent. Erythropoietin should be used only when a severe anemia persists following blood transfusion and other therapies to restore renal function, and it should be discontinued as soon as possible.

- A practical way to administer sodium bicarbonate is to add 17 teaspoons of baking soda to a liter of water, making a 1 mEq $NaHCO_3$/mL solution. One or 2 mL are given SID or BID PO. The dose is adjusted to serum HCO_3 levels. The solution is stable for up to 3 months if capped and refrigerated.

- Renal transplantation has been performed successfully at some veterinary teaching hospitals. This is an expensive and not always successful form of treatment, but it can be recommended for select patients.

Prognosis

It is not possible to make a prognosis on the outcome of a case of chronic tubulointerstitial nephritis at the beginning of therapy. In addition, there is not a serum creatinine level that is considered a sign of absolute therapeutic failure. However, if the kidneys are less than one-third normal size, if the serum creatinine is greater than 10 mg/dL, if hyperphosphatemia is present, or if therapy for 3–4 days fails to achieve significant clinical and laboratory improvement, a guarded prognosis is warranted. Conversely, if response to therapy occurs and aggressive long-term maintenance therapy is provided, many cats will live 1 to 3 years while maintaining quality life.

Suggested Readings

DiBartola SP, Rutgers HC. Diseases of the kidneys. In: Sherding RG, ed. The cat: diseases and clinical management, 2nd ed. New York: Churchill Livingstone, 1994;1711–1767.

DiBartola SP, Buffington CA, Chew DJ, et al. Development of chronic renal disease in cats fed a commercial diet. *J Am Vet Med Assoc* 1993;202:744–749.

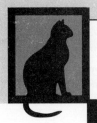

CHAPTER 38

Chylothorax

Gary D. Norsworthy

Overview

C hylothorax is the collection of chylous fluid in the pleural space. Chyle may access the pleural space due to thoracic duct rupture. This is usually trauma-related but accounts for only a small percentage of feline cases. The most common mechanism for chylothorax is lymphangiectasia that is thought to occur when systemic venous pressure increases. Initially, the chylous effusion is reabsorbed through the pleura. However, it is a pleural irritant. After a few days to weeks of exposure to chyle, the pleural surfaces no longer permit reabsorption, and the effusion collects in the pleural space. The most common underlying causes are right heart failure (heartworms and cardiomyopathy) and mediastinal neoplasia (especially lymphosarcoma and thymoma). Following an unsuccessful search for a primary disease, many cats are deemed to have idiopathic chylothorax. Cats with chylothorax are usually presented with a reported sudden onset of dyspnea. They are lethargic, often anorectic, and may cough.

 D i a g n o s i s

Primary Diagnostics

- **Clinical signs:** Dyspnea with systemic signs will occur. Coughing may occur.
- **Auscultation:** Muffled heart and lung sounds are found.
- **Radiography:** Radiographic signs of pleural effusion include visualization of pleural fissure lines and scalloping of the lung borders.
- **Ultrasound:** This should be performed before the fluid is removed from the pleural space. It may be helpful in establishing the presence of an anterior mediastinal mass. Occasionally, heartworms can be visualized in the right side of the heart or in the pulmonary arteries.

- **Thoracentesis:** A few milliliters of fluid may be removed to confirm the presence of pleural effusion and to obtain fluid for laboratory analysis.

- **Pleural fluid analysis:** The protein content and specific gravity will vary depending on the underlying cause; the nucleated cell count is typically less than 10,000 cells/μL. The fluid is milky white in color; if hemorrhage has occurred, it may be pink.

- **Pleural fluid cytology:** Cells may be more than 80% mature lymphocytes, having the same diameter as RBCs. If the disease is chronic, there will be a large number of neutrophils and macrophages, but bacteria are generally absent.

- **Test for FeLV antigen:** A positive test result greatly raises the index of suspicion that lymphosarcoma may be present.

- **Heartworm antigen test:** A positive result is confirmation of heartworm infection.

Ancillary Diagnostics

- **CBC and serum chemistries:** These are usually normal.
- **Radiography:** Note the pulmonary arteries as an indication of heartworm disease and observe for an anterior mediastinal mass.

Diagnostic Notes

- Chylous fluid has a higher triglyceride content than serum. Pseudochylous fluid has a greater cholesterol content than serum and a triglyceride content less than or equal to serum. Pseudochylous fluid has not been reported in the cat; therefore, any milky white pleural effusion should be considered chylous until proven otherwise.

- Dyspneic cats should be handled very carefully because increased stress may be fatal. Extreme care should be taken when doing the physical examination, radiographs, and thoracentesis. It may be necessary to place the cat in an oxygen cage for several minutes prior to diagnostics and between diagnostic procedures. The least stressful radiographic view is the dorsoventral view; it may be the only view that is practical in some cases and is usually sufficient to diagnose the presence of pleural effusion.

- A limited number of diseases cause coughing in cats. Chylothorax should be considered when this occurs.

- Chyle is irritating to the pleura. When chronic, chylothorax causes fibrosing pleuritis. Radiographs will reveal rounded and/or collapsed lung lobes, and inflammatory cells will be present in the effusion.

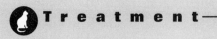

T r e a t m e n t

Primary Therapeutics

- **Thoracentesis:** The least amount of sedation should be employed. If sedation is needed, the use of 2 mg/kg of ketamine IV is generally safe. Aspirate both sides of the chest, and remove as much fluid as possible. Aspirate below the costochondral junction in multiple locations beginning at the fourth to sixth IC space with the cat in ventral recumbency.

Secondary Therapeutics

- **Thoracostomy tube:** This permits continuous or intermittent chest drainage without further stress to the cat. Generally, one tube will drain both sides of the chest; however, some cases require bilateral tube placement. The chest should be aspirated 1 to 2 times per day until less than 2 mL/kg of fluid is removed. (This amount usually is due to the presence of the tube.)
- **Intravenous fluids:** Placement of an intravenous catheter and fluid administration should be delayed until thoracentesis has been performed because of the stress involved.
- **Thoracotomy:** Cats that do not respond to 5–10 days of chest drainage are candidates for surgical ligation of the thoracic duct or pleuroperitoneal or pleurovenous shunts. However, these procedures do not have a high success rate so they should be reserved for the cases in which medical management and thoracostomy tube placement are not successful.

Therapeutic Notes

- Repeated thoracentesis may be used in place of thoracostomy. However, this can be a painful procedure that may be too stressful for many cats that are fragile patients. The use of a chest drain is strongly recommended for all but the most debilitated patients.
- **Rutin:** This drug is in the benzopyrone family and is available at health food stores. Preliminary work with it is promising in resolving the pleural effusion. It should be used when finances prohibit more conventional forms of therapy. It should also be considered as an adjunct to other therapies. Rutin is dosed at 50 mg/kg TID and supplied as 500-mg tablets that are tasteless. They may be crushed and mixed in food. Rutin has no efficacy in resolving fibrosing pleuritis.
- **Low-fat diets and medium chain triglycerides:** These have been used in an attempt to reduce chyle formation; however, their successes are uncommon.

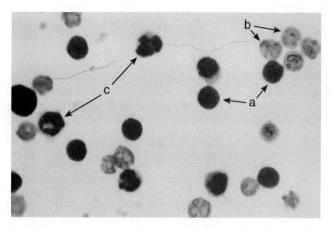

FIGURE 38.1. Chylothorax: The presence of small lymphocytes (*a*) along with the size of mature erythrocytes (*b*) is the classic finding in the effusion of chylothorax. The presence of neutrophils (*c*) signals the possibility of chronic disease leading to fibrosing pleuritis.

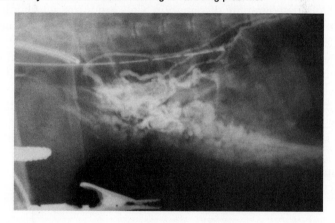

FIGURE 38.2. This lymphangiogram is typical of most cases of feline chylothorax. Instead of the thoracic duct being ruptured, lymphectasia is present with leakage of contrast material and chyle into the pleural space.

Prognosis

This is a serious and potentially fatal disease. However, with aggressive diagnostics and therapeutics, including a thoracostomy tube, most of these cats will recover as long as fibrosing pleuritis has not occurred.

Suggested Readings

Fossum TW, Miller MW, Rogers KS, Bonagura JD, Meurs KM. Chylothorax associated with right-sided heart failure in five cats. *J Am Vet Med Assoc* 1994;204:84–89.

Fossum TW, Evering WN, Miller MW, et al. Severe bilateral fibrosing pleuritis associated with chronic chylothorax in dogs and cats. *J Am Vet Med Assoc* 1992;201:317–324.

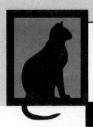

CHAPTER 39

Coccidioidomycosis

Sharon K. Fooshee

Overview

Of all the deep mycotic agents, *Coccidioides immitis* has the most limited geographic distribution. Cats are infrequently infected with this organism outside the endemic area of the dry, southwestern United States. The ecologic lower Sonoran life zone is well suited to support growth of the organism. In this area, dry hot summers are followed by moderately wet winters; the soil is sandy and alkaline. Although only a limited number of cases have been described in cats, it appears that the primary route of infection is by inhalation of small, airborne arthrospores. Infection by direct inoculation of the organism has also been reported. Dissemination occurs through hematogenous and lymphatic routes. A competent cell-mediated immune response must be present to contain infection. Infection with the feline leukemia and feline immunodeficiency viruses does not appear to predispose cats to coccidioidomycosis. Humans are not at risk for the disease from contact with infected cats but may become infected because of shared environmental exposure.

Nonspecific signs of fever, anorexia, and weight loss are common. Ocular inflammation, bony and dermatologic lesions, and lower respiratory signs are the most frequently reported clinical findings. Reported abnormalities include uveitis, detached retinas, lameness, fistulating skin lesions, dyspnea, cough, neurologic signs (paresis, seizures, hyperesthesia), and lymphadenopathy.

Diagnosis

Primary Diagnostics

- **Clinical signs:** Clinical signs are nonspecific; however, cats from the endemic area with signs of systemic disease should be suspected of being infected.

- **Cytology:** Cytologic specimens may be sufficient to make a diagnosis and can be obtained by aspiration of lung parenchyma or lymph nodes, impression smears from draining tracts, or bronchoalveolar lavage. The associated inflammatory response is granulomatous. Routine in-office stains will sometimes fail to stain the organism. Special stains may be requested from commercial diagnostic laboratories.

- **Histopathology:** As with cytologic specimens, special stains may be required to identify the organism in tissue. Grocott-Gomori methenamine silver nitrate and PAS (periodic acid-Schiff) stains are often useful. The laboratory or pathologist should be alerted when coccidioidomycosis is a differential diagnosis.

Ancillary Diagnostics

- **CBC/Biochemical profile/UA/FeLV/FIV:** The minimum database will not provide a diagnosis but is useful as a general health screen for the patient. Nonregenerative anemia is not uncommon. In one retrospective study, hyperproteinemia was found in 52% of cases.

- **Radiography:** Hilar lymphadenopathy, interstitial lung disease, and pleural disease are reported. Infected bone may have osteoproductive or osteolytic lesions.

- **Serologic testing:** Recent studies suggest that serologic testing may be of more value than previously thought. Precipitin antibodies and complement-fixing antibodies were present in most cats tested in one study. False negatives may occur. Serology is a questionable means, at present, for detecting progression of disease and response to therapy. Further evaluation is needed to assess the usefulness of serologic testing.

Diagnostic Notes

- The organism does not typically exfoliate in large numbers so a careful microscopic search may be required to locate it.

- The travel history should always be obtained for any sick cat.

 T r e a t m e n t

Primary Therapeutics

- The potential value of itraconazole in treating this disease remains to be determined. Previous efforts to treat with ketoconazole have met with limited success for long-term resolution of disease. The imidazole drugs, at present, are considered fungistatic, not cidal.

- Itraconazole is safely dosed at 5 mg/kg PO BID and should be given with a meal; an acid environment in the stomach enhances absorption of the drug. The capsule may be opened and the contents divided into gelatin capsules or mixed into canned food.

Therapeutic Notes

- Relapse is fairly common following cessation of therapy, even with very long-term therapy.

- Itraconazole is better tolerated than ketoconazole by most cats. However, it is still recommended to periodically check serum chemistries. For cats with *clinical* evidence of hepatotoxicity (anorexia, jaundice), the drug should be discontinued, at least temporarily. Asymptomatic cats with increased liver enzymes (ALT) do not necessarily need cessation of therapy but should be closely monitored.

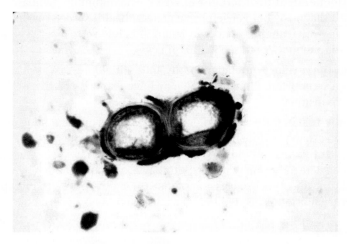

FIGURE 39.1. Coccidioidomycosis: Large (50–100 μm) organisms of *Coccidioides immitis* are found in relatively small numbers. They are most likely to be found in draining tracts or areas of inflammation.

Prognosis

The long-term prognosis for cats with coccidioidomycosis is guarded.

Suggested Readings

Fooshee SK, Woody BW. Systemic fungal diseases. In: Norsworthy GD, ed. Feline practice. Philadelphia: JB Lippincott, 1993;540–550.

Greene RT, Troy GC. Coccidioidomycosis in 48 cats: a retrospective study (1984–1993). *J Vet Intern Med* 1995;9:86–91.

Taboada J, Merchant SR. Treatment of fungal diseases. In: Proceedings of the American College of Veterinary Internal Medicine, Thirteenth Annual Meeting. 1995;800.

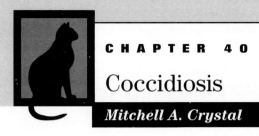

CHAPTER 40

Coccidiosis

Mitchell A. Crystal

Overview

C occidia are small-intestinal and occasionally large-intestinal protozoan parasites of low pathogenicity. Although diarrhea, mucochezia, hematochezia, and even death are occasionally seen with coccidial infections (especially in kittens), most coccidia cause no clinical signs. There are several species of coccidia (Table 40.1). For information regarding *Toxoplasma gondii*, refer to Chapter 119. Coccidia are acquired via ingestion of intermediate hosts (which demonstrate extra-intestinal stages) or from ingestion of infected feces. There is generally no extra-intestinal involvement in the cat, and transplacental and transmammary infection does not occur. Physical examination may be normal or reveal evidence of diarrhea and weight loss. *Cryptosporidium* spp. is of special note. This coccidia can cause severe diarrhea, weight loss, weakness, and dehydration. Cats with *Cryptosporidium* spp. often have a predisposing underlying disease process (such as alimentary lymphoma, inflammatory bowel disease, or FeLV or FIV infections) that should be investigated. Also, as this is a disease of limited zoonotic potential, appropriate handling of feces should be discussed with owners, and immunocompromised individuals should avoid contact with infected animals.

TABLE 40.1.

Species of Coccidia

Coccidia Organism	Intermediate Host
Besnoitia spp.	Cattle, mice, opossum
Cystoisospora spp. (previously *Isospora*)	Cats and various other mammals
Cryptosporidium spp.	Cats and various other mammals
Hammondia hammondi	Cattle
Sarcocystis spp.	Cattle, sheep, goats, pigs, horses, mule deer, and white-tailed deer

Diagnosis

Primary Diagnostics

- **Fecal flotation:** Oocysts are seen on microscopic examination.

Ancillary Diagnostics

- **Direct saline smear:** Oocysts are sometimes seen on microscopic examination.

Diagnostic Notes

Cryptosporidium spp. will not be seen on routine fecal floatation because of the extremely small size of these organisms (1/10 the size of *Cystoisospora* spp.). This diagnosis is usually made via biopsy and histopathology. Fecal ELISA for the detection of *Cryptosporidia*-specific antigens is available, although the accuracy of this test is still being evaluated.

Treatment

Primary Therapeutics

- **Sulfadimethoxine:** Administer 60 mg/kg PO on day one, then 30 mg/kg PO for 10 days.

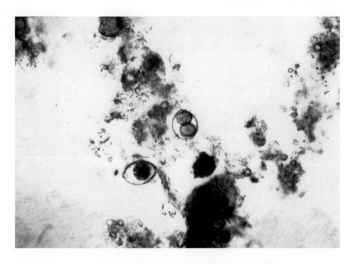

FIGURE 40.1. Coccidiosis: These oocysts are typical of *Isospora* spp.

Secondary Therapeutics

- **Trimethoprim/sulfadiazine:** Administer 15 mg/kg BID PO for 10 days.

Therapeutic Notes

Infections may be self-limiting and thus may not require therapy.

Infections can be avoided by preventing predatory behavior and maintaining appropriate sanitation.

No definitive effective therapy has been determined for *Cryptosporidium* spp. Paromycin at 165 mg/kg BID PO for 5 days was effective in one cat. Clindamycin has been utilized in people and was found to be partially effective in one cat. Another feline case responded to tylosin therapy.

Prognosis

The prognosis is excellent for cure except in cats infected with *Cryptosporidium* spp.

Suggested Readings

Guilford WG, Strombeck DR. Gastrointestinal tract infections, parasites, and toxicoses. In: Strombeck's small animal gastroenterology, 3rd ed. Philadelphia: WB Saunders, 1996;411–432.

Lappin MR. Cryptosporidiosis in the dog and cat. Proceedings of the Eleventh Annual Veterinary Medical Forum 1993;265–268.

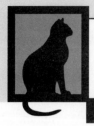

CHAPTER 41

Corneal Ulceration/Keratitis

Gary D. Norsworthy

Overview

Keratitis is an inflammatory disease of the cornea. A corneal erosion is a loss of corneal epithelium. A corneal ulcer is loss of variable amounts of corneal stroma. Feline corneal disease may progress from keratitis to erosion to ulcer within a few hours. Most cases are due to trauma, often from cat fight wounds or foreign bodies; however, the feline herpesvirus can also cause ulcers. A foreign body lodged behind the nictitating membrane can rapidly cause a deep ulcer. Early clinical signs result from pain (excessive tearing, squinting, and rubbing of the eye) and infection (mucopurulent ocular discharge). Later clinical signs include neovascularization, scleral hyperemia, and corneal pigmentation.

 D i a g n o s i s

Primary Diagnostics

- **Clinical signs:** Cats with blepharospasm should be suspected of having a corneal erosion or ulcer.

- **Corneal staining:** Fluorescein stain will illuminate a corneal erosion or ulcer and is confirmatory. Rose bengal stain will demonstrate superficial linear ulcers (dendritic ulcers) caused by the feline herpesvirus.

Ancillary Diagnostics

- **Cytology:** Corneal scrapings may reveal evidence of microbial organisms. This can suggest appropriate initial therapy.

- **Bacterial culture:** This test is recommended with deep, progressive, or nonhealing corneal ulcers.

Diagnostic Notes

- An examination behind the nictitating membrane should be performed to detect a lodged foreign body.

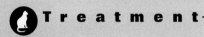T r e a t m e n t

Primary Therapeutics

- **Antibiotics:** Although not all corneal erosions or ulcers are infected, topical antibiotic therapy is appropriate because of the likelihood of secondary infection. Initially, one should consider ophthalmic forms of chloramphenicol, triple antibiotic ointments, gentamicin, or tobramycin.

- **Atropine:** This drug, applied topically, is very effective in relieving intraocular pain associated with corneal erosions or ulcers.

- **Antivirals:** Herpetic ulcers should be treated with trifluridine or idoxuridine.

Secondary Therapeutics

- **Analgesic/anti-inflammatory agents:** The judicious use of aspirin (10 mg/kg q48h PO) should be considered if atropine is not successful in relieving pain.

- **Corneal debridement:** The loose epithelial edges of refractory ulcers should be debrided with a dry, sterile cotton-tipped applicator. This can be performed under general anesthesia; however, topical anesthesia is usually adequate.

- **Conjunctival flap:** A rotational pedicle conjunctival flap should be used on refractory ulcers that do not heal after debridement, deep ulcers, and descemetoceles. Its purpose is to provide corneal support and neovascularization. It should remain in place for 4–6 weeks.

Therapeutic Notes

- An uncomplicated corneal erosion or superficial ulcer should heal in 24–72 hours. Restaining the eye after 24–48 hours of treatment is encouraged to confirm a positive response. If the response is not occurring, culturing and surgical procedures should be considered.

- Topical or systemic corticosteroids are contraindicated when a corneal erosion or ulcer is present.

- Topical atropine is contraindicated if glaucoma or lens luxation is present.

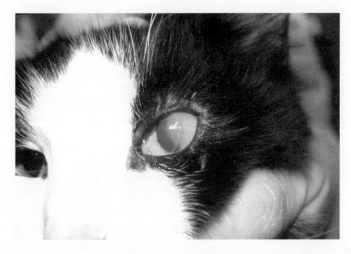

FIGURE 41.1. Corneal ulceration/keratitis: The ulcer in this cornea is readily seen when highlighted with fluorescein stain.

Prognosis

The prognosis for uncomplicated erosions and superficial ulcers is good. Deep, refractory ulcers, especially those with a descemetocele, have a guarded prognosis; however, this prognosis is improved if a conjunctival flap is utilized.

Suggested Readings

Miller PE. Keratitis, ulcerative. In: Tilley LP, Smith FWK, eds. The five-minute veterinary consult. Philadelphia: Williams & Wilkins, 1996;754–755.

Wilkie DA. Diseases and surgery of the eye. In: Sherding RG, ed. The cat: diseases and clinical management, 2nd ed. Philadelphia: WB Saunders, 1994;2011–2046.

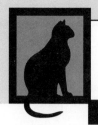

CHAPTER 42

Cryptococcosis

Sharon K. Fooshee

Overview

I nfection with the dimorphic fungus, *Cryptococcus neoformans*, is observed regularly in cats. Cryptococcosis is the only systemic fungal infection observed more commonly in cats than in dogs. The organism is worldwide in distribution and is reportedly associated with the nitrogen-enriched droppings of pigeons, although many infected cats have no known contact with pigeon excreta. There is no known breed or sex predisposition. Inhalation of the large, encapsulated organism is generally regarded as the primary route of infection. Opportunistic infection of the fungus in patients with human immunodeficiency virus infection or other immune-deficient states is well documented. Although cats infected with FeLV and FIV represent comparable states of cell-mediated suppression, the potential for the viruses to predispose to cryptococcal infection has not been clearly defined. It appears that the thick, mucopolysaccharide capsule of *C. neoformans* may induce some degree of immunosuppression in the host cat. Also, antigens hidden beneath the capsule may evade recognition by and stimulation of the immune system. Infected cats do not represent a health hazard to humans but serve as a sentinel to raise awareness of the presence of the organism in the environment.

The organism appears to have the greatest affinity for the upper respiratory system, with the nervous system and integumentary systems also commonly involved. The lower airways are infrequently involved. Sneezing, snuffling, or snorting and progressive respiratory distress (usually inspiratory) are common; nasal discharge is not always present. Some cats may have an obvious swelling across the bridge of the nose or a fleshy mass protruding from one or both nostrils. The submandibular nodes may be enlarged. When the central nervous system is involved, signs are usually chronic in onset and may include seizures, blindness, and behavioral changes. Infection of the skin and subcutaneous tissues is usually a manifestation of disseminated disease. Signs include solitary or multiple nodules, which appear to be ulcerated or draining gelatinous material, as well as nonhealing abscesses. Inflammatory lesions of the posterior ocular chamber are common and may involve one or both eyes.

D i a g n o s i s

Primary Diagnostics

- **Clinical signs:** Cryptococcosis should be suspected when respiratory signs and the other manifestations previously described are present.
- **Cytology:** Cytologic inspection of aspirates, swabs, or exudative material is often sufficient to make a diagnosis. India ink preparations are the "gold standard" for demonstrating the organism, although modified Wright's or new methylene blue stains will often provide the diagnosis.
- **Serologic testing:** The latex agglutination test (LAT) is considered a sensitive and specific test for antigens associated with the fungal capsule. When the test is performed properly, a positive result is usually considered diagnostic of cryptococcosis, although immune-mediated diseases may result in a false positive test. Negative results may occasionally be obtained in cats with transient or localized infection.

Ancillary Diagnostics

- **Radiography:** Skull and thoracic radiographs may be useful to detect respiratory involvement but will not offer a definitive diagnosis.
- **CBC/Biochemical profile/urinalysis/FeLV/FIV:** This minimum data base will not provide a diagnosis but is useful as a general health screen for the patient.

Diagnostic Notes

- Histopathology is usually not needed to make a diagnosis; routine hematoxylin-eosin stains may fail to demonstrate the capsule. In addition, culture is rarely necessary.

 T r e a t m e n t

Primary Therapeutics

- Itraconazole is the antifungal drug of choice. It should be dosed at 5 mg/kg PO BID and given with a meal; an acidic environment in the stomach enhances absorption of the drug. The capsule may be opened and the contents divided into gelatin capsules or mixed into canned food.
- Fluconazole has better penetration into the CNS than itraconazole and may be a useful alternative when the nervous system is involved. It is eliminated by renal excretion and should be used judiciously with impaired renal function.

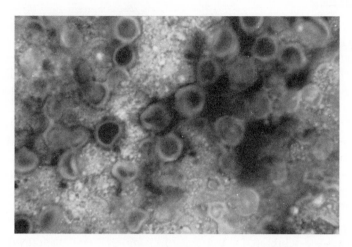

FIGURE 42.1. Cryptococcosis: *Cryptococcus neoformans* is seen readily when stained with a modified Wright's stain and is often present in exudates.

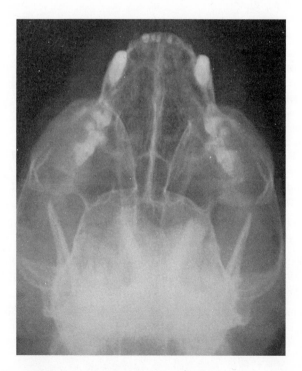

FIGURE 42.2. One of the most common locations for cryptococcosis is the nasal cavity, producing bony lysis and increased density radiographically.

Therapeutic Notes

- Cats should be periodically re-evaluated with the LAT during treatment; a falling titer has potential usefulness in determining a favorable response to therapy. Many cats maintain a positive titer for months after clinical resolution of signs. It is reasonable to suggest that treatment should be continued for at least several months beyond resolution of clinical signs or until a negative LAT is obtained, although it is unknown whether the LAT continues to detect dead organisms.

- Itraconazole is better tolerated than ketoconazole by most cats. However, it is still recommended that the cat's serum chemistries be periodically checked. For cats with *clinical* evidence of hepatotoxicity (anorexia, jaundice), the drug should be discontinued, at least temporarily. Asymptomatic cats with increased liver enzymes (i.e., ALT) do not necessarily need cessation of therapy but should be closely monitored.

- Many cats are debilitated at the time of diagnosis due to prolonged anorexia. Placement of a feeding tube permits the owner to administer proper nutritional support.

P r o g n o s i s

In general, the prognosis for infected cats has improved with the introduction of itraconazole. However, severely debilitated cats with advanced systemic disease still have a guarded prognosis.

S u g g e s t e d   R e a d i n g s

Fooshee SK, Woody BW. Systemic fungal diseases. In: Norsworthy GD, ed. Feline practice. Philadelphia: JB Lippincott, 1993;540–550.

Medleau L, Jacobs GJ, Marks MA. Itraconazole for the treatment of cryptococcosis in cats. *J Vet Intern Med* 1995;9:39–42.

Medleau L, Marks MA, Brown J, Borges WL. Clinical evaluation of a cryptococcal antigen latex agglutination test for diagnosis of *Cryptococcus* in cats. *J Am Vet Med Assoc* 1990;196:1470–1473.

Taboada J, Merchant SR. Treatment of fungal diseases. In: Proceedings of the American College of Veterinary Internal Medicine, Thirteenth Annual Meeting. 1995;800.

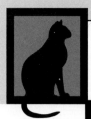

CHAPTER 43

Cytauxzoonosis

Mitchell A. Crystal

Overview

Cytauxzoonosis is caused by the small protozoan hemoparasite *Cytauxzoon felis*. Infection is most common in the south central and southeastern United States. Cytauxzoonosis is nearly 100% fatal; only one domestic cat has been reported to have survived the naturally occurring disease. Infection is acquired by tick vectors (*Dermacentor variabilis* and others), and bobcats serve as an asymptomatic reservoir host. Clinical signs of Cytauxzoonosis include depression, anorexia, fever, pallor, icterus, dehydration, and hypothermia 1 to 2 days prior to death. Cats usually die within 1 week of demonstrating clinical signs. Outdoor cats with exposure to tick vectors are more at risk of developing the disease.

 D i a g n o s i s

Primary Diagnostics

- **CBC:** Abnormalities include a mild to moderate anemia, which may or may not be regenerative. Leukocyte counts vary but are more often decreased and accompanied by occasional left shifts and thrombocytopenia. Piroplasms may be seen within erythrocytes and appear as either signet ring-shaped, bipolar oval safety pin-shaped, or anaplasmoid round dot-shaped bodies. Piroplasms occur near the time of pyrexia, but only 1 to 5% of erythrocytes are affected until near death, when up to 25% of erythrocytes contain piroplasms. There is usually only one piroplasm per erythrocyte, although multiples and chains of piroplasms are occasionally seen. Rarely, large mononuclear phagocytes containing schizonts of developing merozoites are seen.

Ancillary Diagnostics

- **Chemistry profile:** This may demonstrate increased bilirubin or hepatic transaminases and a prerenal azotemia.

- **Spleen, lymph node, or bone marrow aspiration/cytology:** These often reveal large mononuclear phagocytes containing schizonts in various stages of development.

Diagnostic Notes

- *Cytauxzoon felis* must be differentiated from *Hemobartonella felis*. *C. felis* organisms are single, usually signet ring-shaped bodies within the erythrocyte, whereas *H. felis* organisms are usually coccoid or rod-shaped bodies seen on the external periphery of the erythrocyte.
- CBCs should be repeated if *Cytauxzoon* is suspected, as parasitemia may be undetectable one day and then large numbers of organisms may be present the next day.

 T r e a t m e n t

Primary Therapeutics

- **Supportive care:** Administer fluids and nutritional support as needed.

Secondary Therapeutics

- **Thiacetarsamide (anecdotal):** Administer at 1 mg/kg SID IV for 2 days.

Therapeutic Notes

- Cats are likely to die despite therapy.
- Tick control is important in prevention.

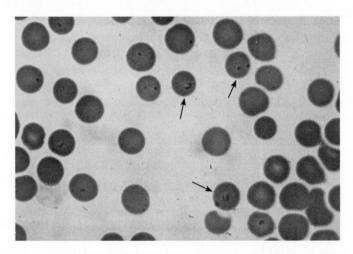

FIGURE 43.1. Cytauxzoonosis: *Cytauxzoon felis* is seen on many of these erythrocytes stained with a modified Wright's stain.

P r o g n o s i s

The prognosis is grave for recovery.

S u g g e s t e d   R e a d i n g s

Cowell RL, Fox JC, Tyler RD. Feline cytauxzoonosis. *Compend Contin Educ Pract Vet* 1988;731–735.

Hoover JP, Walker DB, Hedges JD. Cytauxzoonosis in cats: eight cases (1985–1992). *J Am Vet Med Assoc* 1994;205(3):455–460.

Kier AB. Cytauxzoonosis. In Green CE, ed. Infectious diseases of the dog and cat. Philadelphia: WB Saunders, 1990;792–795.

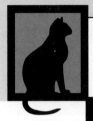

CHAPTER 44

Dermatophytosis

Gary D. Norsworthy

Overview

Dermatophytosis, frequently called ringworm, is a fungal infection affecting cornified areas of the skin and nails, as well as the superficial layers of the skin. About 95% of feline cases are caused by *Microsporum canis.* The cat is also infected by *Trichophyton mentagrophytes* and *Microsporum gypseum.* Direct exposure to a fungus does not necessarily result in an infection, and an infection does not always cause clinical signs. Long-haired cats are more likely to have symptomatic infections. The typical incubation period is 1–4 weeks, but some cats remain asymptomatic carriers for long periods of time. Lesions may have the typical appearance of circular areas of alopecia, but their appearance is so diverse that virtually any cat with skin disease, including those with miliary dermatitis, should be suspected of having dermatophytosis. Risk factors include immunosuppression, multicat facilities, poor nutrition, poor sanitation, and lack of quarantine for new cats entering a multicat facility.

 D i a g n o s i s

Primary Diagnostics

- **Clinical signs:** Dermatophytosis may resemble any feline skin or nail disorder.
- **Wood's lamp examination:** The lamp should be turned on for 5 minutes and the suspected hairs exposed for up to 5 minutes. An apple-green fluorescence of individual hairs is characteristic. However, there can be many false positives and false negatives, so this should be used only as a screening tool. Fluorescing hairs should be cultured.
- **Fungus culture:** This is the best single test. Obtain culture material from the periphery of the lesion and from several sites. Alternatively, a sterile toothbrush may be used to collect hair by brushing the entire cat. This is especially helpful for exposed, asymptomatic cats. Dermatophyte test

medium changes to a red color simultaneously with light-colored, cottony fungal growth within 7 to 14 days.

Ancillary Diagnostics

- **CBC, blood chemistries, urinalysis:** These tests may reveal an underlying disorder that may adversely affect recovery. They should be considered for nonresponsive cases.
- **Skin biopsy:** This test generally is used when another skin disease is suspected, and the finding of a dermatophyte is usually incidental.

Diagnostic Notes

- Because the gross appearance of a dermatophyte infection can be so diverse, it should be considered for any feline skin disease.

 T r e a t m e n t

Primary Therapeutics

- **Quarantine:** This is a contagious and zoonotic disease so, ideally, affected cats should not be in contact with noninfected cats or humans.
- **Topical therapy:** Clotrimazole is reported to be the most effective topical agent. It should be applied BID to lesions.
- **Microsized griseofulvin:** This is the most commonly used systemic product. Dose orally at 40–60 mg/kg SID. A pediatric suspension is available for kittens. Poor gastrointestinal absorption occurs unless it is given with a fatty meal. Treat for at least 30 days and until the patient is asymptomatic and culture negative.
- **Ultramicrosized griseofulvin:** The dose is much lower (2.5–5.0 mg/kg BID) than the microsized form, and good absorption occurs without a fatty meal. The treatment duration is the same for both.
- **Shampoos and dips:** These are used to remove spores from the cat and to kill the fungus. Lime sulfur dip is the most effective; however, it has an odor that most owners find objectionable. The cat should be shampooed and dipped one to two times per week for 1–3 weeks. Exposed, asymptotic cats should also be shampooed and dipped. The use of ineffective shampoos and dips may result in spread of the fungus.
- **Environment:** It is important to prevent further spread or continual reinfection; the organism may persist in the environment for over 1 year. Deep, repeated vacuuming of air conditioning vents, carpet, and furniture, with immediate disposal of the vacuum bag, is important. When possible, dilute bleach (1:10) can be used for decontamination. Grooming equipment, especially clippers and brushes, should be discarded or disinfected.

Secondary Therapeutics

- **Hair clipping:** Clipping may result in the worsening of signs within 7–10 days, presumably due to mechanical spread of the fungus. Clipping short-haired cats with a few lesions is not recommended. Clipping the entire haircoat of any cat is not recommended except when widespread lesions are present.

- **Ketoconazole:** This may be used in place of griseofulvin. It is dosed orally at 5 mg/kg BID.

- **Itraconazole:** This may be used in the place of griseofulvin. It is dosed orally at 10 mg/kg SID and generally has fewer side effects than ketoconazole. However, it is contraindicated in cats with liver disease.

- **Vaccination:** A vaccine is available for use as adjuvant therapy for *M. canis* infections. Currently, it is not recommended for use without the items listed in the Initial Therapeutics section, and production of lasting immunity has not been proved.

Therapeutic Notes

- A dermatophyte-infected cat should be considered contagious to humans. Exposed persons should be instructed to consult their physician. Contagion is more likely in children than adults, and prior infection confers some immunity.

- Griseofulvin can cause a severe leukopenia when given to FIV-infected cats; cats should be tested for FIV prior to administration. Other side effects, including anorexia, vomiting, hepatotoxicity, and bone marrow suppression, have been reported but are considered idiosyncratic. Griseofulvin is teratogenic, so it should not be given to pregnant cats. Some authorities recommend that a CBC (and platelet count) be performed every 2 weeks while a cat is taking this drug.

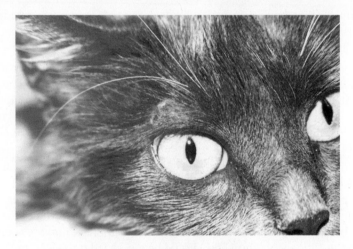

FIGURE 44.1. Dermatophytosis: The classic circular area of alopecia is seen over this cat's right eye.

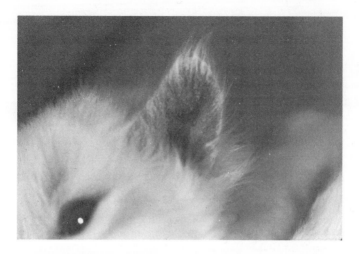

FIGURE 44.2. A less likely presentation is a crusty dermatitis on this cat's pinna. Because there are so many presentations of feline ringworm, it should be suspected in virtually any form of dermatitis or alopecia.

- Captan dip has been widely used to treat and control dermatophytosis. A recent study demonstrated no efficacy as a fungicidal agent for *M. canis*.
- Although hairclipping will ultimately increase the rate of recovery, the owner should be warned that the lesions may appear to worsen immediately following the procedure. If the cat is put on therapy for 14 days prior to clipping, worsening of the lesions is much less likely.

Prognosis

Some cats have self-limiting infections, but the occurrence of a persistent infection, the carrier state, and zoonosis justifies aggressive treatment. The prognosis is generally good if aggressive therapeutic measures are taken.

Suggested Readings

Merchant SR. The skin: fungal diseases. In: Norsworthy GD, ed. Feline practice. Philadelphia: JB Lippincott, 1993;504–510.

Moriello KA. Treatment of feline dermatophytosis: revised recommendations. *Feline Pract* 1996;24(3):32–37.

Moriello KA, DeBoer DJ. Dermatophytosis. In: August JR, ed. Consultations in feline internal medicine, 2nd ed. Philadelphia: WB Saunders, 1994;219–225.

White-Weithers N, Medleau L. Evaluation of topical therapies for the treatment of dermatophyte-infected hairs of dogs and cats. *J Am Anim Hosp Assoc* 1995;31(3):250–253.

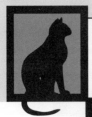

CHAPTER 45

Diabetes Mellitus

Gary D. Norsworthy

Overview

Diabetes mellitus (DM) is a disease resulting from destruction of the beta cells of the pancreas. **Type I** results from immune-mediated destruction of the beta cells. **Type II,** the most common form, is caused by amyloid deposition that destroys the beta cells. **Type III,** or secondary DM, is due to underlying condition (obesity, Cushing's disease, acromegaly, progestin administration, etc.) that causes insulin resistance. **Type IV** is due to chronic pancreatitis and is probably more common than it is recognized. **Insulin-dependent DM** (IDDM) requires insulin injections for control. **Non–insulin-dependent DM** (NIDDM) may be controlled with oral hypoglycemics or insulin injections. The classic clinical signs are polyuria (PU), polydipsia (PD), polyphagia (PP), and weight loss (WL). These are brought about by persistent hyperglycemia. Complicated DM, **diabetic ketoacidosis,** results in ketonuria, acidosis, and various electrolyte imbalances. It is imperative that ketoacidosis be identified, as its treatment is far more urgent and complicated.

Diagnosis

Primary Diagnostics

- **Clinical signs:** PU, PD, PP, and WL should be present in order to distinguish this from other causes of hyperglycemia.
- **Hyperglycemia and glucosuria:** These should be present in order to distinguish this from other causes of these clinical signs and from stress hyperglycemia.
- **Ketonuria:** This is an important finding to identify ketoacidosis, which also produces the clinical signs of anorexia, vomiting, dehydration, and lethargy.
- **Chemistry profile:** In addition to the previously mentioned abnormalities, ketoacidosis may produce hypokalemia, hyperosmolarity, and hypophosphatemia.

Ancillary Diagnostics

- **Fructosamine:** This serum test determines the average glucose level for the past 2 weeks. It can be used to differentiate DM from stress hyperglycemia.

Diagnostic Notes

- In order to justify a diagnosis of DM, it is imperative that the diagnostic triad be satisfied: correct clinical signs, hyperglycemia, and glucosuria.
- It is imperative that ketoacidosis be identified immediately, because these cats may die within a few hours if they are not treated properly and aggressively.
- Ketonuria can be caused by starvation or anorexia. When ketonuria is present, be sure that the other signs of diabetes are or have recently been present before diagnosing diabetic ketoacidosis.
- Exocrine pancreatic insufficiency may coexist with DM if chronic pancreatitis is the etiolgy. Diabetics should be tested with feline TLI test.

 T r e a t m e n t :   K e t o a c i d o s i s

Primary Therapeutics

- **IV normal saline:** Use normal saline; however, if the osmolarity is greater than 350 mOsm/kg, a hypotonic fluid (1/2 strength saline [0.45%]) should be used instead. Give at a rate to correct dehydration in the first 24 hours.
- **For metabolic acidosis:** Unless severe, this will correct itself with fluid and insulin administration. If the total CO_2 is less than 12 mEq/l, give $NaHCO_3$:
  a. Not as an IV bolus
  b. Amount $= 0.3 \times$ body wt in kg $\times (24 - \text{total } CO_2)$
  c. Give half the calculated amount over 6 hours in an IV drip, then the other half over the next 6–24 hours PRN based on total CO_2.
- **For hypokalemia:** Rehydrate the cat first. As intracellular dehydration is corrected, potassium shifts to the extracellular compartment and may correct hypokalemia. However, diuresis can also aggravate hypokalemia by dilution and further renal excretion.
  a. If there is no ECG or serum evidence of hyperkalemia, add 40 mEq to a liter of IV fluids.
  b. Do not exceed KCl administration of 0.5 mEq/kg/hr.
- **For hyperosmolarity:**
  a. If the osmolality is 325–350 mOsm/kg, give isotonic fluids (normal saline).
  b. If the osmolality is greater than 350 mOsm/kg, give hypotonic fluids (1/2 strength saline).

- **For hypophosphatemia:** Although it may be detected in serum tests, it is uncommon for it to manifest clinical signs (confusion, seizures, decreased cardiac contractility, dyspnea, hemolytic anemia, and respiratory arrest). Overzealous treatment with potassium phosphate may cause hypocalcemia, hypotension, and metastatic calcification. Therefore, treatment is not recommended unless the serum phosphate is less than 2.5 mg/dL. If treatment is instituted, give potassium at 0.03–0.12 mmol/kg/hr. Discontinue when the serum phosphate level is greater than 2.5 mg/dL.
- **For hyperglycemia:** Do not overtreat. Intravenous fluids may reduce the blood glucose level by 30% without insulin.
  a. Give regular insulin intramuscularly.
  b. Initial dose: 0.2 units/kg
  c. Thereafter: 0.1 units/kg hourly until the glucose is about 250 mg/dL
  d. Give in the muscles of the rear leg or lumbar area to assure good absorption.
  e. Dilution may be necessary in order to give accurate doses.
  f. After glucose is about 250 mg/dL, change to subcutaneous administration every 4–8 hours at the dose of 0.1–0.4 units/kg and change to 5% dextrose fluids.
  g. Monitor the blood glucose every 1–2 hours.
  h. When the cat is stable (eating; no vomiting; hydrated without IV fluids; not acidotic or azotemic), change to a long-acting or intermediate-acting insulin for 3–5 days, then do a glucose curve.

Therapeutic Notes

- Not all diabetics are hypokalemic; some are hyperkalemic. Hyperkalemia should be ruled out by serum monitoring or ECG evidence before potassium supplementation is given.
- When hyperglycemia is corrected, ketone levels will follow, but they will diminish 1–3 days later. Therefore, do not use urine ketone levels to monitor progress.
- Watch for bacterial cystitis. Glucose-containing urine is an excellent medium for bacterial growth.

Treatment: Nonketoacidosis

Primary Therapeutics

- **Client education:** This disease requires a major committment on the part of the owner. Owners should be informed regarding the financial and personal involvement that is likely to be required. A written client handout is strongly recommended.

- **Oral hypoglycemic drug***: Glipizide or glyburide.

  a. Begin at 2.5 mg BID.

  b. Determine glucose level weekly and monitor for reduction of clinical signs.

  c. Give for 4 weeks (or more). If no response, change to insulin.

- **High-fiber diet:** Slows digestion and reduces postprandial hyperglycemia.

  a. Low-calorie/high-fiber diet for obese cats.

  b. Normal-calorie/high-fiber diet for normal-weight cats.

  c. High-calorie/high-fiber diet for emaciated cats.**

- **Antibiotics:** One to 2 weeks of a broad-spectrum antibiotic can be very helpful in treating undiagnosed bacterial infections, which are common in diabetic cats. The infections' presence makes glycemic control very difficult.

- **Treat EPI if present.** See chapter 51.

Secondary Therapeutics

- **Insulin:** A long-acting or intermediate-acting insulin is chosen and given twice daily. The author's preferred initial dose is based on the glucose level at the time of diagnosis

  a. Glucose < 400 mg/dL: give 1/4 unit/kg subcutaneously

  b. Glucose > 400 mg/dL: give 1/2 unit/kg subcutaneously

- **Glucose curve:** A glucose curve is performed after the cat has been on the initial dose of insulin for 3 to 5 days. It is repeated until the proper dose of insulin can be determined. Alternatively, if the pre-insulin glucose is > 350 mg/dL, the dose of insulin can be increased 1–2 units, and the glucose curve stopped. The cat is to be returned in 3–5 days and the process repeated until the initial glucose is <350 mg/dL. At that time, the

---

* There are no reliable tests to identify responders to oral hypoglycemics. It is not universally accepted that this should be the first approach, and some evidence suggests that these drugs may result in the formation of amyloid in beta cells. However, it is an especially good option for owners who may initially be reluctant to give injections of insulin. If oral hypoglycemics are administered, a high-fiber diet should be fed, and 2 weeks of antibiotics should be administered.
** Powdered psyllium or psyllium tablets (Vetasyl) can be added to food at the rate of 1–2 tsp BID to increase fiber content. Instruct the owner to use the sugar-free variety.

TABLE 45.1

Interpretation of the Glucose Curve.*

1) To determine the dosing interval:
   a) Peak time: time from insulin injection until glucose is at its lowest level
      < 5 hrs: TID or longer-acting insulin
      5–8 hrs: BID
      > 8 hrs: SID
2) To determine the dose:
   a) Nadir: the value at the peak time
      < 100 mg/dL: decrease dose
      The nadir in the hospital is higher than what it will be at home (few exceptions).
   b) Range: lowest to highest glucose levels
   c) Range midpoint
      Determines dose of insulin or if problems exist
      Ideal: 200 mg/dL
      Good: 150–250 mg/dL
      <150 mg/dL: reduce dose of insulin
      150–250 mg/dL: no change if the nadir is above 100 mg/dL
      >250 mg/dL:
         Dose too low: increase dose
         Insulin problem: inactive insulin, insulin not mixed, poor injection technique,
            poor absorption
         Stress
         Insulin resistance: concurrent disease (Cushing's disease, acromegaly, hyper-
            thyroidism, any systemic illness); insulin antibodies

*This interpretation scheme assumes that insulin is being administered twice daily.

glucose curve is completed. The technique for performing a glucose curve is found in Appendix F. Interpretation of the glucose curve is found in Table 45.1.

Therapeutic Notes

- Bacterial infections, including oral infections associated with dental disease, make it difficult to achieve good glycemic control. If regulation proves difficult, consider cleaning the cat's teeth.

- It is reported that about 25–40% of diabetic cats respond to oral hypoglycemic drugs. However, the author's success rate is considerably lower.

- Dysregulation is a major problem in many diabetic cats. Table 45.2 can be used to help identify causes of dysregulation.

TABLE 45.2

Causes of Dysregulation

Independent Dysregulators: any one capable of causing dysregulation
1. Improper measuring of insulin
2. Improper injection technique
3. Improper storage of insulin
4. Estrus
5. Pregnancy
6. Cushing's disease
7. Acromegaly
8. Insulin incompatibility

Contributing Dysregulators: usually requires more than one to cause dysregulation
1. Inconsistent caloric intake
2. Inconsistent activity level
3. Inconsistent dosing interval
4. Poor home monitoring
5. Improper diet (sugar, fiber)
6. Multicat household
7. Boarding
8. Obesity
9. Use of steroids or megestrol
10. Concomitant disease
11. Reuse of insulin syringes

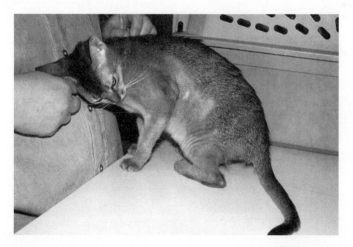

FIGURE 45.1. Diabetes mellitus: Peripheral neuropathy is a fairly common complication of diabetes mellitus. This cat's plantigrade positioning of the hock is the typical presentation. This is a sign of chronicity but is not necessarily associated with ketoacidosis. The truncal alopecia is not associated with diabetes mellitus.

P r o g n o s i s

The prognosis for cats with diabetic ketoacidosis is guarded for the first 24 to 48 hours. However, once the cat is stabilized or if the cat is diagnosed as having uncomplicated (nonketotic) DM, the prognosis is good. The likelihood of frequent dysregulation varies with the understanding of the clinician, the commitment of the owner, and several undefined variables with the cat. It is not unusual for owners to elect euthanasia when recurrent regulation problems occur because of financial limitations or the personal commitment required.

S u g g e s t e d   R e a d i n g s

Joseph RJ, Allyson K, Graves TK, et al. Evaluation of two reagent strips and three reflectance meters for rapid determination of blood glucose concentrations. *J Vet Intern Med* 1987;10:87–92.

Lutz TA, et al. Fructosamine concentrations in cats. Proceedings of the American College of Veterinary Internal Medicine. Washington, DC. 1993;927.

Lutz TA, Rand JS. Pathogenesis of feline diabetes mellitus. *Vet Clin North Am* 1994;25:527–552.

MacIntire DK. Emergency therapy of diabetic crises: insulin overdose, diabetic ketoacidosis, and hyperosmolar coma. *Vet Clin North Am* 1995;25:639–650.

Norsworthy GD. A rational approach to feline blood glucose curves. *Vet Med* 1995;90(11):1064–1069.

Wolf AM. Management of geriatric diabetic cats. *Compend Contin Educ Pract Vet* 1989;11:1088–1095.

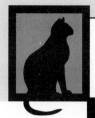

Diaphragmatic Hernia

Gary D. Norsworthy

Overview

A diaphragmatic hernia (DH) is a rent in the diaphragm through which one or more abdominal organs may pass. The most common cause is **trauma,** usually associated with automobile-related injury or a fall from several stories. A sudden increase in abdominal pressure directed cranially can tear the diaphragm at any point. It may also occur in a **congenital** form with communication between the abdomen and the pleural space or between the abdomen and the pericardium. Other congenital defects involving the heart may also occur with congenital DH. Clinical signs may include tachypnea and orthopnea, especially if accompanied by pulmonary contusion or bleeding or marked lung compression, and pain, especially if accompanied by rib fractures. Cats may become dyspneic immediately or a few hours later as more viscera enter the pleural space. Without treatment, some cats will stabilize in a few days, adhesions will form between the viscera and the diaphragm, and clinical signs will only be associated with increased activity. This is the **chronic** form. These cats often become sedentary but may live for many years without surgical correction. The **acute** traumatic form produces dyspnea, which may increase over 1–2 days as more abdominal organs are displaced into the thorax. The congenital form is often diagnosed incidentally, but gaseous distention of organs within the pericardium may produce acute signs of dyspnea. The chronic form may produce only marked lethargy and shortness of breath upon exercise.

Diagnosis

Primary Diagnostics

- **Clinical signs:** Dyspnea or tachypnea should cause one to consider DH, especially if there are other clinical signs or history of trauma.
- **Auscultation:** Muffled lung and heart sounds occur on one or both sides of the chest.

- **Radiography:** Typical findings are loss of the diaphragmatic line and abdominal viscera in the thoracic cavity, including gastrointestinal (GI) gas patterns. The abdomen will appear smaller in size if several organs are displaced into the thorax.

Ancillary Diagnostics

- **Abdominal palpation:** Palpation may reveal an "empty" feeling due to organ displacement.
- **Ultrasound:** This may reveal abdominal viscera within the pleural space or pericardium.
- **Celiogram:** Positive contrast organic iodine material is injected into the abdomen, and the cat is gently tilted to encourage flow of contrast into the thorax. If the contrast agent is found in the thorax on a lateral radiograph, a diaphragmatic hernia is present. This may be nondiagnostic for chronic or pericardial hernias.
- **Positive contrast study of the GI tract:** Barium is instilled in the stomach and a series of radiographs taken. The stomach or loops of the bowel may be visualized in the pericardium if a congenital pericardial DH is present. If the liver but not the stomach has herniated, the stomach will be in close proximity to the diaphragm.
- **ECG:** Myocardial trauma often produces arrhythmias, especially ventricular tachyarrhythmias.

Diagnostic Notes

- Radiographs made immediately after trauma will not be diagnostic for DH if abdominal organs have not migrated into the thorax. If a DH is suspected, the cat should be re-radiographed in 12–24 hours, or a celiogram should be performed.
- Chronic DH may produce pleural effusion classified as a modified transudate or nonseptic exudate containing 2.5–6.0 g/dL of protein, fibrin, nondegenerate neutrophils, macrophages, and mesothelial cells. This type of fluid can be confused with that of feline infectious peritonitis or chronic heart failure.
- Dyspneic cats should be handled very carefully because increased stress may be fatal. Extreme care should be taken when doing the physical examination, radiographs, and thoracentesis. It may be necessary to place the cat in an oxygen cage or tent for several minutes prior to diagnostics and between diagnostic procedures. The least stressful radiographic view is the dorsoventral (DV) view; it may be the only view that is practical in some cases and often is sufficient to diagnose the presence of diaphragmatic hernia.

🐱 T r e a t m e n t

Primary Therapeutics

- **Patient stabilization:** In cases involving trauma, treat for shock, improve cardiac output and ventilation, and manage concurrent injuries. Failure to do this prior to surgery may result in anesthetic death. Cage confinement for several hours, especially in an oxygen-enriched atmosphere, can be a useful part of patient stabilization.

- **Surgical repair of the diaphragm:** This should be attempted after patient stabilization unless one or more of the following occur: a) persistent hypotension in spite of IV fluid therapy; b) severe lung compression; c) liver failure due to entrapment; or d) enlarging stomach or bowel due to gas entrapment. The death rate is greater if surgical repair is attempted within the first 24 hours following trauma.

Secondary Therapeutics

- **Thoracentesis:** This procedure may improve respiration, especially if pneumothorax is present. The cat's forequarters should be elevated and the chest aspirated in the dorsal two-thirds of the thorax in the 7th to 9th intercostal spaces. The needle is inserted just deeply enough to enter the pleural space to avoid penetrating the lungs or displaced abdominal viscera.

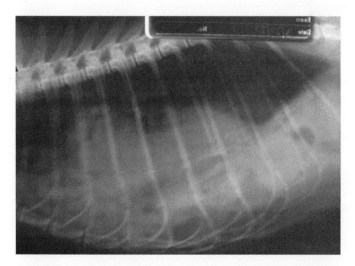

FIGURE 46.1. An incomplete diaphragmatic line and the presence of abnormal soft tissue and gas densities cranial to the diaphragm are characteristic signs of diaphragmatic hernia. The gas densities are due to gas accumulations within the small intestine.

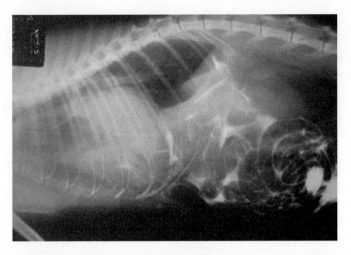

FIGURE 46.2. A celiogram can be used to confirm a diaphragmatic hernia. Contrast material is injected into the abdomen. If it migrates cranial to the normal diaphragmatic line, a hernia is confirmed.

Therapeutic Notes

- The arrhythmias associated with DH are usually seen 24–72 hours after trauma and are difficult to control with anti-arrhythmics. They usually resolve spontaneously within 5 days.
- Surgical repair of congenital and chronic DH may be more difficult due to adhesions present between entrapped organs and the diaphragm or pericardium.

Prognosis

The prognosis for all forms of DH is good as long as shock and arrhythmias resolve and successful surgical repair can be accomplished. However, cats with traumatic DH may be poor surgical risks, especially if other traumatic injuries are present.

Suggested Readings

Boudrieau RJ, Muir WW. Pathophysiology of traumatic diaphragmatic hernia in dogs. *Compend Contin Educ Pract Vet* 1987;9(4):379–385.

Sherding RG. Diseases of the pleural cavity. In: Sherding RG, ed. The cat: diseases and clinical management. 2nd ed. New York: Churchill Livingstone, 1994;1053–1116.

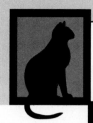

CHAPTER 47

Dilated Cardiomyopathy

John-Karl Goodwin

Overview

D ilated cardiomyopathy (DCM) is characterized by severe left and right ventricular dilatation and poor systolic function, resulting in backward (pulmonary edema, pleural effusion, and ascites) and forward (decreased cardiac output) heart failure.

After the discovery in 1987 that taurine deficiency was a significant cause of DCM, the incidence of this disease decreased dramatically following provision of adequate taurine in commercial foods. Dietary taurine supplementation reverses the pathology if cardiomyopathy is secondary to taurine deficiency.

Currently, most cases of feline DCM are primary or idiopathic. A diagnosis of idiopathic DCM is made only after other causes of myocardial failure (such as nutritional or taurine deficiency, long-standing congenital or acquired left ventricular volume overload, toxic, ischemic, or metabolic-induced myocardial failure) have been ruled out.

Dilated cardiomyopathy results in heart failure secondary to severe left and right ventricular volume overload and poor systolic function. Typical physical examination abnormalities include weak femoral pulses, cardiogenic shock, increased respiratory sounds, cardiac murmurs, gallop rhythms, jugular distention or pulses, and ascites.

Diagnosis

Primary Tests

- **Echocardiography:** Typical findings include severe left and right ventricular eccentric hypertrophy (dilation), left and right atrial dilation, and left ventricular systolic dysfunction, as demonstrated by a reduced fractional shortening.

- **Thoracic radiography:** Expected findings are moderate-to-severe cardiomegaly, patchy mixed interstitial-alveolar pulmonary patterns, and pulmonary venous congestion.
- **Electrocardiography:** This reveals increased R-wave amplitude, suggesting left ventricular enlargement, and arrhythmias, such as sinus tachycardia, atrial premature complexes, and ventricular tachyarrhythmias.

Ancillary Diagnostics

- **Taurine analysis:** Decreases in plasma and whole blood taurine levels can be seen.
- **Chemistry profile and urinalysis:** Concurrent renal and hepatic dysfunction should be ruled out prior to initiation of drug therapy.
- **Fundic examination:** This may reveal evidence of central retinal degeneration in cats with taurine deficiency.

Diagnostic Notes

- Ascites seems to be more commonly associated with DCM than with other forms of cardiomyopathy.
- Hyperthyroidism should be ruled out in all cats with dilated cardiomyopathy.
- Cats with severe left atrial enlargement are more likely to form thrombi.

 T r e a t m e n t

Primary Therapeutics

- **Diuretic therapy:** Give furosemide at 1–4mg/kg IV q1hr PRN or IM q2hr PRN.
- **Thoracentesis:** This should be considered if pleural effusion is present.
- **Oxygen:** Supplement as needed.
- **Stress:** Provide a low-stress environment.
- **Pericardiocentesis:** Perform if significant pericardial effusion is present (rare).

Secondary Therapeutics

- **Vasodilator therapy:** Use a) topical nitroglycerin (1/8 to 1/4 inch TID-QID for 24–36 hours) in selected cases with severe acute congestive heart failure; b) ACE-inhibitor therapy (enalapril 0.25–0.50 mg/kg PO SID-BID) or benazepril (0.2–0.5 mg/kg PO SID-BID).

- **Positive inotropic agents:** Consider a) digoxin (¼ of a 0.125 tablet PO SID-EOD) or b) intravenous agents such as dobutamine as needed for cardiogenic shock.
- **Taurine supplementation:** Give to maintain normal plasma taurine levels (>60 nmol/ml). The normal dose is 250–500 mg BID.
- **Anticoagulation:** Give aspirin (25 mg PO q2–3 days) or warfarin (0.05–0.5mg/cat PO SID) to prevent blood clots.

Therapeutic Notes

- Aggressive diuretic therapy is continued until respiratory distress resolves and is followed by a reduction in dose to maintain a normal respiratory rate (usually less than 40 bpm).
- Maintenance furosemide doses usually range from 6.25 mg PO SID to 12.5 mg PO TID.
- Diuretic therapy should not precede pericardiocentesis if significant pericardial effusion is present.
- Taurine supplementation may be discontinued once echocardiographic values return to within normal limits and dietary taurine intake is deemed satisfactory.

P r o g n o s i s

Cats with a taurine–deficiency-induced dilated cardiomyopathy have a good to excellent prognosis with taurine supplementation if they survive the congestive

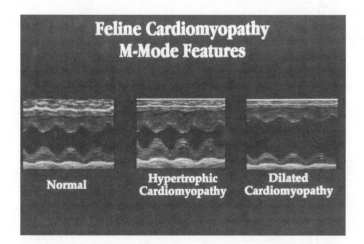

FIGURE 47.1. Dilated CM: M-mode echocardiogram showing left ventricular dilation and reduced fractional shortening compared with normal and hypertrophic cardiomyopathy.

heart failure crisis. Cats with congestive heart failure secondary to idiopathic dilated cardiomyopathy have a guarded to poor prognosis. They may survive 1–3 months; therapy should stabilize the patient but probably does not alter the progression of the failure.

Suggested Reading

Pion PD, Kienle RD. Feline cardiomyopathy. In: Miller MS, Tilley LP, eds. Manual of canine and feline cardiology, 2nd ed. Philadelphia: WB Saunders, 1995.

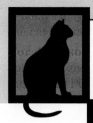

CHAPTER 48

Ear Mites

Sharon K. Fooshee

Overview

Otoacariasis, or infestation with ear mites (*Otodectes cynotis*), is common in cats and is responsible for at least half of all cases of feline otitis externa. Kittens are most frequently infested by the queen or other kittens. The mites live on the skin surface; they are nonburrowing but irritate the ceruminous glands of the ear, filling the canal with cerumen, blood, and mite exudate. As the mite feeds on the host's lymph and blood, the cat may be exposed to mite salivary antigen and become sensitized. Wheal and flare reactions (Type I hypersensitivity) and Arthus-type reactions (Type III hypersensitivity) were noted in large numbers of random cats following exposure to mite antigen. Sensitized cats develop intense otic pruritus with the presence of only a few mites. The immune system appears to limit infestations in most mature cats. Infested cats will often shake the head and twitch or rub the ears. Brownish-black debris is usually evident in the external canals. Miliary lesions are occasionally present.

 D i a g n o s i s

Primary Diagnostics

- **Clinical signs:** The presence of a brownish ear discharge and evidence of scratching at the ears is highly suggestive.

- **Otic examination:** The white mites are often seen moving in response to the warmth of the otoscope. Although they are relatively large in comparison to some other mites, they cannot be seen in the ear canal without otoscopic magnification. The canals should be thoroughly examined; when possible, the patency of the tympanic membrane should be determined.

Ancillary Diagnostics

- **Cytology:** Some of the debris from the ear canal may be rolled onto each of two microscope slides with a cotton swab.

1. Two or three drops of mineral oil can be applied to the first slide. On a scanning (4X) or low (10X) power, mites will be observed "swimming" in the oil. Mites' eggs can sometimes be found, even when adult mites are not present.

2. The second slide may be stained with an in-office modified Wright's stain to determine the presence of yeasts or bacteria.

Diagnostic Notes

- Although some cats have an extreme response to the presence of ear mites, others are relatively asymptomatic.

 T r e a t m e n t

Primary Therapeutics

- **Topical:** Many parasiticides are available for instillation into the ear canal. These medications may contain glucocorticoids, antimicrobials, cerumenolytics, and antifungal agents.

- **Systemic:** Although not approved for use in cats, ivermectin may be helpful. It is dosed at 300–400 µg/kg orally or subcutaneously at 1–2 week intervals for a total of 3–5 treatments. The likelihood of cure increases with the number of treatments. *Always seek owner's consent prior to administration.*

Secondary Therapeutics

- **Cleaning:** If the ear canal is full of dried debris, thorough irrigation and cleaning of the external canal will improve penetration of topical medication. However, in most cases, aggressive cleaning is not necessary.

- **Ectopic treatment:** Insecticidal dips, sprays, and shampoos may be useful in eliminating ectopic mites, although this is usually not necessary.

- **Premises:** Cleaning and insecticidal treatment of the premises may be appropriate.

Therapeutic Notes

- Ear mites are highly contagious. All exposed animals should be identified and treated. Insecticidal collars have shown little utility in preventing infestation.

- The use of ivermectin as a sole treatment does nothing to remove the debris from the ear canals. If this is chosen because of the personality of the cat, sedation for cleaning should occur either before or after treatment.

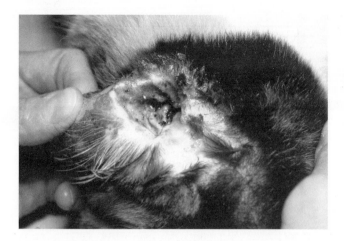

FIGURE 48.1. Ear mites: A black otic discharge is typical of ear mite infection. However, yeast infections can create similarly appearing debris.

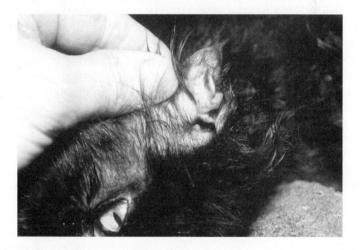

FIGURE 48.2. A "cauliflower" ear may be the result of an untreated hematoma that can form as a result of violent head shaking caused by chronic ear mites.

Prognosis

The prognosis is good with appropriate treatment.

Suggested Readings

Merchant SR. The skin: parasitic diseases. In: Norsworthy GD, ed. Feline practice. Philadelphia: JB Lippincott, 1993;511–517.

Scott DW, Miller WH, Griffin CE, eds. Muller and Kirk's small animal dermatology, 5th ed. Philadelphia: WB Saunders, 1995.

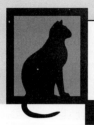

CHAPTER 49
Eosinophilic Granuloma Complex ·

Sharon K. Fooshee

Overview

Eosinophilic granuloma complex (EGC) is a syndrome of three cutaneous reaction patterns that develop in response to underlying allergy (insects, food, atopy) or other immune-mediated factors; bacteria, viruses, and stress are proposed to play a role in some cases. The three forms of this syndrome are eosinophilic plaque, linear (collagenolytic) granuloma, and indolent (rodent) ulcer. Although each reaction pattern has histologic distinctions, there may be overlap between them, and some cats may have more than one form. These are the reasons that the three forms are grouped into a complex. Linear granuloma is most common in younger female cats. Indolent ulcers are more common in female cats of all ages.

Diagnosis

Primary Diagnostics

- **Clinical signs:** Linear granuloma most commonly presents as an alopecic, well-circumscribed band of tissue on the caudal thighs. Related lesions may also occur on the footpads, in the pharynx, and on the tongue. Some cats have a swollen lower chin or lip. Peripheral lymphadenopathy is often present, and pruritus is variable. Lesions of eosinophilic plaque are well-demarcated raised areas of alopecia and ulceration, usually on the ventral abdomen and medial thighs. Associated lesions are extremely pruritic and remain moist because of constant licking. Indolent ulcers are usually well-circumscribed areas of ulceration on the upper lip; lesions may be bilateral or unilateral. Often they have a crater-like appearance. Pruritus is not associated with this form.

- **Cytology:** Intracellular bacteria indicate primary or secondary bacterial involvement. Eosinophils will be present in the plaque and granuloma forms.

- Histopathology: Biopsy of the skin offers the most valuable tool for pathologic classification of lesions.

Ancillary Diagnostics

- **CBC:** Eosinophilic plaques are frequently accompanied by a peripheral eosinophilia. The oral form of linear granuloma may occasionally have a peripheral eosinophilia. The indolent ulcer is not associated with either peripheral or tissue eosinophilia.

 T r e a t m e n t

Primary Therapeutics

- **Identification of underlying cause:** A thorough history should be taken and detailed attention given to the potential for underlying flea allergy, atopy, or food allergy. Other hypersensitivities are also potentially involved. Removal of the causative agent may eliminate the disorder or greatly aid in effective management.

- **Corticosteroids:** Systemic glucocorticoids are the most commonly employed treatment for all forms of EGC. Cats have fewer glucocorticoid receptors than dogs and demonstrate fewer complications with high-dose steroid therapy, although adrenal suppression can occur. Options include:
  - Oral prednisone or prednisolone once daily at 4 to 5 mg/kg. Treatment is continued until the lesions are in remission and then tapered to a lower alternate day dose for chronic management, if needed.
  - Methylprednisolone acetate at 4 mg/kg SC (usually requiring at least 20 mg in the average-sized cat) is generally the most effective therapy. Some cats require several injections initially; these should be spaced several weeks apart. When lesions are in remission, treatment should be given no more often than every 2 months.

- **Antibiotics:** Trimethoprim-sulfa, cefadroxil, and amoxicillin-clavulanate are potentially valuable when bacterial involvement is suspected. Occasionally, improvement or even total remission can occur with antimicrobial therapy. Because the response is unpredictable, a therapeutic trial is recommended.

Secondary Therapeutics

- Immunomodulating agents, such as levamisole and thiabendazole, have been used in refractory cases; side effects may occur.
- Megestrol acetate, a progestational agent, is also a less desirable treatment because of the great potential for significant side effects. It is not the drug

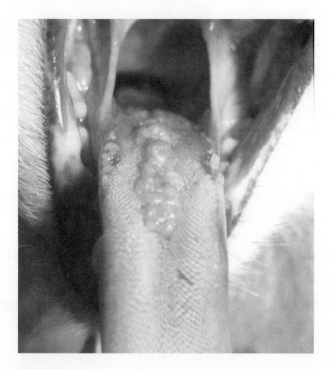

FIGURE 49.1. Eosinophilic granuloma complex: Eosinophilic granuloma in the oral cavity can have the gross appearance of a tumor. This mass at the base of the tongue was confirmed as an eosinophilic granuloma.

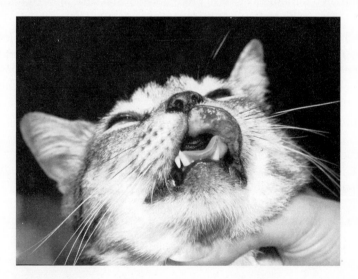

FIGURE 49.2. The ulceration on the upper lip is a severe "rodent ulcer". These lesions are usually unilateral.

of choice, but it may be used in refractory cases to induce remission, to be followed by corticosteroids.

Therapeutic Notes

Lesions of linear granuloma may resolve spontaneously, especially in younger cats.

Prognosis

The prognosis is good in most cats, although continuous or repeated therapy may be needed. The prognosis is better if an underlying condition can be identified and treated.

Suggested Readings

Song MD. Diagnosing and treating eosinophilic granuloma complex. *Vet Med* 1994;89: 1141–1145.

Rosenkrantz WS. Feline eosinophilic granuloma complex. In: Griffin CE, Kwochka KW, MacDonald JM, eds. Current veterinary dermatology. St. Louis: Mosby Yearbook, Inc., 1993;319–324.

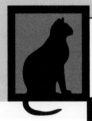

CHAPTER 50

Ethylene Glycol Toxicosis

Gary D. Norsworthy

Overview

E thylene glycol is a common ingredient in antifreeze, but it is also found in photographic developing fluid, some cosmetics, and some plants. It is used as an industrial solvent for lacquers and paints. Ethylene glycol has a sweet taste that appeals to many cats. Several toxic metabolites are produced including glycolate, glycoaldehyde, glyoxylate, and oxalate. The first three cause renal tubular damage, resulting in severe metabolic acidosis. The last one combines with calcium to form calcium oxalate crystals, which lead to renal tubular blockage, renal epithelial necrosis, and hypocalcemia. Hypocalcemia results in seizures. The toxic dose is 1–1.5 mL/kg or as little as one-and-one-half teaspoons for an adult cat of average size. Vomiting, depression, seizures, and coma develop in one-half to 12 hours after ingestion. Tachypnea and tachycardia develop within the next 12 hours, and renal failure occurs within 24 to 72 hours after ingestion. Therefore, early diagnosis and therapy are essential in reversing this potentially fatal toxicity.

Diagnosis

Primary Diagnostics

- **History:** Often, there is a history of exposure to a puddle of antifreeze. This is especially true in the fall as people winterize their cars.
- **Clinical signs:** Ethylene glycol toxicity should be suspected when acute renal failure and neurologic signs are present.
- **Blood test:** A test is commercially available for rapid identification of ethylene glycol in whole blood (EthylenGlycol Test Kit, PRN Pharmacol Inc., Pensacola, FL).
- **Ultrasound:** Within a few hours, the renal medulla will be hyperechoic due to the presence of calcium oxalate crystals. This echo pattern may extend into the cortex. Later, the medullary rim sign and halo sign may develop. At this point, therapy is unlikely to be successful (Figure 50.2).

Ancillary Diagnostics

- **Urinalysis:** When renal failure occurs, the urine specific gravity will be low or in the fixed range. Calcium oxalate crystals are usually present.

Diagnostic Notes

Successful treatment requires rapid diagnosis.

 T r e a t m e n t

Primary Therapeutics

- **Induce vomition and lavage stomach:** This should only be done within the first 4 hours of ingestion and only if the cat is conscious.

- **Ethanol 20%:** This drug should be administered as soon as the diagnosis is made. Five intraperitoneal injections are made at 6-hour intervals at the rate of 5.5 mL/kg. Four more treatments are given at 8-hour intervals. To be effective, this must begin within 6 hours after ingestion.

- **Sodium bicarbonate:** This is given primarily to counter metabolic acidosis. Administer according to serial plasma bicarbonate and base deficit determinations with monitoring every 4–6 hours. If this is not possible, administer at approximately 5 mEq/kg/h.

- **Fluid therapy:** Aggressive fluid therapy is important to maintain tissue perfusion and renal function and to correct metabolic acidosis.

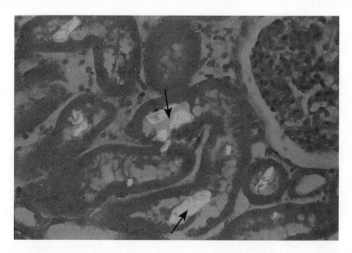

FIGURE 50.1. Ethylene glycol toxicosis: Calcium oxalate crystals within the renal tubules cause renal tubular blockage and renal epithelial necrosis.

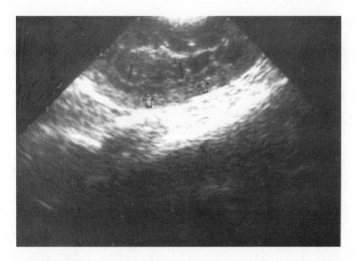

FIGURE 50.2. The medullary rim sign (small closed arrows) is a line of hyperechogenicity in the outer zone of the renal medulla that parallels the corticomedullary junction. The halo sign (open arrows) is a thin hypoechogenic zone at the corticomedullary junction. Both can occur as a result of ethylene glycol toxicity, but neither are specific for it.

Secondary Therapeutics

- **Peritoneal dialysis:** When this is feasible, it can be important in maintaining the cat until renal function can be reestablished. This should be done only by those persons experienced with this technique.
- **Osmotic diuresis:** Dextrose 20% (20 mL/kg q6–8h IV) or mannitol 20% (1.25–2.5 mL/kg q6–8h IV) can be helpful in reestablishing renal output.

Therapeutic Notes

- It is unusual for a cat to recover if treatment does not begin within 6 hours of ingestion.
- Electrolytes and acid-base balance should be monitored as frequently as possible.

P r o g n o s i s

The prognosis for ethylene glycol toxicity is always guarded. However, if treatment is not begun within 6 hours of ingestion, the prognosis is grave.

S u g g e s t e d   R e a d i n g s

Groff RM, Miller JM, Stair EL, et al. In: Norsworthy GD, ed. Feline practice. Philadelphia: JB Lippincott, 1993;551–569.

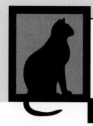

CHAPTER 51
Exocrine Pancreatic Insufficiency
Gary D. Norsworthy

Overview

D estruction of exocrine pancreatic acinar cells usually occurs secondary to chronic pancreatitis. Because the latter disease also destroys beta cells, diabetes mellitus may occur concurrently. Other causes of exocrine pancreatic insufficiency (EPI) include neoplasia, pancreatic flukes, and proximal duodenal resection. Based on the disease in other species, it is presumed that feline EPI produces abnormal intestinal enzyme action and impaired absorption of sugars, amino acids, and fatty acids. Subsequently, small intestinal bacterial overgrowth, steatorrhea, malabsorption of fat-soluble vitamins, cobalamin deficiency, and vitamin-K responsive coagulopathy may occur. Affected cats typically have soft, pale, voluminous stools with weight loss. The steatorrhea may cause oily material to collect on the haircoat, especially in the region of the perineum.

 ## Diagnosis

Primary Diagnostics

- **Feline trypsin-like immunoreactivity (TLI):** This feline-specific test is the most reliable test for EPI.*

Ancillary Diagnostics

- **Fecal proteolytic activity:** This test will identify most affected cats. However, it will give false positive or equivocal results in some cats with small intestinal disease. The test is cumbersome to perform. Three fecal samples are needed, and the samples must be frozen immediately following collection and during transit to the laboratory.
- **Serum cobalamin:** The level of serum cobalamin is markedly subnormal in most EPI cats, although this test alone is not adequate evidence for a diagnosis of EPI.

*Feline TLI is performed by: GI Lab, Texas A&M University, College Station, TX

Diagnostic Notes

- Hyperthyroidism and inflammatory bowel disease cause clinical signs similar to EPI. These conditions are much more common, so they should be ruled out before testing for EPI.
- In contrast to dogs, cats with EPI do not have elevated serum folate levels.

 Treatment

Primary Therapeutics

- **Pancreatic enzyme replacer:** Powdered pancreatin is recommended. A dose of 1 teaspoon with each meal is the recommended amount, but the dosage should be determined by patient response.
- **Cobalamin:** Parenteral administration of 250 µg SC every 7 days for 1–2 months is recommended if cobalamin levels are documented to be low.

Secondary Therapeutics

- **Antibiotics:** These are indicated for possible small intestinal bacterial overgrowth.
- **Glucocorticoids:** These are given for possible inflammatory bowel disease.
- **Diet:** A high-protein, low-fat diet may be beneficial; however, high-fat diets are often advantageous to cats with diarrhea.

Therapeutic Notes

The items mentioned under Secondary Therapeutics should be instituted if use of a pancreatic extract is unsuccessful in relieving clinical signs.

Prognosis

The prognosis generally is good.

Suggested Readings

Hardy RM. Diseases of the exocrine pancreas. In: Sherding RG, ed. The cat: diseases and clinical management, 2nd ed. Philadelphia: WB Saunders, 1994;1287–1296.

Steiner JM, Williams DA. Validation of a radioimmunoassay for feline trypsin-like immunoreactivity (FTLI) and serum cobalamin and folate concentrations in cats with exocrine pancreatic insufficiency (EPI). *J Vet Int Med* 1995;9:193–196.

Williams DA. Feline exocrine pancreatic disease. *Fel Health Topics* 1995;10(4):1–8.

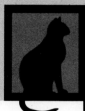

CHAPTER 52

Feline Immunodeficiency Virus Infection

Sharon K. Fooshee

Overview

Feline immunodeficiency virus (FIV) is a member of the lentivirus subfamily of retroviruses. Since it was first isolated in the late 1980s from a cattery in northern California, it has remained a focus of research interest. Cats infected with FIV have served as excellent animal models for the study of human immunodeficiency virus and AIDS. Bite wounds appear to provide the major mode of transmission, although the role of transmission by close physical contact alone (without bite wounds) is under study. Queens who become infected during gestation may transmit the virus in utero or later through colostrum or saliva. Five phases of infection have been determined: a) acute; b) asymptomatic carrier; c) persistent generalized lymphadenopathy; d) feline AIDS-related complex; and e) terminal feline AIDS. Older, free-roaming outdoor male cats are at the highest risk of infection. Lentiviruses are species-specific and pose no apparent public health risk. During the acute phase, signs may consist only of peripheral lymphadenopathy. As an asymptomatic carrier (stage 2), the cat is usually free of clinical disease. In later stages, signs include weight loss, persistent diarrhea, gingivitis/stomatitis, chronic respiratory disease, lymphadenopathy, and chronic skin disease. Profound oral/dental disease is a common finding in the late stages of FIV; in some cats, the mucosa is ulcerated and necrotic. Neurologic dysfunction has been seen in a small percentage of infected cats. Inflammatory ocular disease, nonspecific renal disease, and neoplastic disorders are occasionally reported.

Diagnosis

Primary Diagnostics

- **Clinical signs:** Chronic disease states and seemingly minor infections that do not respond well to treatment should alert one to FIV infection.
- **Antibody tests:** Because infected cats may have no circulating viral antigen, commercially available enzyme-linked immunosorbent assay (ELISA) kits

test for the presence of lentivirus antibody. Sensitivity is equivalent to indirect fluorescent antibody (IFA) methodology but is less specific.

- **Western blot:** Positive tests should be verified by the more specific Western blot assay.

Ancillary Diagnostics

- **CBC:** Hematologic abnormalities are common with FIV infection. Leukopenia, neutropenia, and nonregenerative anemia are frequently observed. Occasionally, neutrophilia or thrombocytopenia are reported.

Diagnostic Notes

- The relative difficulty of recovering virus from blood cells and body fluids varies with the stage of infection. As noted above, assays for viral antigen have been unreliable for diagnosis of FIV, and current commercial tests screen for antibody.

- *Maternal FIV antibody may cause kittens to have a positive ELISA test result for up to 4 months after birth. Positive kittens should be retested after 6 months of age.*

- FIV-infected cats often have a profound leukopenia when griseofulvin is administered. Leukopenic cats on griseofulvin should be tested for FIV.

 T r e a t m e n t

Primary Therapeutics

- **Supportive:** Treatment of FIV is supportive and is directed toward management of related complications. No specific antiviral therapy for FIV is available at present. It is recommended that FIV-positive cats be examined by a veterinarian every 4–6 months to facilitate early intervention when problems arise. Special care should be given to periodontal disease.

Secondary Therapeutics

- **Interferon:** Low-dose oral interferon-alpha is an immune stimulant that can be beneficial to many FIV-infected cats. It is dosed at 30 units per day orally. However, it is not viricidal. See Table 55.5.

- **Stress avoidance:** To prolong the life of FIV-positive cats, stressful situations should be avoided, a good quality diet fed, and appropriate bactericidal antibiotics administered when necessary. Fecal exams should be performed at 6–12 month intervals.

- **Isolation:** FIV-infected cats should be isolated from other cats to avoid transmission of the virus and to avoid exposure to secondary pathogens. Clients should be counseled to keep FIV-positive cats indoors.

Therapeutic Notes

- Opportunistic infections are associated with the later stages of FIV infection and should be anticipated. Problems that may develop include viral and bacterial respiratory infection, toxoplasmosis, mycobacteriosis, and hemobartonellosis.

- Some authorities recommend that FIV-positive cats should receive only killed vaccines if vaccinated at all. At present, no vaccine exists to protect against FIV infection.

- The use of AZT is being investigated.

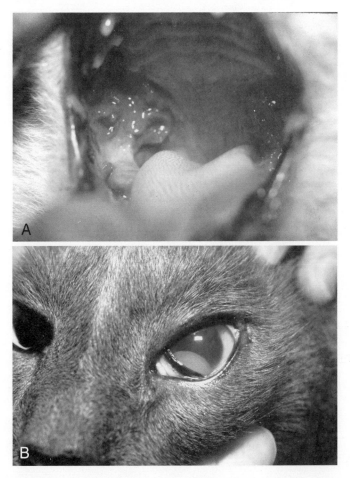

FIGURE 52.1. Feline immunodeficiency virus: The immunosuppressive effects of the FIV result in several seemingly unrelated diseases. Lymphoplasmacytic gingivitis (*A*) and hypopyon (*B*) have been associated with the FIV, as seen in these two cats.

P r o g n o s i s

The prognosis is variable and dependent upon clinical stage at diagnosis.

S u g g e s t e d   R e a d i n g s

Sparger EE. Current thoughts on feline immunodeficiency virus. In: Hoskins JE, Loar AS, eds. Feline infectious diseases. Philadelphia: WB Saunders, 1993;173–191.

Sparkes AH, Hopper CD, Millard WG, Gruffyd-Jones TJ, Harbour DA. Feline immunodeficiency virus. *J Vet Intern Med* 1993;85–90.

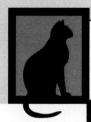

CHAPTER 53
Feline Infectious Enteritis (Panleukopenia)
Sharon K. Fooshee

Overview

F eline infectious enteritis (FIE), or panleukopenia, is caused by a nonenveloped parvovirus. As with canine parvovirus, FIE has an affinity for rapidly dividing cells of the bone marrow and intestinal epithelium. A fecal-oral route of transmission is most likely; the attendant incubation period is 2 to 9 days. Large quantities of the virus are shed into the feces during the acute phase of illness. Prenatal infection of kittens may occur in mid to late gestation; the queen usually remains clinically unaffected. Panleukopenia has the potential to cause significant disease in unprotected cats of all ages. Kittens and young cats frequently present with fever, peracute or acute onset vomiting, prostration, and dehydration. Liquid diarrhea may not occur initially. The abdomen may be painful upon palpation. Bowel loops are sometimes thickened and often contain fluid and gas. Profound fluid loss may result in death. Kittens infected in utero may abort or, if they survive, demonstrate nonprogressive cerebellar dysfunction: ataxia and hypermetria with a wide-based stance. The disease is most prevalent in cats less than 1 year of age, where fatalities may reach 50 to 90%. Subclinical infections do occur, usually in adult cats or older kittens. Inapparent carriers of the disease may serve as reservoirs of the virus. Routine vaccination has made FIE less prevalent than in the past; it is usually found in unvaccinated cats living in conditions of stress or overcrowding, such as animal shelters.

 ## Diagnosis

Primary Diagnostics

- **Clinical signs:** Kittens and young cats presented with fever and vomiting should be suspected. Kittens born with cerebellar disease should be highly suspected.

- **CBC:** Panleukopenia is a consistent finding on the complete blood count. A nadir of 100–200 white cells/μL may occur within a few days of infection. More severe leukopenia is associated with a poorer prognosis.

Ancillary Diagnostics

- Kittens suspected of having FIE should be tested for FeLV and FIV.
- The stool should be examined for parasites because heavy parasitism may worsen the prognosis.
- Because the history, clinical signs, and profound leukopenia are very suggestive of FIE, more elaborate testing, such as electron microscopy of stool, is rarely necessary.

Diagnostic Notes

- A history of recent vaccination in the young kitten does not eliminate the possibility of FIE because maternal antibodies may interfere with early vaccination efforts.
- Clinical signs of FIE may be consistent with poisoning, toxoplasmosis, and bacterial enteritis. Toxoplasmosis usually has an associated respiratory component and rarely causes profound leukopenia. Primary bacterial enteritis (*Escherichia coli*, salmonellosis) may present with similar clinical signs and leukopenia.

 Treatment

Primary Therapeutics

- **Fluid therapy:** Intravenous fluid therapy should be directed at supplying maintenance needs and correcting ongoing losses due to vomiting and diarrhea. Maintenance needs are approximately 60 mL/kg/day; the deficit is estimated as a percentage of body weight. A balanced electrolyte solution such as lactated Ringer's solution with 5% dextrose is acceptable in most situations. Subcutaneous fluids would be sufficient in only the mildest cases.
- **Antibiotics:** Broad-spectrum antimicrobial therapy with a cephalosporin antibiotic is often employed due to leukopenia and associated bacterial infections. Aminoglycosides should be used if gram-negative sepsis is considered likely. However, potential nephrotoxicity in the dehydrated patient increases the risk of drug-induced renal failure. Quinolone antibiotics may also be considered for gram-negative infections, but there may be limitations posed by potential routes of administration.
- **NPO:** Oral antibiotics should be avoided initially because of vomiting. Water may be offered after 24–48 hours as long as it does not induce more

vomiting. Feeding should be delayed until the cat is able to drink water; a bland diet is recommended.

- **Antiemetics:** Metoclopramide can be used in cases of intractable vomiting. It may be administered by continuous infusion at 1–2 mg/kg/24 hours. Phenothiazines should be avoided because of hypotension.

Secondary Therapeutics

- Fever may be present initially. As the disease progresses, some kittens will become hypothermic due to fluid loss and endotoxemia. Body temperature should be monitored.

- Intestinal protectants and motility modifiers are not routinely necessary, and results are variable.

Therapeutic Notes

The vaccination status of all cats in the household should be reviewed.

Prognosis

With appropriate supportive care, most kittens and cats can survive FIE. Complications that would worsen the prognosis include gram-negative sepsis and endotoxic shock.

Suggested Readings

Pedersen NC. Feline panleukopenia. In: Pedersen NC, ed. Feline infectious diseases. Goleta, CA: American Veterinary Publishing, 1988;15–20.

Pollock RVH, Postorino NC. Feline panleukopenia and other enteric viral diseases. In: Sherding RG, ed. The cat: diseases and clinical management. Philadelphia: WB Saunders, 1994:479–487.

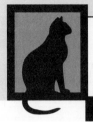

CHAPTER 54

Feline Infectious Peritonitis

Gary D. Norsworthy

Overview

Feline infectious peritonitis (FIP) is a progressive, immune-mediated viral disease that is, with few exceptions, fatal within a few weeks. It is caused by a coronavirus, the FIP virus (FIPV), which many authorities consider to be an in vivo mutation of the widespread and mildly pathogenic feline enteric coronavirus (FECV). The FIPV is relatively unstable in the environment but may remain infectious for as long as 7 weeks within dried organic matter or on dry surfaces. It is susceptible to most commonly used veterinary disinfectants. The virus is transmitted via oral and nasal secretions; prolonged contact with an infected cat is usually required for transmission. The incidence of virus-infected cats in a closed population is typically found to be either zero or 80 to 90%. The outcome of an infection may not be known for months or years, as the virus may remain dormant. The outcome is influenced by the cat's immune response. Antibodies produced against the virus may promote the disease rather than cause immunity. Recently, it was reported that there is a genetic influence on susceptibility to FIP. It appears that certain breeding toms may pass this trait to offspring. The **wet** or **effusive form** results in pyogranulomatous lesions within single or multiple organs and the formation of effusive fluid within the thoracic or abdominal cavity. The **dry** or **noneffusive form** causes the same organ lesions, but effusion does not occur. The most commonly affected organs are the kidneys, liver, visceral lymph nodes, intestines, lungs, eyes, and brain. The clinical signs are referable to the affected organ or organs, but all cases generally include weight loss, inappetence, and refractory fever. Icterus and pale mucous membranes are common. Abdominal distention or dyspnea occur when abdominal or pleural effusions develop.

Diagnosis

Primary Diagnostics

- **Clinical Signs:** The clinical signs are not unlike many infectious or inflammatory diseases; however, the presence of persistent, antibiotic-resistant fever should raise one's index of suspicion for FIP. Retinal hemorrhages are found in a limited number of diseases and are not consistently present in FIP, but they should also put FIP on one's differential list.

- **Histopathology:** This is the only way to confirm FIP; however, biopsy is not always feasible.
- **Coronavirus titer:** This test is meaningful only if it is high (greater than 1:1600) and if appropriate clinical signs are present. It is positive at low levels in FIPV infections without disease, in some cases of FIP, or with FECV infections. It may also be negative in clinical cases of FIP.
- **Serum protein level:** Many cats with FIP have an elevated total serum protein level (>7.8 mg/dL) and a decreased A:G ratio (<0.6). This pattern is also present in other chronic, inflammatory diseases.
- **Combination testing:** The positive predictive value is about 90% if all of these are present: hyperglobulinemia, lymphopenia, and a coronavirus titer greater than 1:100. The negative predictive value is nearly 100% if none of these findings are present.
- **Fluid analysis:** The typical effusion is clear to straw-colored, viscous, and contains fibrin strands. It has a specific gravity greater than 1.018 and is sterile. When stained with a modified Wright's stain, the background stains pink due to the high level of protein.

Ancillary Diagnostics

- **PCR testing:** This test is offered by some commercial veterinary laboratories. It is extremely sensitive; however, its specificity has not been documented.
- **Protein electrophoresis:** When hypergammaglobulinemia is detected, serum protein electrophoresis may be requested. The typical pattern with FIP is a polyclonal gammopathy.

Diagnostic Notes

- Dry FIP is one of the most difficult antemortem diagnoses to make, even for experienced practitioners. It should be on the differential list for any cat with chronic weight loss, poor appetite, and fever.
- The use of organ biopsy should be pursued when feasible.
- Feline leukemia virus (FeLV) testing should be part of the minimum data base for cats with fever of unknown origin. Many cats with FIP are infected with the FeLV.

 T r e a t m e n t

Primary Therapeutics

- **Euthanasia:** There is no proven successful treatment for FIP. When FIP is confirmed or when the evidence is considerable, euthanasia is the logical course.

Secondary Therapeutics

- **Chemotherapy:** Prednisolone, cyclophosphamide, and other immune suppressants have provided temporary response when combined with supportive care.

- **Supportive Care:** Nutritional support, fluid therapy, and removal of effusive fluids should be part of any therapeutic effort.

Therapeutic Notes

A few apparent cases of spontaneous remission have been reported. However, clients should not be told to expect this.

Prevention

- **Vaccination:** An attenuated, live-virus, intranasal vaccine is available. Its efficacy is only about 70%; however, it is indicated in known exposure situations. Its widespread use is controversial owing to the low incidence of this disease in most practice populations.

- **Cattery control:** Maternal antibodies protect most kittens until they are about 6–7 weeks of age. The most effective plan is to remove kittens from exposure to any seropositive cat, including their mother, at 5 weeks of age and to keep them isolated until removed from the cattery. Minimizing environmental stress and overcrowding, cleanliness, and optimum nutrition are also important. FeLV-infected cats should be removed from the cattery.

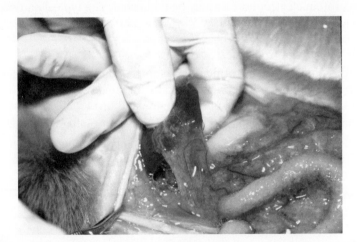

FIGURE 54.1. Feline infectious peritonitis: The wet, abdominal form of FIP results in ascites and the formation of fibrin adhesions between abdominal organs. The dry form may affect almost any organ.

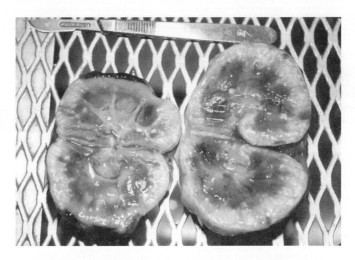

FIGURE 54.2. Granulomas and hemorrhage are common in renal FIP.

Prognosis

The prognosis for cats with FIP is grave. However, seropositive cats should not be euthanized, as many will not develop the disease.

Suggested Reading

Weiss RC. Feline infectious peritonitis and other coronaviruses. In: Sherding RG, ed. The cat: diseases and clinical management, 2nd ed. Philadelphia: WB Saunders, 1994;449–477.

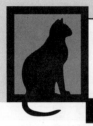

CHAPTER 55

Feline Leukemia Virus Diseases

Gary D. Norsworthy

Overview

The feline leukemia virus (FeLV) is a retrovirus that is transmitted horizontally via salivary contact with other cats; known routes of transmission include biting, licking, and grooming and via in utero and transmammary routes. However, virus contact does not assure infection, and infection does not ensure persistent viremia or disease. The four possible outcomes to exposure are listed in Table 55.1. Once introduced into the cat, the virus progresses through various tissues. The ability of the immune system to halt this progression determines the ultimate outcome and influences the results of various antigen tests (See Table 55.2). The virus produces several proliferative diseases (lymphosarcoma [LSA], leukemias), several degenerative diseases (nonregenerative anemias, thymic atrophy, panleukopenia-like syndrome, stillbirths, abortions), and immunosuppression. Clinical signs vary widely depending on the disease type and the organs involved. Diagnostic tests detect the presence of the viral antigen. Test results vary depending on the form of disease present and the target organs involved. For example, over 90% of cats with anterior mediastinal LSA are virus positive; less than 50% of cats with alimentary LSA are virus positive.

Because the virus is environmentally labile, household disinfection is easily accomplished. Without treatment, the virus is gone within a week. The FeLV can be removed from the household by a test and removal program. New cats introduced into a household should be tested for FeLV prior to admission. Vaccination is recommended for all cats that have exposure to free-roaming cats or to known FeLV-infected cats. Exposure produces solid immunity in 80–90% of vaccinated cats, but the rate is lower when cats are continuously exposed to infected cats. Public health aspects of this virus have been the subject of numerous studies, but none have found a link between the FeLV and any human disease. However, it is recommended that neonates and immunocompromised individuals avoid exposure to cats with the FeLV.

TABLE 55.1

Possible Outcomes of Exposure to the FeLV

1. **Virus neutralization:** The cat mounts an immune response; some immunity is produced, making the cat resistant to future infections for an undetermined period of time.
   Tests: PCR test is positive during Stages 1 and 2, and serum ELISA test is positive during Stage 2. Then both become negative.
   Occurrence rate: About 30% of exposures
2. **Persistent viremia:** The virus progresses through all six stages.
   Tests: All tests become positive in the following order: PCR, Serum ELISA, IFA, Tears/saliva ELISA.
   Occurrence rate: About 40% of exposures
3. **Latency:** The cat does not produce immunity, but it does not become persistently viremic. Viral DNA is hiding in the cat's genome, but no viral replication is occurring. This is a transient stage that lasts an average of 30 months. Ultimately, it results in virus neutralization or persistent viremia.
   Tests: PCR is positive. Others are negative.
   Occurrence rate: About 30% of exposures
4. **Immune carrier:** The whole virus is sequestered in epithelial tissue and is replicating, but it does not leave the cells due to antibody production.
   Tests: PCR and serum ELISA are positive; IFA and tears/saliva ELISA are negative.

TABLE 55.2

Progression of the FeLV Through the Cat and Test Results at Each Stage

Pos Tests	Stage	Duration	Disease Progression
P	1.	(1–4 days)	Replication of FeLV occurs in lymphoid tissues surrounding the site of exposure (tonsils and pharyngeal LNs via oronasal exposure).
P/E1	2.	(2–14 days)	Small numbers of circulating lymphocytes and monocytes are infected.
P/E1	3.	(3–12 days)	FeLV replication is amplified in the spleen, LNs, and gut-associated lymphoid tissue.
P/E1 I	4.	(7–21 days)	Replication progresses to include bone marrow neutrophils and platelets and intestinal crypt epithelial cells.
P/E1	5.	(14–28 days)	Peripheral viremia occurs once FeLV has been incorporated into bone marrow-derived neutrophils and platelets.
P/E1 I/E2	6.	(28–56 days)	Widespread epithelial infection causes excretion of virus in saliva and urine.

P = PCR; E1 = ELISA of blood or serum; I = IFA; E2 = ELISA of saliva or tears

Diagnosis

Primary Diagnostics

- **Clinical signs:** These vary widely but often include dyspnea, lethargy, anorexia, fever, gingivitis/stomatitis, and nonhealing abscesses.
- **Physical examination:** Findings often include evidence of pleural effusion, pale mucous membranes, intraocular abnormalities, palpable intra-abdominal masses, and organomegaly (spleen, liver, kidneys).
- **CBC and chemistry profile:** Common findings include nonregenerative anemia, azotemia, increased liver enzymes, and increased serum bilirubin. Many FeLV-infected cats have nucleated RBCs on a blood smear but not a truly regenerative anemia. A reticulocyte count can identify these cats.
- **FeLV antigen tests:** The tests will be positive in varying incidence depending on the form of the disease and the organs involved.

Ancillary Diagnostics

- **Bone marrow aspirate:** It may reveal marrow dysplasia even when the peripheral blood smear is normal.
- **Pleural fluid analysis:** This often reveals lymphoblasts in a fluid with high protein content and high total cell count.
- **Aspiration cytology:** It often reveals lymphoblasts in enlarged organs and unidentified abdominal masses.

Diagnostic Notes

- Because the FeLV causes such a wide variety of diseases, any seriously ill cat should be tested for it.
- The serum ELISA antigen test should be part of feline health panels; a positive test means that the virus is present. However, its presence does not necessarily mean that it is the cause of the cat's current illness or that the cat is contagious.

Treatment

Primary Therapeutics

- **Chemotherapy:** Various drugs are used for treating cats with LSA. Commonly used drugs are listed in Table 55.3, and a commonly used protocol is listed in Table 55.4.
- **Blood transfusion:** Because many FeLV-related diseases are accompanied by nonregenerative anemia, transfusion of whole blood may

TABLE 55.3

Drugs Used for Treating LSA*

Cyclophosphamide: 50 mg/m^2 BSA PO
Vincristine: 0.5 mg/m^2 BSA IV
Cytosine arabinoside: 100 mg/m^2 BSA/day IV or SC
Prednisolone: 40 mg/m^2 BSA PO
L-Asparaginase: 10,000–20,000 IU/m^2 BSA SC
Chlorambucil: 2 mg/m^2 BSA PO
Methotrexate: 2.5 mg/m^2 BSA PO
Adriamycin: 20–30 mg/m^2 BSA IV

* Consult with an oncology reference book for the appropriate protocol for these drugs and see Appendix B.

TABLE 55.4

Drug Protocol for Treating LSA

Induction (for 6 weeks)
Vincristine: 0.5 mg/m^2 BSA, IV, once weekly
Cyclophosphamide: 50 mg/m^2 BSA, PO, on alternating days
Cytosine arabinoside: 100 mg/m^2 BSA, SC, on first 2 days only
Prednisolone: 40 mg/m^2 BSA, PO, once daily for 7 days and then 20 mg/m^2, PO, on alternating days
Maintenance
Methotrexate: 2.5 mg/m^2 BSA, PO, three times per week
Chlorambucil: 20 mg/m^2 BSA, PO, every 14 days
Prednisolone: 20 mg/m^2 BSA, PO, on alternating days
Vincristine: 0.5 mg/m^2 BSA, IV, once monthly

BSA = body surface area

be necessary to stabilize the cat for diagnostics or as an adjuvant to other forms of therapy.

Secondary Therapeutics

- **Low-dose oral interferon:** This drug is used to stimulate the cat's immune system, resulting in clinical improvement and enhanced quality of life. However, it is not virucidal. See Table 55.5.

- **Prednisolone:** The drug can produce appetite stimulation and short-term reduction in the size of lymphosarcomatous masses.

TABLE 55.5

Low-dose Interferon-alpha for Use in FeLV-infected Cats

Product:
  Roferon-A by Hoffman LaRoche; 3,000,000-unit vial
  Note: Several concentrations are available through local pharmacies.
Preparation:
  a. Mix one vial with one liter of saline (makes 3000 units/mL solution).
  b. Freeze this in 10-mL aliquots that will keep for 1–2 years.
  c. One 10-mL aliquot is diluted with one liter of saline; this will keep for at least 2 months
      under refrigeration. (Makes 30 units/mL solution.)
Protocol:
  a. Give 0.88 mL per 4-kg cat PO: 7 days on and 7 days off, other equivalent schedule,
      or daily. Note: Some clinicians give it at twice this dose.
  b. Tell owner to keep the drug refrigerated.
  c. Some cats do best if treated long term.
  d. Another approach is to treat until the cat is clinically normal, then discontinue the
      drug until it is needed again.

Therapeutic Notes

Successful treatment of LSA and nonregenerative anemia results in
remission but not cure. The FeLV remains viable within the cat, so future
relapse is common, and contagion is present.

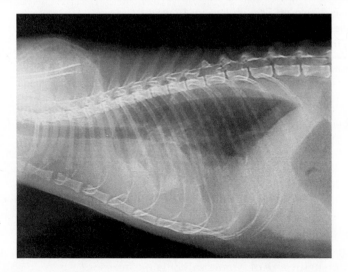

FIGURE 55.1. Feline leukemia virus diseases: The FeLV causes many forms of disease. Pleural
effusion frequently accompanies anterior thoracic lymphosarcoma.

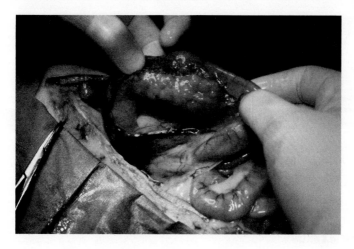

FIGURE 55.2. LSA can also affect the intestinal tract, but affected cats usually test negative for the FeLV antigen.

P r o g n o s i s

Cats that are infected with the FeLV but show no clinical signs may remain asymptomatic for several years. They may be healthy, but they are contagious to other cats. Cats with any FeLV disease have a guarded prognosis. Those with proliferative diseases have an average survival rate of 6 months when aggressive chemotherapy is used.

S u g g e s t e d   R e a d i n g s

Couto CG, Hammer AS. Oncology. In: Sherding RG, ed. The cat: diseases and clinical management, 2nd ed. Philadelphia:WB Saunders, 1994;755–818.

Rojko JL, Hardy WD, Jr. Feline leukemia virus and other retroviruses. In: Sherding RG, ed. The cat: diseases and clinical management, 2nd ed. Philadelphia:WB Saunders, 1994;263–432.

Norsworthy GD. Feline leukemia virus diseases. In: Norsworthy GD, ed. Feline practice. Philadelphia:JB Lippincott, 1993;360–368.

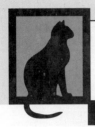

CHAPTER 56

Feline Urologic Syndrome

Gary D. Norsworthy

Overview

The term "feline urologic syndrome" (FUS) is used to describe a syndrome of hematuria and dysuria that is not caused by bacterial infection, uroliths, or neoplasia. Although the term has found disfavor with some, it is accepted by others as a functional designation, allowing discussion of a common form of cystitis and urethritis with an unknown etiology. Another name commonly used for this disease is feline lower urinary tract disease (FLUTD). Affected cats often urinate frequently in small amounts and frequently outside the litterbox, and bright red blood is usually present. Male cats frequently lick the penis. Crystalluria is often present, almost always composed of struvite ("triple phosphates"). If a large amount of mucoid material combines with this crystalline material, a plug forms that may lodge in the tapering distal urethra, resulting in urethral obstruction. Obstructed cats will die if urine flow is not reestablished within 2–4 days. This disease does not appear to be contagious and affects male and female cats, although female cats are extremely unlikely to experience a urethral obstruction. This disease has recently been likened to interstitial cystitis of women.

 Diagnosis

Primary Diagnostics

- **History:** The most common findings include hematuria and dysuria. Inappropriate urination in also common. Many male cats will lick the penis.
- **Physical examination:** Dysuria causes most cats to empty their bladders when only a small amount of urine is present. Upon presentation, most cats have an empty bladder. Cats with urethral obstruction present with pain in the abdomen; abdominal palpation is resisted and reveals a large, firm urinary bladder. These cats become dehydrated and very depressed with increasing duration.

- **Urinalysis:** The most common findings include hematuria, crystalluria, and alkaline pH. Bacteria ($<2\%$ incidence) and pyuria are rarely present. Crystals are typically struvite; however, it should be noted that many normal cats have struvite crystals present. Calcium oxalate crystals are also common, especially in cats over 8 years of age.

Ancillary Diagnostics

- **Chemistry profile:** Cats without urethral obstruction have normal values. Urethral obstruction results in several changes largely related to duration. These include hyperkalemia, elevated BUN and creatinine, and metabolic acidosis evidenced by a decreased anion gap and an increased TCO_2.
- **ECG:** Changes consistent with hyperkalemia are found when the duration of urethral obstruction exceeds 24–36 hours.

Diagnostic Notes

- Inappropriate urination is the most common behavior problem of cats. It can be confused with the loss of litterbox training common in cats with FUS.
- Because the nonobstructed form of this disease is self-limiting in 1 week or less, cats that are still dysuric or hematuric after 1 week (with or without therapy) should receive further diagnostics looking for other diseases that may cause the same symptoms. These tests include culture and sensitivity, urethrogram, multicontrast cystogram, and ultrasound.

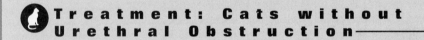

Treatment: Cats without Urethral Obstruction

Primary Therapeutics

- **Antispasmodics:** Drugs in this category can provide symptomatic relief. Commonly used drugs include propantheline bromide (7.5 mg/cat SID PO), flavoxate (50 mg BID), and dantrolene (1 mg/kg TID PO).
- **Anti-inflammatories:** These drugs can help relieve dysuria. Prednisolone, megestrol acetate, and amitriptyline have been used in this manner.

Secondary Therapeutics

- **DMSO:** Some cats respond to intravesicular instillation of 10–20 mL of 10% DMSO. The drug should be left in the bladder for about 10 minutes with the cat under general anesthesia. Do not use a stronger solution.

Therapeutic Notes

- Most cats have a spontaneous remission within 7 days. It is important that treatment not create a secondary disease that requires specific treatment.

- Products containing methylene blue and phenazopyridine have been used for symptomatic relief of these cats. However, both can cause methemoglobinemia and Heinz-body anemias, so they should be avoided.

- The use of megestrol acetate is controversial. The author uses it for only 5 days at a dose of 5 mg SID PO and feels it is the most effective drug for relieving dysuria.

- Antibiotics are often used but are rarely indicated.

🐱 Treatment: Cats with Urethral Obstruction

Primary Therapeutics

- **Catheterization:** This should be attempted as soon as possible using as little sedation as possible. Some cats can be catheterized without any sedation; others require sedation, such as 2 mg/kg of ketamine IV or mask induction with isoflurane.

- **Bladder irrigation:** Repeated irrigation of the bladder with 20-mL aliquots of a sterile, isotonic solution helps to remove crystals from the bladder. If hematuria is severe, the use of a chilled fluid may reduce bleeding by causing vasoconstriction.

- **Intravenous fluids:** An alkalinizing, balanced electrolyte solution, such as lactated Ringer's solution (LRS), should be given. Three-fourths of the calculated volume needed to correct dehydration should be given within the first 24 hours, followed by maintenance rate administration. Postobstructive diuresis often occurs for 1–3 days. Fluid administration should continue so that dehydration does not recur. After the first 24 hours of fluid administration, fluids can be given subcutaneously.

- **Potassium:** When renal function and urine flow are restored, hypokalemia may occur. When needed, 30 to 40 mEq of potassium chloride can be added to a liter of IV fluids. Potassium administration should not exceed 0.5 mEq/kg/h.

Secondary Therapeutics

- **Cystocentesis:** This procedure can relieve intravesicular pressure, which may make catheterization easier to perform.

- **Perineal urethrostomy:** This procedure is indicated if catheterization is not possible following cystocentesis or if repeated obstruction occurs. Because cats undergoing this procedure are then predisposed to bacterial cystitis and urolith formation, perineal urethrostomy should not be considered a first-choice procedure.

- **For overdistention bladder atony:** This is best treated with bethanechol chloride (1.25–2.5 mg/cat BID PO). The use of an indwelling catheter for

1–3 days may be needed to prevent continued overdistention, especially if the cat is receiving IV or SC fluids.

- **For detrusor-urethral sphincter dyssynergia:** To relax the bladder sphincter, give diazepam (2.5–5.0 mg/cat BID-TID PO) dantrolene (0.5–1.0 mg/kg TID PO) or phenoxybenzamine (2.5–10 mg/cat SID PO).

- **Indwelling catheterization:** This should be done only if there was great difficulty catheterizing the cat, there is a tiny urine stream following bladder flushing, the cats reobstructs within 24 hours, or bladder atony occurs.

- **DMSO:** Some cats respond to intravesicular instillation of 10–20 mL of 10% DMSO. The drug should be left in the bladder for about 10 minutes with the cat under general anesthesia. Do not use a stronger solution.

Therapeutic Notes

The use of an indwelling catheter predisposes the cat to bacterial cystitis. If this is necessary, the use of antibiotics during or after removal is recommended.

Prevention

- **Urine acidification:** This has been shown to have significant benefit in preventing struvite crystallization. It may be accomplished with diet or medication (ammonium chloride [300 mg/kg/day PO] or DL-methionine [500 mg/cat BID PO]). It is contraindicated in calcium-oxalate crystallization.

- **Weight management:** Obesity appears to be a predisposing factor for this disease.

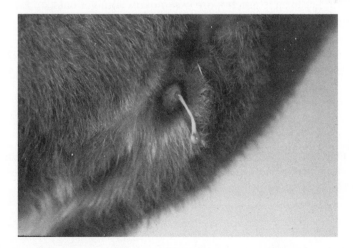

FIGURE 56.1. Feline urologic syndrome: The combination of a mucoid matrix and crystalline material results in the plug that causes urethral obstruction.

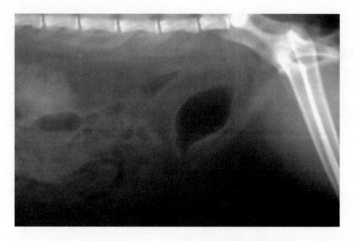

FIGURE 56.2. A diverticulum at the cranial end of the bladder may be associated with chronic or recurrent cystitis and can be demonstrated with a pneumocystogram.

Prevention Notes

Urine acidification and low-magnesium diets increase the risk of calcium oxalate urolithiasis. Crystal-type determination is recommended prior to dietary prescription.

Prognosis

- Struvite crystalluria is much more common in younger cats, and calcium-oxalate cystalluria is much more common in older cats. The prognosis for nonobstructed cats is good, even without treatment. Cats that have urethral obstruction and uremia have a guarded prognosis. Recovery is likely if urine flow occurs normally and renal function returns.

Suggested Reading

Barsanti JA, Finco DR, Brown SA. Diseases of the lower urinary tract. In: Sherding RG, ed. The cat: diseases and clinical management, 2nd ed. New York:Churchill Livingstone, 1994;1769–1823.

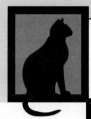

CHAPTER 57

Fight Wound Infections

Gary D. Norsworthy

Overview

T he territoriality of the cat is largely responsible for its fighting behavior. The typical feline bite wound is due to a tooth that penetrates the skin and underlying tissue, leaving a lesion of minimal diameter but substantial depth. Within a few hours, the skin puncture closes, entrapping bacteria from the cat's mouth and debris carried into the wound. Aerobic and anaerobic bacterial and fungal infections are common. The lesion progresses from swelling to pain and lameness (if on a leg) to abscessation. Abscess formation occurs about 3 to 5 days after the bite. If not lanced, it will usually rupture by 7 days. Some cats develop chronic draining tracts due to resistant bacteria, mycoplasma, mycobacterium, or fungal infections, the presence of foreign bodies or bone sequestra within the wound, or immunosuppressive states usually associated with the feline immunodeficiency virus (FIV) or the feline leukemia virus (FeLV). Cellulitis is a variant of this process. If a bite wound occurs in a location that does not have loose skin, such as a distal extremity, the infection will dissect through fascial and muscle planes, resulting in diffuse swelling instead of an abscess. Lethargy, inappetence, fever, and lameness are the early signs. Areas of swelling anywhere on the body of a cat showing the appropriate clinical signs should arouse suspicion. Draining tracts, especially if the material has a putrid odor, indicates an advanced stage of the process.

Diagnosis

Primary Diagnostics

- **History:** Outdoor cats or cats in multicat households with a history of fighting are at highest risk.
- **Clinical signs:** The presence of a painful swollen area or a draining tract should arouse one's suspicion for a bite wound abscess.

Ancillary Diagnostics

- **Culture and sensitivity:** This is generally not necessary; however, chronic draining wounds should be cultured for aerobes, anaerobes, fungi, and mycobacteria.
- **CBC:** A marked neutrophilic leukocytosis with a left shift is typical.
- **Viral tests:** Cats with recurrent or nonresponsive abscesses should be tested for FeLV and the FIV.

Diagnostic Notes

- Because of the high incidence of this disease, a bite wound infection should be suspected first for draining tracts, especially if fever and a history of fighting are present.

 T r e a t m e n t

Primary Therapeutics

- **Antibiotics:** The high incidence of *Pasteurella multocida* makes the penicillins the drugs of choice. If given within the first 48 hours after the bite, they may be curative. Antibiotic therapy is the treatment of choice for cellulitis.
- **Surgical drainage:** Lancing an abscess enhances rapid resolution. A drainage hole should be made in the ventral aspect to facilitate drainage of purulent material. Flushing or swabbing the abscess with an antibacterial solution is appropriate. Suturing should not occur for 3–4 days; however, abscesses generally granulate and close well without suturing. Surgical drainage is not appropriate for cellulitis.

Secondary Therapeutics

- **Surgical exploration and excision:** Abscesses that do not heal promptly should be surgically explored to identify and remove foreign material. Chronic fistulous tracts should be excised, if surgically feasible.
- **Alternative antibiotics:** Bite wound infections that are not responsive to penicillins or aminoglycosides may be due to unusual organisms, including mycobacteria. It has been shown that enrofloxacin or doxycycline may be effective in abscesses resistant to other antibiotics.

Therapeutic Notes

Castration should be recommended because the nature of the tom cat is to enlarge his territory by fighting. Fighting often leads to abscesses and FeLV or FIV infections.

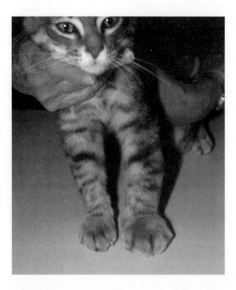

Figure 57.1. Fight-wound infections: Fight wounds result in cellulitis in locations in which the skin is taut, such as in an extremity.

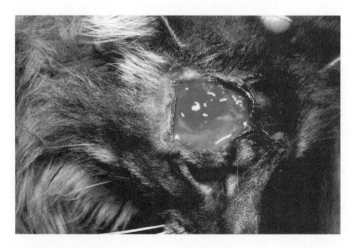

Figure 57.2. An abscess has formed over this cat's eye. The purulent material is exposed when the overlying skin is removed.

P r o g n o s i s

The prognosis for fight wound infections is excellent with proper diagnosis and antibiotic therapy. Cats with nonhealing wounds should be cultured and tested for FeLV and FIV. These viral organisms make the cat susceptible to repeated and resistant infections.

S u g g e s t e d   R e a d i n g s

Greene CE. Feline abscesses. In: Greene CE, ed. Infectious diseases of the dog and cat, 2nd ed. Philadelphia: WB Saunders, 1990;595–598.

Studdert VP, Hughes KL. Treatment of opportunistic mycobacterial infections with enrofloxacin in cats. *J Am Vet Med Assoc* 1992;201(9):1388–1390.

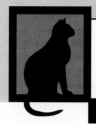

CHAPTER 58

Fleas

Sharon K. Fooshee

Overview

The cat flea, *Ctenocephalides felis*, is the most common ectoparasite of cats. This blood-sucking parasite spends its entire adult life on the unwilling host. When the female flea lays her eggs on the cat, they eventually hatch into larvae. The larvae pupate by spinning a cocoon and may remain in this stage for up to 140 days. Emergence occurs when ideal environmental conditions develop. In humid, warm parts of the country, the life cycle may be completed every 2–4 weeks. When all the life stages of the flea are considered as a single population, the egg comprises 50% of the total, leaving the larvae at 35%, the pupae at 10%, and the adult flea at only 5%. As such, effective flea control programs usually focus on control of juvenile (pre-emergent) fleas, instead of on the relatively small population of adults.

Diagnosis

Primary Diagnostics

- **Clinical signs:** In most cases, flea infestation is readily diagnosed by the presence of fleas crawling through the pet's haircoat. Occasionally, owners may first notice the problem when entering the home after the pet has been removed for some time; fleas seeking a food source will bite the pet and, perhaps, humans.
- Heavily parasitized cats may develop anemia due to blood loss. Flea-allergic dermatitis and tapeworms are other problems associated with flea infestation.

Ancillary Diagnostics

The presence of flea feces (flea dirt) indicates flea infestation. This may be demonstrated to the owner by combing the dark material out of the pet's haircoat and onto a moistened paper towel. The red stain of resuspended digested blood can be easily visualized.

219

Diagnostic Notes

- Ectoparasitism may result in peripheral eosinophilia.
- Papulocrusting lesions of miliary dermatitis are often found on the tailhead and around the neck of flea-allergic cats.

T r e a t m e n t

Primary Therapeutics

- Cats are quite sensitive to organophosphate pesticides. Chlorpyrifos is particularly toxic and is commonly found in over-the-counter adulticide treatments. For additional details, see Chapter 93.
- Botanical insecticides, such as pyrethrins and pyrethroids, may be applied to the cat as well as in the environment. They have no activity against juvenile stages of the flea. Caution is required because some of these products are associated with toxicity (including death) in cats. Over-the-counter products containing a combination of fenvalerate and DEET are of particular concern.
- Borates are used for indoor flea control and are considered relatively safe. Primarily the larval stage of the flea is affected by these products.
- Insect growth regulators (IGRs) are geared toward control of the juvenile stages of the flea. One advantage to IGRs is that they may result in less chemical treatment of the home and yard, as well as less total exposure of the cat to insecticides.
- The recent introduction of monthly products (Advantage, Program, and Frontline) is making flea control easier and more effective.

Secondary Therapeutics

- Flea collars, combs, shampoos, sprays, and dips have nominal value as the sole agents in a flea control program because they primarily kill adult fleas (5% of the population). Clients should be counseled as to a reasonable expectation of success if these are the only products used in their flea control program.
- Ultrasonic flea collars are of no proven value in flea control.
- Environmental flea control (both indoors and outdoors) should be emphasized as an important part of total flea control.

Therapeutic Notes

Significant risk for insecticide exposure to the cat (especially cumulative exposure) may occur when the premises are treated.

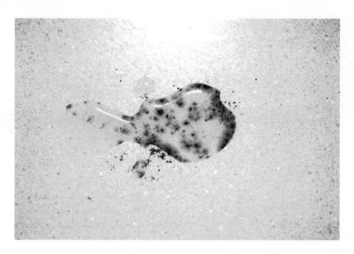

FIGURE 58.1. Fleas: "Flea dirt" is composed of digested blood. It is a sure sign that fleas are or have been present on the cat, and it can be differentiated from other material on the cat's skin by putting it in a drop of water. When wet, the material is resuspended, making a reddish-colored pool.

Prognosis

Successful flea control can be achieved safely with careful attention to the products used. Extensive client education is the key to a successful outcome.

Suggested Readings

Dryden MW. Biology of fleas of dogs and cats. *Compend Contin Educ Pract Vet* 1993; 15:569–579.

Merchant SR. The skin: parasitic diseases. In: Norsworthy GD, ed. Feline practice. Philadelphia: JB Lippincott, 1993;511–517.

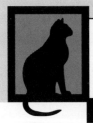

C H A P T E R   5 9

Flea-Allergic Dermatitis

Gary D. Norsworthy

Overview

The most common allergic skin disease of cats is due to type I and type IV hypersensitivity reactions and a cutaneous basophil hypersensitivity to allergens found in flea saliva. The reaction causes local edema, eosinophilia, and perivascular infiltration of lymphocytes and histiocytes. These produce clinical signs of pruritus, excessive licking, and scratching. Some cats are secretive in these activities, so many owners will deny their existence. Papular, crusty eruptions, known as miliary dermatitis, and varying amounts of alopecia often result. The pattern may be generalized, localized to the head and neck, localized to the caudal aspects of the rear legs, or localized to the tailhead region, as with the dog. However, the tailhead pattern is much less common in the cat than in the dog. Flea-allergy dermatitis is one of the causes of eosinophilic plaques and eosinophilic ulcers. In dogs, it has been observed that intermittent exposure to fleas is more likely to result in the allergic state than in dogs with constant flea exposure, and that any dog with enough exposure to fleas can become flea allergic. It is also known that dogs whose initial exposure to fleas occurs in the adult years are more likely to develop a flea allergy. These theories are unproved but suspected in the cat as well.

 D i a g n o s i s

Primary Diagnostics

- **Clinical signs:** The presence of pruritus, alopecia, and miliary dermatitis in cats with fleas or flea feces (flea dirt) should cause one to suspect flea-allergic dermatitis.
- **Hypersensitivity to flea antigen:** This test is specific for flea-allergic dermatitis. Intradermal testing using an aqueous flea antigen is recommended. It is important that a positive and negative control be used to validate the test results. A positive test results in erythema or induration, which may sometimes be subtle.

Ancillary Diagnostics

- **Response to steroids:** This is not a specific test because the same positive response may occur with atopy. However, it can be helpful in differentiating it from food-allergic dermatitis. Most cats with food-allergic dermatitis will have no response or very short response to steroids, although the gross skin lesions may be identical.

Diagnostic Notes

- This disease is very common in climates that are warm enough to support a year-round flea population.
- Positive flea antigen testing results in a skin reaction within 5 to 15 minutes. The intensity of the reaction is less severe than that seen in dogs. Delayed reactions are rare.

 T r e a t m e n t

Primary Therapeutics

- **Flea control:** Because the flea's eggs fall off of the cat and hatch off of the cat, successful treatment requires treatment of every aspect of the cat's environment, as well as the cat itself. Even though total flea control is not possible for outdoor cats in warm climates, every effort should be made to reduce flea exposure to a minimal level. Some of the newer monthly flea-control products have the ability to kill fleas before they bite the cat. These are effective in preventing the reaction.
- **Anti-inflammatory drugs:** Corticosteroids are the main drugs to block the allergic reaction. Short-term therapy is preferred, but long-term alternating day prednisolone (0.5–1.0 mg/kg PO) or injections of a long-acting corticosteroid (methylprednisolone, 20 mg/cat SC q2–6w) may be required in some climates and environmental situations.

Secondary Therapeutics

- If a flea-allergic cat can be completely removed from flea exposure, this disease will go into remission. This should be achievable in indoor-only cats. It is often not possible for outdoor cats, especially in warm, humid climates.
- See Chapter 58 for recommendations on flea control.

Therapeutic Notes

- There is not a direct correlation between the severity of the disease and the number of fleas present. Only a few fleas will produce marked pruritus when the allergic state is severe.

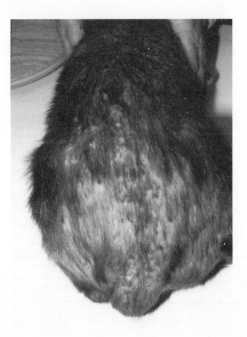

FIGURE 59.1. Flea-allergic dermatitis: A flea-allergic cat that is bitten by a flea experiences intense pruritus. Chewing and scratching may cause alopecia and scab formation.

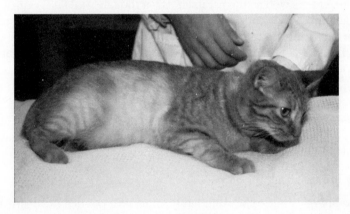

FIGURE 59.2. However, some flea-allergic cats respond by intense licking that removes substantial amounts of hair but creates minimal dermatitis.

- Hyposensitization is usually not successful in treating this disease in cats.
- Many flea-allergic cats also have atopy, which may produce the same clinical signs. Strict flea control alone will be ineffective in relieving clinical signs in these cats.
- Antihistamines and fatty-acid therapy have not been found very beneficial for cats with flea-allergy dermatitis.

P r o g n o s i s

This is not a fatal disease. However, the goal of therapy is to restore quality life to the cat. The prognosis for doing so is good with either good flea control or the use of corticosteroids.

S u g g e s t e d   R e a d i n g s

Merchant SR. The skin: hypersensitivity diseases. In: Norsworthy GD, ed. Feline practice. Philadelphia: JB Lippincott, 1993;518–525.

Moriello KA. Diseases of the skin. In: Sherding RG, ed. The cat: diseases and clinical management, 2nd ed. Philadelphia: WB Saunders, 1994;1907–1968.

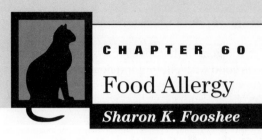

CHAPTER 60

Food Allergy

Sharon K. Fooshee

Overview

Food hypersensitivity, or food allergy, is an adverse reaction to a component of the diet; protein is the most consistent offender. The reaction is immune-mediated and usually manifests as a dermatologic disorder. Food allergy has a fairly classic presentation but can sometimes be confused with other dermatologic conditions. Diagnosis is relatively easy with strict adherence to specific dietary recommendations.

 Diagnosis

Primary Diagnostics

- **Clinical signs:** Feline food allergy most commonly presents as alopecia and severe nonseasonal pruritus of the face and neck; classic miliary lesions may be present. Some cats will self-mutilate, leading to ulcerative lesions. Occasionally, generalized pruritus may be found. Otitis externa is also reported.

- **Food trial:** Elimination diet testing remains the only reliable method for confirming food allergy in the cat. Some improvement is noted in most cats after 6 weeks of a food trial. The diagnosis can be confirmed with provocative testing. Distilled water is preferred during the food trial.

Ancillary Diagnostics

- **Other tests:** Skin scraping and fungal culture should be performed to eliminate ectoparasites and dermatophytosis as the cause of pruritus. Intradermal testing with flea antigen may identify coexistent flea allergy.

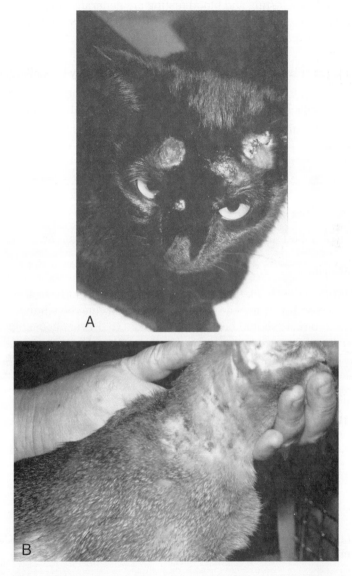

FIGURE 60.1. Food allergy: Intense pruritus on the head (*A*) and neck (*B*) is the characteristic finding in food-allergic cats. The resulting scratching causes alopecia and dermatitis in these locations.

Diagnostic Notes

- Intradermal skin testing and blood testing are generally considered unreliable for diagnosis of food allergy. With these tests, a cat may have a positive reaction to foods it has never eaten.
- Many lamb-based commercial diets contain potentially allergenic substances, including other sources of protein. Lamb is not inherently hypoallergenic.
- Most cats with food allergy are poorly responsive or nonresponsive to corticosteroids. Lack of response should raise one's index of suspicion.
- Atopy and flea allergy frequently coexist with food allergy.

 ## T r e a t m e n t

Primary Therapeutics

Avoidance of the offending food is the only effective treatment.

Therapeutic Notes

- In a multicat household, the food-allergic cat should not have access to the other pets' food. This may necessitate feeding all cats the elimination diet. Also, outdoor cats should be confined indoors to prevent consumption of potentially allergenic prey or cat foods at neighbors' houses.
- Some cats will eventually become allergic to the new protein source.

P r o g n o s i s

The prognosis is good as long as the offending allergen can be avoided.

S u g g e s t e d   R e a d i n g

MacDonald JM. Food allergy. In: Griffin CE, Kwochka KW, MacDonald JM, eds. Current veterinary dermatology. St. Louis: Mosby Yearbook, 1993;121–132.

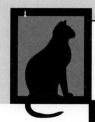

CHAPTER 61

Giardiasis

Mitchell A. Crystal

Overview

G *iardia* is a small intestinal and occasionally large intestinal protozoan parasite that causes acute and/or chronic diarrhea and occasionally malabsorption. *Giardia* exists in two forms: a) a cyst form, which is shed in the feces, can survive for months in the environment, and is infective to other animals, and b) a trophozoite form that develops in the small intestine from ingested cysts and causes clinical signs. *Giardia* is acquired via ingestion of infected feces or contaminated food or water. There is no extra-intestinal migration, and transplacental and transmammary infections do not occur. Once ingested, *Giardia* cysts may be shed in the feces 5 to 16 days later. Clinical signs include small intestinal diarrhea, occasionally large or mixed intestinal diarrhea, steatorrhea, borborygmus, and weight loss. Rarely, an infection is severe and causes dehydration, lethargy, and anorexia. Infection may also be asymptomatic. Physical examination may be normal or reveal evidence of diarrhea and weight loss. Rarely, dehydration may be detected.

Giardia may also accompany other intestinal diseases; in this case, clinical signs will reflect the underlying disease process. *Giardia* is considered of zoonotic importance, and appropriate handling of feces should be discussed with owners. Immunocompromised individuals should avoid contact with infected animals.

 D i a g n o s i s

Primary Diagnostics

- **Zinc sulfate fecal flotation:** Cysts may be seen on microscopic examination.
- **Direct saline smear:** Cysts and/or trophozoites are sometimes seen on microscopic examination.

Ancillary Diagnostics

- **Fecal ELISA for *Giardia*-specific antigens:** This test is still in the evaluation stage. It appears to be reasonably sensitive and specific.

- **Duodenal aspiration via endoscopy or during exploratory laparotomy:** Instill 10 mL of saline into the duodenum via a polypropylene tube passed through the biopsy channel (at endoscopy) or via needle and syringe (at exploratory laparotomy) and aspirate material back for immediate microscopic examination for motile trophozoites.
- **Response to fenbendazole:** When other tests are inconclusive or not feasible, this can be utilized.

Diagnostic Notes

- Flotation in saturated sugar solutions will cause distortion of cysts, making them unrecognizable.
- Performing zinc sulfate fecal flotation on three different fecal samples will maximize the chances of finding *Giardia* cysts in an infected cat.
- Trophozoites seen on direct smear or duodenal aspiration have a concave ventral surface and rapid, nonrolling motility. Trichomonads are the only other motile protozoan similar in size to *Giardia* and are nonpathogenic. Trichomonads lack a concave surface and demonstrate rolling motility.
- Cats with *Giardia* should be screened for FeLV and FIV.

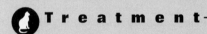 **T r e a t m e n t**

Primary Therapeutics

- **Fenbendazole:** Administer 25 mg/kg SID PO for 3 days.

Secondary Therapeutics

- **Metronidazole:** Administer 25 mg/kg BID PO for 5 days.
- **Albendazole:** Administer 25 mg/kg BID PO for 2 days.

Therapeutic Notes

- Infections may be self-limiting and thus may not require therapy.
- Cysts in the environment are susceptible to drying and most disinfectant solutions.

P r o g n o s i s

The prognosis is excellent for cure, although cysts may persist in the environment and lead to reinfection. This may be a problem in outdoor cats. Occasionally, infections are difficult to clear and may need prolonged therapy. *Giardia* infections associated with underlying immunosuppressive diseases (FeLV and FIV) may be more difficult to eliminate.

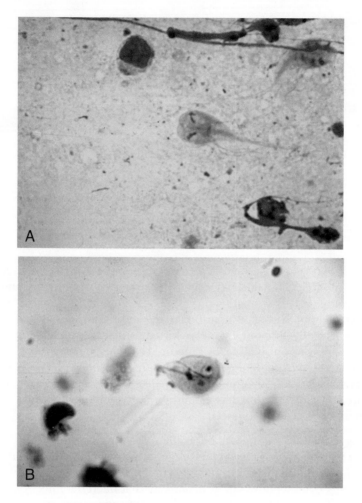

FIGURE 61.1. Giardiasis: Trophozoites can be found on direct saline smears. They have a characteristic face-like appearance (A, B).

Suggested Reading

Leib MS, Zajac AM. *Giardia:* diagnosis and treatment. In: Bonagura JD, ed. Kirk's current veterinary therapy XII small animal practice. Philadelphia: WB Saunders, 1995;716–720.

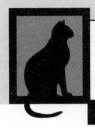

CHAPTER 62

Gingivitis/Stomatitis/Pharyngitis

Mitchell A. Crystal

Overview

Feline gingivitis-stomatitis-pharyngitis complex (GSPC), also known as lymphocytic-plasmacytic gingivitis-stomatitis-pharyngitis and plasma cell gingivitis-stomatitis-pharyngitis, is a common disease causing inflammation, ulceration, and proliferation of the soft tissues of the mouth. Middle-aged cats are usually affected; 1 study reported median age of affected cats as 7.1 years and age range from 4–17 years. Pure-bred cats may be over-represented. The area of the mouth most commonly affected is the glossopalatine arches. The gingiva, pharynx, soft palate, lips, and tongue are less commonly affected. The lesions present are associated with a dense infiltration of lymphocytes and plasma cells into the oral mucosa and submucosa.

The etiology of GSPC is unknown but is felt to be multifactoral with an immune-mediated component, possibly representing a hypersensitivity to oral bacterial antigens. *Bacteroides* spp. are commonly cultured from the oral cavity in association with this disease; however, it is unlikely that bacterial infection is the primary cause, as antibiotic therapy does not eliminate the disease and immunomodulating therapy is often helpful in improving lesions. Dental disease is also a likely contributing factor to GSPC, although many cats with GSPC do not have significant periodontal changes, and most cats with GSPC and concurrent periodontal disease do not respond to dental therapy alone.

Clinical signs of GSPC vary depending on the severity of the lesions. Cats may demonstrate no clinical signs; the disease is noted incidentally at the time of physical examination. Clinical abnormalities present may include ptyalism, halitosis, pain on opening of the mouth, difficulty prehending food, change in food preference from a dry to a soft diet, anorexia, and weight loss. Physical examination reveals the lesions of GSPC and may reveal submandibular lymphadenopathy. Differential diagnoses for GSPC include periodontal disease, retroviral infection, Calicivirus infection, eosinophilic granuloma complex, neoplasia, and systemic diseases such as renal failure and disorders leading to protein-calorie malnutrition or a predisposition to infection (e.g., diabetes mellitus).

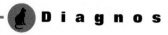

Diagnosis

Primary Diagnostics

- **Oral biopsy/histopathology:** This reveals a dense infiltration of lymphocytes and plasma cells into the oral mucosa and submucosa, although some lesions appear as predominantly plasmacytic. Some neutrophils and eosinophils may be present.

- **FeLV/FIV test:** Retroviral infections can lead to inflammatory oral disease. Approximately 15–20% of GSPC cats test positive for FeLV. Cats with GSPC that test positive for FIV vary in reports from 25–80%.

- **Chemistry profile and urinalysis:** Hyperproteinemia due to hyperglobulinemia is seen in about half of the cats with GSPC. The presence of azotemia with a low urine specific gravity suggests renal failure as a cause.

Ancillary Diagnostics

- **CBC:** This may reveal evidence of systemic disease.

Diagnostic Notes

It is important to exclude systemic diseases as a cause or contributing factor in GSPC.

Treatment

Primary Therapeutics

- **Dental therapy:** Cats with periodontal disease should have their teeth cleaned frequently, as periodontal disease may cause or contribute to GSPC.

- **Antibiotics:** Effective antibiotics include amoxicillin (22 mg/kg PO BID), amoxicillin/clavulanic acid (22 mg/kg PO BID), and metronidazole (10–20 mg/kg PO BID).

- **Corticosteroids:** These are beneficial in 70–80% of the cases treated. Begin prednisone at 1–2 mg/kg PO BID, then gradually, over 4–6 months, taper its use to the lowest effective dose. Indefinite therapy is often required. If oral therapy is difficult, methylprednisolone acetate may be used at 2–5 mg/kg IM, SQ every 2 weeks until a significant response is seen, then every 6–8 weeks.

Secondary Therapeutics

- **Aurothioglucose (gold salts, chrysotherapy):** This is beneficial in 75% of the patients treated. Dose at 1 mg/kg IM every 7 days for 16–20 weeks until a response is seen. A response is seen on the average in 8 weeks. Then, reduce the dose to every 14 days for 2 months, then monthly for 8 months. Therapy should be discontinued at that time. Side effects of therapy are uncommon but include thrombocytopenia, pancytopenia, and renal failure. CBC, chemistry profile, and urinalysis should be performed monthly while the cat is on therapy.

- **Alpha interferon:** Many anecdotal reports of improvement exist. Dose at 30 IU PO SID (see Table 55.5).
- **Other immunosuppressive drugs:** Use azathioprine at 0.3 mg/kg PO QOD until a response is seen, thereafter every 3 days; chlorambucil at 0.1–0.2 mg/kg PO SID until a response is seen, then QOD; or cyclophosphamide at 50 mg/m^2 PO 4 days on, followed by 3 days off, may be attempted if the above measures are unsuccessful.
- **Teeth extractions:** This should be considered when other modalities fail. It has been effective in some cats when lesions are adjacent to or associated with teeth with dental disease.

Therapeutic Notes

- Antibiotic therapy alone has provided only temporary improvement in a low percentage of cats.
- Aurothioglucose can be used in combination with glucocorticoids and antibiotics to help achieve a faster response.
- Megestrol acetate has proven beneficial in cases of GSPC; however, side effects (diabetes mellitus) warrant its use only after other therapies have failed. The dose is 1 mg/kg PO QOD until a response is seen, then change to prednisone for maintenance. Megestrol acetate can be reinstituted for short periods when relapse occurs.

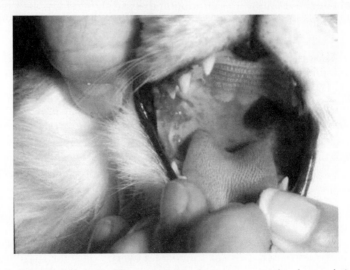

Figure 62.1. Gingivitis/stomatitis: The most obvious lesions occur at the glossopalatine arches.

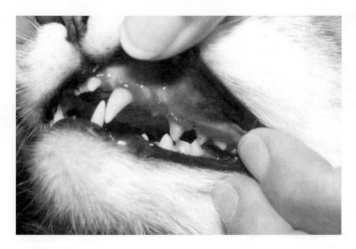

Figure 62.2. Many cats also have lesions at the margin where the gingiva contacts the teeth.

Prognosis

Cats with GSPC will rarely achieve total resolution of the lesions. Response to therapy is poor, and relapses are common. The goal of therapy should be the best possible control of clinical signs.

Suggested Readings

Diehl K, Rosychuk RAW. Feline gingivitis-stomatitis-pharyngitis. In: Hoskins JD, Loar AS, eds. *Vet Clin North Am:* Small animal practice. Philadelphia: WB Saunders, 1993;23(1): 139–153.

White SD, Rosychuk RAW, Janik TA, Denerolle P, Schultheiss P. Plasma cell stomatitis in cats: 40 cases (1973–1991). *J Am Vet Med Assoc* 1992;200(9):1377–1380.

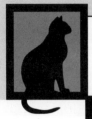

CHAPTER 63

Glomerulonephritis

Gary D. Norsworthy

Overview

Glomerulonephritis is an immune-mediated glomerular disease. Although it may occur in some species due to antibodies reacting to antigens within the glomeruli, the only form documented in the cat is due to circulating immune complexes being filtered out by the glomeruli. The clinically significant causes of these antigen- antibody complexes are diseases due to the feline leukemia virus (FeLV), the feline immunodeficiency virus (FIV), or the feline infectious peritonitis virus (FIPV); chronic progressive polyarthritis; lupus; pancreatitis; and incompatible insulin (usually of human origin). Most cases begin long before clinical presentation, and the etiologic agent is not present at the time of presentation, so diagnosis is not possible; thus, they are classified as idiopathic. Affected cats, which are usually young adult males, have two clinical forms of the disease. The first is the nephrotic syndrome. These cats often develop extensive subcutaneous edema and ascites but are otherwise reasonably healthy. They often have mild weight loss and a depressed appetite. The second form is renal failure. These cats have more pronounced weight loss and appetite depression, polyuria, and polydipsia, and they may be vomiting. Cats with both forms of glomerulonephritis have small, firm kidneys. The nephrotic syndrome is thought to represent an early stage of the disease, and the renal-failure form is believed to be the latter stage.

 D i a g n o s i s

Primary Diagnostics

- **Clinical signs:** Signs of the nephrotic syndrome are typical of the first form of this disease. Signs of renal failure occur in the second form but do not differ from renal failure due to other causes. If polyarthritis is the cause of the disease, multiple joints will be swollen and painful.
- **CBC/Chemistry profile:** The common findings are proteinuria, hypoalbuminemia, hypercholesterolemia, and nonregenerative anemia. Azotemia

occurs as the disease causes renal failure. The urine protein:creatinine ratio is greater than 1.0, which is consistent with glomerular disease.

Ancillary Diagnostics for Underlying Disease

- **Feline viral testing:** These cats should be tested for the FeLV, FIV, and feline coronavirus (FCoV).
- **Serum insulin level:** If the cat is receiving exogenous insulin, insulin injections should be discontinued for 24 hours. A serum-insulin level at that time will be four-fold or more elevated above normal if incompatibility is present.
- **Serum TLI:** The feline-specific form of this test is the most reliable for pancreatitis in the cat.*

Diagnostic Notes

Because glomerulonephritis is often due to an underlying disease, it is important to perform a thorough diagnostic workup.

 T r e a t m e n t

Primary Therapeutics: Nephrotic Syndrome without Azotemia

- **Furosemide:** This drug is to reduce edema and ascites. It is dosed at 2–4 mg/kg/day.
- **Corticosteroids:** An anti-inflammatory dose of prednisolone (2–4 mg/kg/day) may be tried. Some cats respond well and others not at all. If it is successful, it should be continued until the underlying disease is cured. After 2–3 weeks of therapy, a reduced, alternating day schedule should be used for long-term therapy.
- **Diet:** Due to the protein loss occurring, a dietary level of protein should be fed to maintain normal body weight and serum albumin levels. A low-salt diet should be fed to minimize fluid retention.
- **Hypotensive agent:** Amlodipine (0.625 mg SID/cat initially, then adjusted to response) is indicated if hypertension is present.

Primary Therapeutics: Azotemia

- **Fluid therapy, potassium supplementation, etc:** See Chapter 37.

Secondary Therapeutics: Underlying Diseases

See appropriate chapters under Part 2.

---

*This test can be performed by Dr. David A. Williams, College of Veterinary Medicine, Texas A&M University, College Station, TX 77843; phone: 409-862-2861, fax: 409-862-2864.

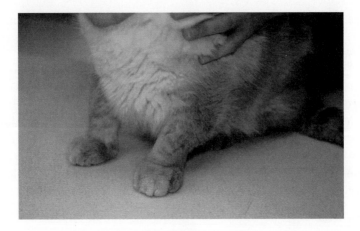

Figure 63.1. Glomerulonephritis: Cats with the nephrotic syndrome present with pitting edema in the extremities.

Therapeutic Notes

Azotemic cats should not receive salt supplementation, furosemide, or corticosteroids.

Prognosis

The prognosis depends on the form of glomerulonephritis, the stage of diagnosis, and the underlying disease. Nonazotemic cats with the nephrotic syndrome diagnosed early can often be managed for months or years, especially if an underlying disease can be cured. Cats in end-stage renal failure have a poor prognosis.

Suggested Reading

DiBartola SP, Rutgers HC. Diseases of the kidney. In: Sherding RG, ed. The cat: diseases and clinical management, 2nd ed. Philadelphia: WB Saunders, 1994;1711–1767.

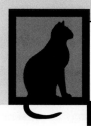

Heartworm Disease

John-Karl Goodwin

Overview

Heartworm disease has been increasingly recognized as an important cardiovascular disease of the cat, particularly in endemic areas where prevalence rates as high as 12% have been reported. In general, the incidence of feline heartworm disease parallels that of canine heartworm disease.

Cats naturally infected with *Dirofilaria immitis* usually harbor an average of three to five adult worms within the heart and pulmonary arteries, with a range of 1 to 31 worms reported. Aberrant migration of *D. immitis* larvae to the brain (lateral ventricles) and skin occurs more commonly in the cat than in the dog.

The mean age of affected cats is between 3 and 6 years. Males may be predisposed to this disease. Although an important risk factor is exposure to infected mosquitoes, it has been determined that the rate of infection of indoor cats is equal to that of outdoor cats. Indeed, indoor cats may be at higher risk, as immune-mediated resistance to infection is lower.

Endarteritis lesions induced by adult heartworms are similar to those found in affected dogs. Larger pulmonary arteries, especially the right caudal lobar artery, are more severely affected with characteristic lesions including villous myointimal proliferation and muscular hypertrophy. The immune response to migrating larvae and adult heartworms tends to be greater in the cat than the dog.

Clinical signs vary greatly from none to severe cardiopulmonary or neurologic complications. The most commonly reported clinical signs include cough, dyspnea, weight loss, malaise, and chronic and sporadic vomiting.

Diagnosis

Primary Tests

- **CBC, chemistry profile:** Typical findings include eosinophilia (transient), basophilia (transient), and hyperglobulinemia.

- **Radiography:** A mixed bronchointerstitial pattern is consistently present. Generalized cardiomegaly and enlargement of the cranial and caudal lobar pulmonary arteries are also fairly consistent. Other abnormalities may include pleural effusion and pulmonary hyperinflation.
- **Serologic testing:** Antigenemia can be detected in approximately 30% of infected cases using commercial test kits. Antibodies against *D. immitis* are present in approximately 95% of affected cats, but also may be present in cats that have cleared previous infections.

Ancillary Diagnostics

- **Modified Knott's test:** It is unusual to find circulating microfilaria in affected cats.
- **Echocardiography:** Adult heartworms may be visualized as short, hyperechoic bilinear objects within the right heart and/or main pulmonary artery.
- **Angiography:** Nonselective angiography may be used to visualize adult heartworms, which appear as linear filling defects within the pulmonary arteries and blunted or tortuous pulmonary arteries.

Diagnostic Notes

- Most cases are presented in the fall and winter.
- Radiographic and transtracheal cytologic features of heartworm disease may be very similar to feline asthma.
- Heska Corporation (Fort Collins, CO, Ph: 1–800-464–3752) and Animal Diagnostics (St. Louis, MO, Ph: 314–647-3348) offer heartworm antibody and antigen testing.

 T r e a t m e n t

Primary Therapeutics

- **Prednisone:** Give 1–2 mg/kg/day to reducing clinical signs and controlling pneumonitis.
- **Furosemide:** Give 1–2 mg/kg BID PO to control pleural effusion.

Secondary Therapeutics

- **Diltiazem:** Give 1–2 mg/kg TID to reduce clinical signs and pulmonary hypertension.
- **Oxygen:** This is used to manage acute cardiopulmonary collapse, if present.
- **Ivermectin:** Give 50 µcg/kg PO or SC as a microfilaricide, if needed.

- **Thiacetarsamide:** Give 2.2 mg/kg IV BID for 2 days; there is a significant risk of toxicity and acute thromboembolism with adulticide therapy in the cat. Some advocate pretreatment with diphenhydramine prior to thiacetarsamide administration; others discourage its use completely.

Therapeutic Notes

- Adulticide therapy should be reversed for cats exhibiting significant clinical signs. In cats with no or mild clinical signs, supportive care rather than adulticide therapy is indicated.
- Preventative: Ivermectin (24 µcg/kg) and milbemycin (500 µcg/kg) once monthly have been used.
- There is an increased interest in the use of heartworm prevention in cats due to a) unknown incidence; b) difficulty in diagnosis; c) difficulty in treatment; d) sudden death occurring in some cats; and e) lack of toxicity for monthly prevention products.

P r o g n o s i s

The prognosis of affected cats is dependent upon the severity of disease. Mildly affected cats are expected to naturally clear infection within 1-1/2 years and to respond well with supportive therapy during this time frame. Prognosis is guarded to poor in cats with significant cardiovascular or cerebral signs.

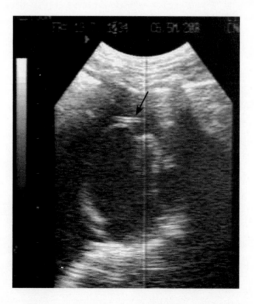

FIGURE 64.1. Heartworm disease: Heartworms can often be visualized with ultrasound as two parallel lines.

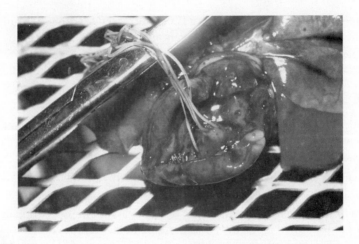

FIGURE 64.2. Heartworms are often in small numbers, i.e., one to two per cat, but this cat had 15 adults at the time of acute death due to embolization of the main pulmonary arteries.

Suggested Readings

Atkins C, De Francesco T, Miller M, Meyers K, Keene B. Prevalence of heartworm infection in cats with cardiorespiratory abnormalities. (In Press, 1997.)

McCall JW, Calvert CA, Rawlings CA. Heartworm infection in cats: a life-threatening disease. *Vet Med J* 1994;89:639–647.

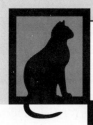

Helicobacter

Mitchell A. Crystal

Overview

*H*elicobacter spp. are spiral-shaped bacteria that inhabit the stomach and have the potential to cause gastritis, gastric ulcer disease, and gastric neoplasia both in humans and animals. There are many different types of *Helicobacter* organisms, each having various unique characteristics. The organisms considered to be potential pathogens at this time are listed in Table 65.1 along with their host species. It is felt that *Helicobacter* organisms can survive in the acidic environment of the stomach by residing within and below the gastric mucus layer. They also break down urea into ammonia and bicarbonate and thus create a less acidic microenvironment that is more conducive to survival. There is much debate on the pathogenicity of these organisms in both humans and animals. Infections may be asymptomatic or may have mild clinical signs, signs of nonulcer gastritis, or signs of ulcer disease. There is also information in the human literature suggesting that infection may predispose to gastric carcinoma or gastric lymphoma. Clinical findings may include chronic vomiting, weight loss, abdominal pain, anorexia, and

TABLE 65.1.

Helicobacter Organisms Currently Considered to Be Potential Pathogens

Organism	wHost
Helicobacter pylori	Human, cat
Helicobacter felis	Cat, dog
Helicobacter acinonyx	Cheetah
Helicobacter mustelae	Ferret
Helicobacter heilmannii (formerly *Gastrospirillum* spp.)	Human, cat, dog, cheetah, pig

borborygmus. It is unknown whether animals transmit infection to people or other animals (and vice versa). Many *Helicobacter* species seem to colonize a specific host, suggesting that transmission between people and animals or between animals and other animals is unlikely. Also, studies suggest that humans acquire *H. pylori* at an early age and have a lifelong infection rather than transmitting the organism from adult to adult. Nevertheless, there is currently not enough information to determine if *Helicobacter* is a zoonotic threat. Differential diagnoses for *Helicobacter* gastritis include those of chronic vomiting (see Chapter 23).

 D i a g n o s i s

Primary Tests

- **Gastric biopsy and histopathology:** Histopathologic evaluation of mucosal (endoscopic) or full thickness (laparotomy) biopsies can detect spiral-shaped bacteria, although a special silver stain (Warthin-Starry) is needed to see smaller *Helicobacter* organisms (hematoxylin-eosin stains often reveal *H. heilmannii* but not other *Helicobacter* species).

Ancillary Tests

- **Urea test (campylobacter-like organism [CLO] test** [Delta West PTY LTD, Perth, Australia; distributed in the United States by Tri-Med Specialists Inc., Overland Park, KS]**) on gastric biopsies:** The test media is an agar that contains urea, sodium azide (a preservative to help prevent positive reactions due to growth of urease-positive contaminates), and phenol red (an indicator that is yellow at a low pH and changes to a red color as the pH increases). The agar assay is inspected visually for 8 hours, then intermittently for another 16 hours. A positive test result occurs if the media changes from yellow to a deep pink; this often occurs within minutes of adding the tissue sample. The rapidity of the change in color estimates the number of organisms that are present.

Diagnostic Notes

Because spiral bacteria are present in normal animals, exclusion of all other diagnoses and confirmation of typical pathologic changes in addition to the organism are necessary before a diagnosis of *Helicobacter* gastritis can be made.

Endoscopic *Helicobacter* lesions may have a wide variety of appearances, including diffuse rugal thickening, mucosal flattening, punctate hemorrhages, erosions, and crateriform ulcers. The body and fundus are often more severely affected than the pyloric antrum. Some cats will have a normal endoscopic examination.

Culture is a very insensitive and difficult-to-perform procedure for the diagnosis of *Helicobacter* spp. The organisms require special handling (20% glucose- or phosphate-buffered saline (PBS) solution kept at 4°C until inoculation), special media (*Brucella* agar with 10% blood, vancomycin, and polymyxin), and a special growing environment (microaerophilic). *Helicobacter* in general has a low culture rate, and *H. heilmannii* has never been successfully cultured on artificial media.

Serologic assays for IgG are effective in the diagnosis of *H. pylori* in humans and *H. mustelae* in ferrets, but at this time they are unreliable for use in cats.

 T r e a t m e n t

Primary Therapeutics

- **Triple Therapy:** Give bismuth subsalicylate or bismuth subcitrate 5 mg/kg TID PO, amoxicillin 20 mg/kg TID PO (or tetracycline 20 mg/kg QID PO), and metronidazole 12.5 mg/kg BID PO.

Secondary Therapeutics

Decreasing the gastric pH with proton pump blockers (omeprazole: 0.7 mg/kg SID PO) or H_2-receptor antagonists (ranitidine: 1.0 mg/kg BID PO; cimetidine: 10 mg/kg TID PO; or famotidine 0.5 mg/kg SID PO) may improve antibiotic efficacy.

Therapeutic Notes

- The pathogenicity of *Helicobacter* has not been firmly established in animals (except for the ferret and cheetah). Positive CLO tests have been documented, and gastric spiral bacteria have been seen in gastric biopsy samples in both normal animals and in animals with clinical signs which might be referable to *Helicobacter* infection. Therefore, recommendations for when and if to treat remain uncertain until further information is gathered.
- Protocols effective in the treatment of *Helicobacter* spp. include two antibiotics (such as bismuth subsalicylate or bismuth subcitrate 5 mg/kg TID PO, amoxicillin 20 mg/kg TID PO, tetracycline 20 mg/kg QID PO, doxycycline 5 mg/kg BID PO, metronidazole 12.5 mg/kg BID PO, and/or azithromycin 5 mg/kg PO SID) along with an antacid (such as omeprazole 0.7 mg/kg SID PO, famotidine 0.5 mg/kg SID PO, ranitidine 1.0 mg/kg BID PO, or cimetidine 10 mg/kg TID PO).

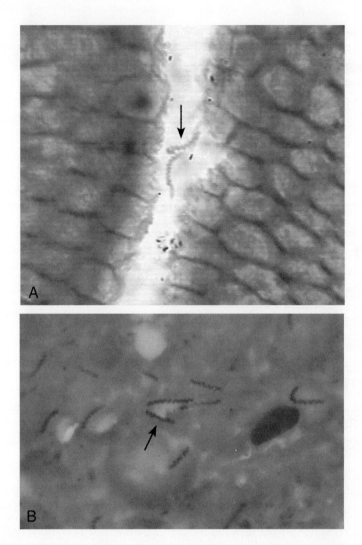

FIGURE 65.1. *Helicobacter* gastritis: The spiral-shaped organisms are seen in a biopsy specimen of the gastric mucosa (*A*) (H&E stain) and from an impression smear of vomitus (*B*) (modified Wright's stain).

Prognosis

Whereas therapy has proven successful in treatment of *Helicobacter* infection (negative testing and improvement of clinical signs), recurrence is a problem to some degree. It is not known whether recurrence is due to reinfection or to recrudescence.

Suggested Readings

DeNovo RC, Magne ML. Current concepts in the management of *Helicobacter*-associated gastritis. Proceedings of the Thirteenth Annual Veterinary Medical Forum, 1995;57–61.

Eaton KA. Gastric bacteria in dogs and cats. In: Burrows CF, ed. Veterinary previews. Princeton, NJ: Ralston Purina Co, 1995;2:3–6.

Fox JG. *Helicobacter*-associated gastric disease in ferrets, dogs, and cats. In: Bonagura JD, ed. Kirk's current veterinary therapy XII small animal practice. Philadelphia: WB Saunders, 1995;720–723.

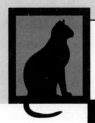

CHAPTER 66

Hemobartonellosis

Gary D. Norsworthy

Overview

Hemobartonellosis is also known as feline infectious anemia. It is caused by the parasite *Hemobartonella felis*, which attaches to the surface of mature red blood cells. When identified by the immune system as abnormal, affected cells are lysed in the spleen. It is believed that there is no breed or sex predilection; however, males seem to be over-represented in the affected populations, presumably due to lifestyle differences. Affected cats are generally presented for lethargy and anorexia of 1–2 days duration. Physical examination usually reveals pale and icteric mucus membranes, normal body temperature, tachypnea, and palpable splenic enlargement. Because of the acute onset, weight loss is generally not apparent. The mode of transmission is not fully understood but is suspected to be via any means of passing blood from one cat to another. Transfusions with infected blood have been shown to be effective in transmission, but blood-sucking parasites, such as mosquitoes and fleas, have not been conclusively shown to be adequate vectors.

 Diagnosis

Primary Tests

- **CBC:** packed cell volume (PCV), red blood cell (RBC) count, and hemoglobin (Hb) are below normal (anemia). A marked bone-marrow response is present as evidenced by polychromasia, anisocytosis, Howell-Jolly bodies. *H. felis* is present on RBCs and appears as small, blue-staining cocci, rings, or rods on RBCs.

- **Reticulocyte count:** It is substantially increased unless performed immediately after a precipitous fall in the hematocrit or if a bone marrow-suppressing disease is concurrent. It takes 4–6 days for the reticulocyte count to increase following RBC destruction.

Ancillary Diagnostics

- **Coombs' test:** This test usually is positive but does not represent true autoimmunity.
- **FeLV antigen test:** This test result is positive about 20% of the time. This is not directly related to the *H. felis* infection but probably represents a lifestyle that increases exposure to both pathogens and signals a poor long-term prognosis.
- **Chemistry profile:** The values are usually normal except for an elevation in total bilirubin.

Diagnostic Notes

- The presence of *H. felis* on RBCs is cyclic. Its presence coupled with a regenerative anemia is justification for a diagnosis of hemobartonellosis. Its presence in a nonanemic cat is probably incidental, because it is often found in a nonpathogenic state. The absence of *H. felis* in a cat with a regenerative anemia is not justification for dismissing this disease as a possibility; subsequent blood samples should be examined. There are few causes of regenerative anemia in cats.
- The presence of *H. felis* in a cat with a nonregenerative anemia can be confusing. *H. felis* results in RBC destruction but not bone marrow suppression. When a nonregenerative anemia exists, a cause of bone marrow disease should be sought. Bone marrow aspiration or biopsy is indicated.
- *H. felis* is a commonly found organism in many asymptomatic cats. It is thought that this disease may occur secondary to another stress-producing disease or event. Look for an underlying cause.
- The *H. felis* organism will detach from the RBC surface with prolonged exposure to EDTA in purple top tubes. It is best to submit fresh blood smears made at the time of blood collection.
- Precipitated blood stain may be confused with *H. felis*.

 T r e a t m e n t

Primary Therapeutics

- **Cage confinement:** Minimizing stress is important in anemic cats.
- **Whole blood transfusion:** This should be employed for cats with PCVs less than 15%.
- **Doxycycline:** Give 4 mg/kg initially, then 2 mg/kg 12 hours later, then 2 mg/kg q24h PO.
- **Prednisolone:** Give 1–2 mg/kg BID or TID PO to reduce hemolysis, stimulate the bone marrow, and increase appetite.

- **IV glucose:** Moribund cats may be severely hypoglycemic and need IV glucose.
- **Nutritional support:** Following blood transfusion, the cat should be supported nutritionally via orogastric or nasogastric tube feeding.

Secondary Therapeutics

The following drugs have been used in place of doxycycline.

- **Enrofloxacin:** A dose of 2 mg/kg BID PO has been reported to be effective against *H. felis*.
- **Chloramphenicol:** A dose of 15 mg/kg PO BID is effective.
- **Thiacetarsamide:** A dose of 1 mg/kg is given IV once each on days 1 and 3.

Therapeutic Notes

- The PCV of treated cats should be rechecked every other day and should show a steady increase.
- Doxycycline induces fever in some cats. Chloramphenicol may cause appetite depression, lethargy, and erythroid hypoplasia. Thiacetarsamide has been associated with acute pulmonary failure.
- All of these drugs are inconsistent in their ability to free the cat of the organism. A carrier state generally exists following successful treatment, although relapse seldom occurs.

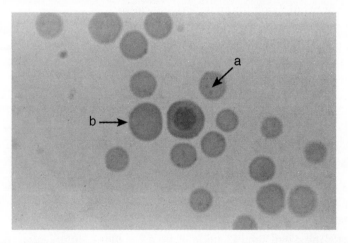

FIGURE 66.1. Hemobartonellosis: A confirmed diagnosis of hemobartonellosis requires that the cat be anemic, have the organism on its erythrocytes (a), and have a regenerative anemia. The presence of early red blood cells, especially macrocytes (or reticulocytes) (b), indicates that the bone marrow is responding.

Prognosis

The prognosis of hemobartonellosis is generally good if the anemic crisis can be quickly averted, but some cats develop fatal anemias due to very low PCVs. The carrier state that often occurs leaves the cat susceptible to recurrence. This cat should not be used as a blood donor, but otherwise it is considered noncontagious to other cats, even in the carrier state. There is no evidence that dogs are affected by *H. felis*.

Suggested Readings

Harvey JW. Haemobartonellosis. In: Green CE, ed. Infectious diseases of the dog and cat. Philadelphia: WB Saunders, 1990;434–442.

Norsworthy GD. Hemobartonellosis. In: Norsworthy GD, ed. Feline practice. Philadelphia: JB Lippincott, 1993;389–391.

Van Steenhouse JL, Tabada J, Millard JT. Feline hemobartonellosis. *Compend Contin Educ Pract Vet* 1993;15(4):535–541.

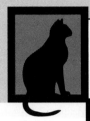

CHAPTER 67

Hepatic Lipidosis

Gary D. Norsworthy

Overview

H epatic lipidosis, also called fatty liver syndrome, is the most common liver disorder of cats in North America. (It is not commonly reported elsewhere.) It is characterized by an accumulation of triglycerides or neutral lipid within the liver and is associated with prolonged anorexia. Obesity is a predisposing factor. It may be a primary, idiopathic disease or secondary to other diseases that cause anorexia. The most commonly reported primary diseases are cholangiohepatitis, biliary obstruction and inflammation, and intrahepatic or extrahepatic neoplasia. The most common clinical signs are anorexia, weight loss, icterus, and vomiting.

Diagnosis

Primary Diagnostics

- **History and clinical signs:** An icteric, obese cat that has been anorectic for at least 1 week should be suspected of having hepatic lipidosis.
- **Chemistry profile:** The most consistent biochemical finding is a 2–5-fold increase in alkaline phosphatase accompanied by a normal or minimally increased (γ-glutamyltransferase (GGT or GGTP).
- **Cellular level study:** Confirmation requires a study of hepatic tissue. Copious amounts of intracellular and extracellular lipid will be seen. Hepatic tissue may be collected by fine-needle aspirate, fine-needle biopsy, cone-needle biopsy, or wedge biopsy.

Ancillary Diagnostics

- **Chemistry profile:** Other common biochemical findings include increased serum, ALT, AST, fasting and postprandial bile acids and bilirubin, bilirubinuria, and a mild nonregenerative anemia.

- **Radiography:** Radiographs may reveal hepatomegaly, but this is inconsistent.
- **Ultrasound:** Ultrasound may reveal a diffusely hyperechoic liver.

 T r e a t m e n t

Primary Therapeutics: Phase I—Stabilization (Up to 7 days)

- **Fluids:** Rehydrate with nonlactated fluids. Normal saline is the fluid of choice.
- **Potassium:** Add 20–40 mEq to each liter of fluids but do not exceed administration of 0.5 mEq/kg/hr. Oral potassium may also be given (2–4 mEq/day/cat).
- **Nutritional support:** Administer a balanced diet via orogastric tube beginning with 20–30 mL TID and adding 10–15 mL to each feeding on each subsequent day until 50–65 mL TID is given.
- **Antibiotics:** Amoxicillin (10 mg/kg BID) or metronidazole (10–15 mg/kg BID) should be given due to the incidence of suppurative cholangiohepatitis that causes anorexia and induces this disease.

Secondary Therapeutics: Phase II—Long-term Care (4–8 weeks)

- **Food:** Feed a balanced diet with the same nutritional goals as above. Feed in small quantities 4–6 times per day. An indwelling feeding tube, such as an esophagostomy or a gastrostomy tube, is needed.

Therapeutic Notes

- The goal of nutritional support is 60–80 kcal/kg and 3–4 g/kg of protein per day supplied by a balanced feline diet.
- The author's preferred diet is composed of:

  Three 5.5-oz. cans of CNM-CV (Ralston Purina, St. Louis, MO)

  8 oz. of water

  2 oz. of vegetable oil (Wesson Oil, Hunt-Wesson, Inc., Fullerton, CA)

  16 mEq of potassium gluconate (Tumil-K, Daniel's Pharmaceuticals, St. Louis, MO)

The ingredients are blenderized. After refrigeration, the food is heated to body temperature in a microwave oven before feeding. The heated food should be mixed or shaken, as microwave ovens produce uneven heating.

- Vomiting should be controlled with reduced feeding volumes (with compensatory increased frequency) and famotidine (0.1 mg/kg BID PO).
- The end point of treatment is when the cat returns to normal eating. Do not remove the feeding tube until the cat has been eating well for at least 3 days.

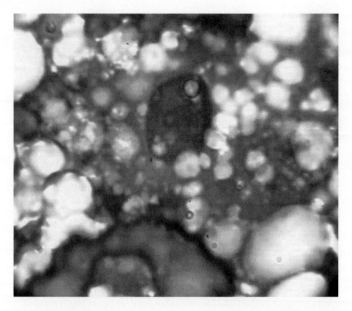

FIGURE 67.1. Hepatic lipidosis: The diagnosis is confirmed by finding intracellular and extracellular fat on a liver aspirate or biopsy.

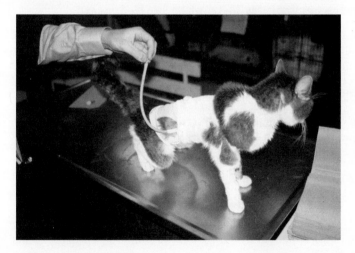

FIGURE 67.2. Because the average treatment time is about 6 weeks, it is necessary to place a feeding tube so that the cat can be treated at home. Gastrostomy tubes or esophagostomy tubes are effective tube-feeding methods.

- Various additives have been recommended, including taurine, arginine, carnitine, vitamin K, and thiamine. However, evidence of improved survivability is lacking when these products have been used.
- Appetite stimulants such as benzodiazepines are not indicated. Many require hepatic biotransformation and their appetite stimulating effects typically do not produce adequate food intake.

Prognosis

The commonly reported survival rate is 50–60%. However, the author's rate is greater than 90%. Almost all deaths occur during Phase I. Increased survival occurs if stress can be minimized during that time. This can be achieved if the diagnosis is made by fine-needle aspiration, the cat is fed with an orogastric tube, and anesthesia for feeding tube placement is delayed until the cat is stabilized. Recurrence is possible if prolonged anorexia recurs, but this seldom happens.

Suggested Reading

Day DG. Diseases of the liver. In: Sherding RG, ed. The cat: diseases and clinical management, 2nd ed. Philadelphia: WB Saunders, 1994;1297–1340.

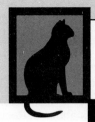

CHAPTER 68

High-Rise Syndrome

Mitchell A. Crystal

Overview

High-rise syndrome describes the collection of injuries sustained by any animal that falls from a substantial height, usually greater than or equal to two stories (about 12 feet/story). This syndrome is most common in younger cats living in urban areas. The term high-rise refers to the tall buildings from which these animals have fallen. About 90% of the cats affected by high-rise syndrome will survive. In a recent feline high-rise syndrome retrospective study, 3% were dead on arrival, 37% required life-sustaining treatment, 30% required nonemergency treatment, and 30% did not require treatment. Cats surviving 24 hours after falling rarely died from high-rise syndrome-related causes. The common injuries incurred in high-rise syndrome cats are listed in Table 68.1 with their approximate frequencies of occurrence.

There is a linear increase in injuries sustained from falling from distances up to about seven stories. Above this height, the number of injuries (especially fractures) either levels off or decreases. This is believed to occur because cats falling greater than seven stories have reached their terminal velocity of fall (due to body mass and drag, about 60 miles per hour), at which point the vestibular apparatus is no longer stimulated. Prior to reaching terminal velocity (less than seven stories), continued vestibular stimulation is believed to result in limb rigidity and failure to maximally prepare for a horizontal landing. The latter causes an uneven and smaller area of distribution of the force of impact which, along with rigid extremities, causes a greater number of injuries. After reaching maximum velocity (greater than seven stories), it is believed that cats assume a less rigid, more horizontal posture. These cats are more prepared for landing and have the force of impact evenly distributed throughout the body, preventing an increase, and in some cases causing a decrease, in the number of injuries.

TABLE 68.1.

Common Injuries Incurred In High-Rise Syndrome Cats and Their Approximate Frequencies of Occurrence

Injury	Approximate Occurrence
Thoracic trauma	90%
Pulmonary contusions	68%
Pneumothorax	63%
Wounds (face, extremity, or trunk)	56%
Extremity fractures	39%
Single	22%
Multiple	17%
Luxations (extremity, pelvic, or TMJ)	17%
Dental fractures	17%
Hard palate fractures	17%
Mandibular fractures	9%
Hematuria without bladder rupture	4%
Rib fractures	3%
Pelvic fractures	3%
Vertebral fractures	2%
Ruptured bladder	2%
Hemoabdomen	2%
Abdominal wall hernia	2%

 D i a g n o s i s

Primary Diagnostics

- **History:** Most cats involved in a high-rise fall are not observed falling, indicating the need to question the client as to the possibility of this occurrence.

- **Physical examination:** Examine for common injuries associated with high-rise syndrome.

- **Thoracocentesis (diagnostic and therapeutic):** Any cat with respiratory distress should undergo this procedure prior to thoracic radiographs to assess for pneumothorax and/or hemothorax.

- **Quick assessment tests (PCV, total protein, blood glucose, BUN, urine dipstick, and urine specific gravity):** These help to identify cats in shock and cats with blood loss or compromised urinary tracts.

Ancillary Diagnostics

- **Thoracic radiography:** This should be performed once the cat is stable to investigate for thoracic trauma.
- **Abdominal radiographs:** This should be performed if abdominal trauma/abdominal effusion is suspected.
- **Abdominocentesis:** This should be performed if abdominal trauma/abdominal effusion is suspected. Any fluid collected should be submitted for fluid analysis.

Diagnostic Notes

If the patient is dyspneic or stressed, thoracocentesis and oxygen administration should be performed prior to any diagnostics.

The PCV does not fall for several hours after blood loss. It should not be used to determine the presence of internal bleeding.

 T r e a t m e n t

Primary Therapeutics

- **Thoracocentesis (diagnostic and therapeutic):** This procedure should be performed in all high-rise syndrome cats with dyspnea.
- **Oxygen therapy:** This is indicated for cats with respiratory difficulty.

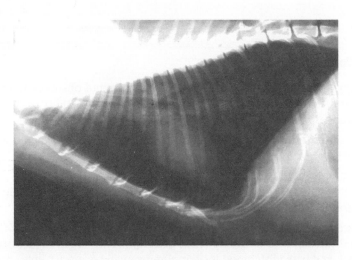

FIGURE 68.1. High-rise syndrome: Typical injuries that occur when cats fall from substantial heights include pneumothorax (shown here), abdominal organ fractures, fractures of the radius, ulna, tibia, and fibula, and facial injuries such as dental and hard palate fractures.

- **Fluid support:** Administer if needed for shock or dehydration. Prolonged fluid support may be needed if oral trauma is present.

Secondary Therapeutics

- **Fracture, wound, and other injury repair:** These should occur after the cat is stable.
- **Nutritional support:** This may be needed once the cat is stabilized if oral trauma is present. An esophagostomy or gastrostomy tube should be used.

Prognosis

The prognosis is good to excellent for recovery and long-term survival as long as initial emergency therapy is provided and successful.

Suggested Reading

Whitney WO, Mehlhaff CJ. High-rise syndrome in cats. *J Am Vet Med Assoc* 1987;191(11): 1399–1403.

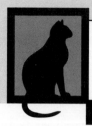

CHAPTER 69

Histoplasmosis

Sharon K. Fooshee

Overview

Cats appear fairly susceptible to infection with the dimorphic fungal organism *Histoplasma capsulatum;* however, most probably develop only a transient, clinically inapparent infection. In North America, the St. Lawrence, Missouri, and Mississippi River valleys and their related tributaries are areas of endemic infection. The organism is commonly associated with topsoil enriched by the nitrogen of bird and bat droppings. Most evidence supports a respiratory route of infection with hematogenous and lymphatic routes of dissemination, although primary gastrointestinal infection has been reported. Histoplasmosis is essentially a disease of the reticuloendothelial system. A competent cell-mediated immune response must be present to contain infection. Infection with the feline leukemia and feline immunodeficiency viruses does not appear to predispose cats to histoplasmosis. Humans are not at risk for the disease from contact with infected cats but may become infected because of similar environmental exposure.

 D i a g n o s i s

Primary Diagnostics

- **Clinical signs:** Diagnosis can be a challenge because the presenting complaints are vague: fever, weight loss, depression, and anorexia. Less than half of infected cats demonstrate organ-specific dysfunction. When signs are localizing, the respiratory system is commonly affected. Hepatosplenomegaly, dyspnea, subcutaneous nodules, lameness secondary to osteomyelitis, diarrhea, and inflammatory ocular disease have been reported.

- **Cytology:** Bone marrow and lymph node aspiration/cytology appear to be high-yield diagnostic procedures. Subcutaneous nodules or an enlarged liver should also be aspirated. Organisms may be found on peripheral blood smears, especially when 1000 white blood cells are examined (versus the normal 100 cells on a differential count) or when a buffy coat smear can be evaluated. The phagocytic cells (monocytes, neutrophils) should be closely examined for engulfed organisms. Bronchoalveolar lavage, rectal scraping, or colonic biopsy can also be considered when organ-specific involvement warrants these tests. A lung aspirate may be helpful, but it is a somewhat invasive procedure; as such, it should be performed only when clinical signs or radiographic findings warrant.

Ancillary Diagnostics

- **Radiography:** A fine, diffuse, or linear interstitial pattern in the lungs is common; the disease may also appear as a more prominent nodular pattern. When osteomyelitis is present, the lesions are most often osteolytic; concurrent osteoproduction may also be found.
- **CBC:** Nonregenerative anemia is common.
- **Serologic and intradermal skin testing:** These *are not* reliable indicators of infection. Although they are potentially useful adjunctive diagnostic tools, a diagnosis of histoplasmosis should not be based on serology alone. *Identification of the organism is essential for confirmation of a diagnosis.*

Diagnostic Notes

- The travel history should always be obtained for any sick cat.
- The organism does not always stain well with hematoxylin/eosin stain; as such, cytology using a modified Wright's stain may be a superior tool for organism identification.
- Indoor-only cats may contract histoplasmosis through potting soil.

T r e a t m e n t

Primary Therapeutics

- **Itraconazole**
  This is the antifungal drug of choice. It should be dosed at 5 mg/kg PO BID and given with a meal; an acid environment in the stomach enhances absorption of the drug. The capsule may be opened and the contents divided into gelatin capsules or mixed into canned food; however, the contents are not readily dissolved.

Therapeutic Notes

Itraconazole is better tolerated than ketoconazole by most cats. However, it is still recommended to periodically check serum chemistries. For cats with *clinical* evidence of hepatotoxicity (anorexia, jaundice), the drug should be

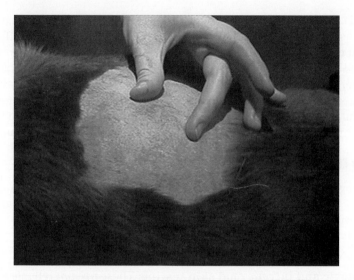

FIGURE 69.1. Histoplasmosis: Seemingly innocent lumps anywhere on the cat should be aspirated, because *Histoplasma capsulatum* can be the cause.

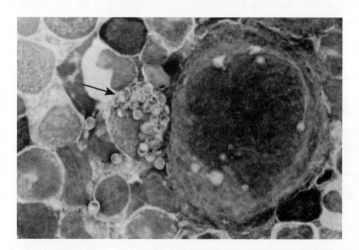

FIGURE 68.2. The organism is easily identified with a Wright's stain. These organisms were found on a bone marrow aspirate.

discontinued, at least temporarily. Asymptomatic cats with increased liver enzymes (ALT) do not necessarily need cessation of therapy but should be closely monitored.

These cats are frequently debilitated and anorectic. Placing of a feeding tube may be necessary until the cat's appetite returns.

Prognosis

In general, the prognosis for infected cats has improved with the introduction of itraconazole. However, severely debilitated cats with advanced systemic disease still have a guarded prognosis.

Suggested Readings

Clinkenbeard KD, Cowell RL, Tyler RD. Disseminated histoplasmosis in cats: 12 cases. *J Am Vet Med Assoc* 1987;190:1445–1448.

Fooshee SK, Woody BW. Systemic fungal diseases. In: Norsworthy GD, ed. Feline practice. Philadelphia: JB Lippincott, 1993;540–550.

Taboada J, Merchant SR. Treatment of fungal diseases. In: Proceedings of the American College of Veterinary Internal Medicine, 13th Annual Meeting, 1995;800.

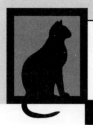

CHAPTER 70

Horner's Syndrome

Sharon K. Fooshee

Overview

Horner's syndrome is a disorder resulting from loss of sympathetic innervation to the eye and adnexa. Sympathetic innervation is responsible for maintenance of smooth muscle tone to the periorbita and eyelids, including the membrana nictitans. It is also important in balancing pupillary dilation (via the iris dilator muscles) against the parasympathetic effect of pupillary constriction (via the iris constrictor muscles). The causative lesion may lie anywhere along the sympathetic chain. Preganglionic lesions involve the pathway from the brainstem to the termination of the cervical sympathetic trunk at the cranial cervical ganglion. Postganglionic lesions lie along the path of the cranial cervical ganglion, course through the middle ear, and terminate in the eye. In cats, trauma to the pathway is the most common cause of Horner's syndrome. Such injuries include bite wounds, thyroidectomy, and cervical or brachial plexus avulsion. Other causes include otitis media (including iatrogenic injury with ear cleaning), nasopharyngeal polyps, and cranial thoracic neoplasia. In a number of cases, the cause cannot be determined. Signs of Horner's syndrome include miosis, enophthalmos, prolapse of the third eyelid, and ptosis. In some cases, all of the signs will not be present; miosis is the most consistent finding in the absence of other signs. Visual deficits would not be typical. A complete physical examination should be performed, with special attention given to evaluation of cranial nerve function and level of mentation, identification of proprioceptive deficits, examination of the ear canal, and recognition of recent trauma.

D i a g n o s i s

Primary Diagnostics

- **Clinical signs:** One or more of the signs of miosis, enophthalmos, prolapse of the third eyelid, and ptosis should raise one's index of suspicion.

Ancillary Diagnostics

- **Radiographs:** Thoracic radiographs may be useful to identify thoracic masses. Bulla films may provide evidence of a soft-tissue density in the bulla (middle-ear polyp or otitis media).
- **Pharmacologic testing:** Testing with ocular medications may aid in distinguishing preganglionic from postganglionic lesions. An indirect-acting sympathomimetic agent (1% hydroxyamphetamine) instilled into *each eye* results in dilation of the miotic pupil when the lesion is preganglionic. This response occurs because the nerve endings of the postganglionic neuron are intact and able to respond. When the lesion is postganglionic, the miotic pupil dilates incompletely or not at all. A direct-acting sympathomimetic agent (10% phenylephrine) should be administered in *each eye* if mydriasis is not achieved on the first test.

Diagnostic Notes

- Anisocoria may be more pronounced in a dark room when the normal pupil is allowed to dilate.
- The eye is nonpainful with Horner's syndrome. Painful conditions, such as uveitis and corneal injury, may result in miosis and should not be confused with Horner's syndrome.
- Results of pharmacologic testing are variable and cannot be used to predict the underlying cause or the attendant prognosis.

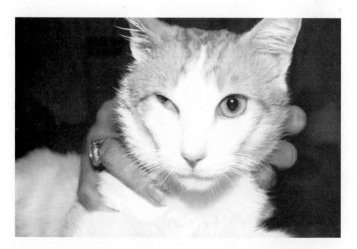

FIGURE 70.1. Horner's syndrome: The signs of Horner's syndrome include miosis, enophthalmos, prolapse of the third eyelid, and ptosis. This cat shows all but enophthalmos, although this photograph does not clearly demonstrate the miosis because of the prolapsed third eyelid.

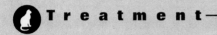

Treatment

Primary Therapeutics

No specific treatment is available for Horner's syndrome.

Prognosis

Horner's syndrome serves as a marker for an underlying disorder. The prognosis is entirely dependent upon identification of the cause and a positive response to treatment.

Suggested Readings

Collins BK. Disorders of the pupil. In: August JR, ed. Consultations in feline internal medicine 2. Philadelphia: WB Saunders, 1994;421–428.

Neer TM. Horner's syndrome. *Compend Contin Educ Pract Vet* 1984;6:740–747.

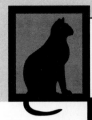

CHAPTER 71

Hydronephrosis

Gary D. Norsworthy

Overview

Hydronephrosis develops when one or both ureters are obstructed, resulting in collection of urine within the renal pelvis. The pelvis dilates, resulting in pressure and ischemic atrophy of the renal cortex. If unilateral disease occurs, the normal kidney functions long enough to allow the abnormal kidney to enlarge to enormous proportions. If bilateral disease occurs, the cat will become azotemic and die before renal enlargement is great. Hydronephrosis may occur due to congenital malformations, or it may be acquired due to conditions such as trauma, ligation during ovariohysterectomy, urolithiasis, or neoplasia. However, the etiology is often not determined. Cats with unilateral disease are often presented for abdominal distention. If pyelonephrosis develops, lethargy, fever, anorexia, and hematuria occur. Cats with bilateral disease are generally presenting with signs of renal failure.

 Diagnosis

Primary Diagnostics

- **Physical examination:** Abdominal palpation will reveal mild to marked renal enlargement.
- **Ultrasound:** An ultrasound examination will reveal a dilated, anechoic, fluid-filled kidney with varying amounts of renal parenchymal tissue present.

Ancillary Diagnostics

- **Excretory urogram:** This study reveals little or no contrast material in the affected kidney. The cortex will be seen as a thin rim of tissue, and the renal pelvis and ureter will be dilated. If unilateral disease is present, the other kidney will be normal.

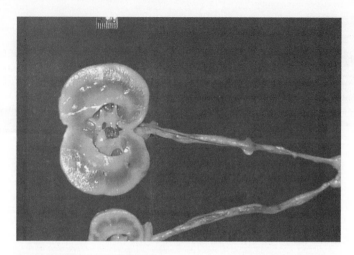

FIGURE 71.1. Hydronephrosis: Hydronephrosis causes the renal pelvis to dilate, as seen in the top kidney.

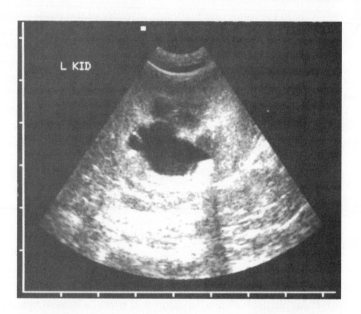

FIGURE 71.2. An ultrasound of a hydronephrotic kidney reveals the dilated pelvis.

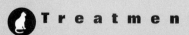

Treatment

Primary Therapeutics

- **Underlying disease:** When possible, the underlying disease causing the obstruction should be treated. In most cases, this is not possible; however, if treatment occurs quickly, renal function may return to a near-normal state.

- **Nephrectomy:** If renal function is lost, the kidney should be removed as long as the other kidney is reasonably normal. Its function should be confirmed with an excretory urogram.

Therapeutic Notes

- Systemic antibiotic therapy is indicated if the affected kidney is infected with bacteria.

- A perinephric pseudocyst may be mistaken for hydronephrosis. However, the former is a fluid-filled sac surrounding a normal kidney. The two can be differentiated with ultrasound or an excretory urogram.

Prognosis

The prognosis is good for unilateral disease. Cats with bilateral disease without a treatable underlying disease have a grave prognosis once azotemia occurs.

Suggested Reading

DiBartola SP, Rutgers HC. Diseases of the kidney. In: Sherding RG, ed. The cat: diseases and clinical management, 2nd ed. Philadelphia: WB Saunders, 1994;1711–1767.

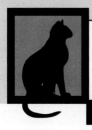

Hypereosinophilic Syndrome

Sharon K. Fooshee

Overview

Feline hypereosinophilic syndrome (FHS) is a rare disorder character-ized by peripheral eosinophilia and an associated eosinophilic infiltrate in various organs.

The infiltrate eventually leads to dysfunction or failure of the involved organ(s). Although FHS has been reported in young cats, most cases involve middle-aged to older cats. No breed predisposition is apparent; females may be more frequently affected.

Diagnosis

Primary Diagnostics

- **Clinical signs:** In the few cases reported, the most consistent signs were vomiting, diarrhea (sometimes bloody), weight loss, and anorexia. Pruritus, seizures, and fever are additional, less common findings. Cutaneous involvement is reported but rare. Abnormalities on physical examination include thickened bowel loops, lymphadenopathy, and hepatosplenomegaly.
- **CBC:** Persistent, unexplained eosinophilia is a hallmark of FHS. The absolute eosinophil count is frequently in excess of 3000 cells/μL. The mean count in one report was approximately 42,000 cells/μL.

Diagnostic Notes

Because the cause of FHS remains unknown, diagnosis of the disorder necessitates eliminating other possible causes of peripheral and tissue eosinophilia.

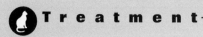 T r e a t m e n t ─────────────────────

Primary Therapeutics

- **Steroids:** Prednisone is the primary therapeutic agent for FHS. High doses are required to induce remission (4–6 mg/kg/day for 2–4 weeks). The dose may then be halved for an additional 2–4 weeks and tapered, if possible.

Secondary Therapeutics

- **Chemotherapy:** Alkylating agents, such as azathioprine, may be considered for refractory cases. Use extreme caution and closely monitor for myeloid suppression. Hydroxyurea has also been used, but experience with the drug is limited due to the rarity of the disorder.

Therapeutic Notes

It should be expected that most cases will require treatment indefinitely.

P r o g n o s i s

In most cases, the relentless progression of the disease leads to a grave prognosis.

S u g g e s t e d   R e a d i n g s

Neer TM. Hypereosinophilic syndrome in cats. *Compend Contin Educ* 1991;13:549–555.

Sherding RG. Diseases of the intestine. In: Sherding RG, ed. The cat: diseases and clinical management. Philadelphia: WB Saunders, 1994;1247–1248.

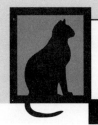

CHAPTER 73

Hyperthyroidism

Mitchell A. Crystal and Gary D. Norsworthy

Overview

H yperthyroidism is the most common endocrinopathy of cats. It is caused by excess production of thyroxine (T_4). Ninety-eight to 99% of cats with hyperthyroidism have functional adenomatous hyperplasia (or adenoma), and 1–2% have thyroid carcinomas. The pathogenesis of the adenomatous or carcinomatous changes seen in the thyroid glands of hyperthyroid cats is unknown.

The normal thyroid gland consists of two lobes located adjacent to the fifth or sixth tracheal ring, just caudal to the larynx. Small amounts of ectopic thyroid tissue are also present in the caudal cervical area and in the mediastinum. A small, pale external parathyroid gland is located in the fascia, usually at the cranial pole of each thyroid lobe. An internal parathyroid gland is located within each thyroid lobe and is not grossly visible. The thyroid gland is not palpable in the normal animal. In hyperthyroidism, bilateral lobe (70%), unilateral lobe (25–30%), or ectopic tissue (3–5%) enlargement may occur. Unilateral or bilateral lobe enlargement is palpable in up to 95% of affected cats depending on the expertise of the veterinarian. Enlarged thyroid lobes sometime descend caudally and, thus, may be detected in their normal location or in the caudal cervical area. Enlarged thyroid lobes will be undetectable if they descend through the thoracic inlet.

Hyperthyroidism occurs in cats 4 to 22 years of age (median age 13 years), and 95% of affected cats are over 10 years old. There is no breed or sex predilection. Common clinical signs include weight loss (88–98%), polyphagia (49–67%), polyuria/polydipsia (36–45%), vomiting (33–44%), increased activity (31–34%), and diarrhea (15–45%). Occasionally cats will present with lethargy, depression, anorexia, and/or weakness. This is known as apathetic hyperthyroidism and occurs in 5–10% of affected cats. Dyspnea/congestive heart failure (CHF) is also an uncommon presenting sign (<5%), and a small number of cats will present with ventral neck flexion (1–3%). Common physical examination findings include emaciation (65–97%), enlarged thyroid lobe(s) (75–95%), tachycardia (42–57%), unkempt hair coat (9–52%), and gallop rhythm (15–17%).

The main differential diagnoses for hyperthyroidism include diseases causing polyphagic weight loss (diabetes mellitus, inflammatory bowel disease, alimentary lymphoma, and, uncommonly, chronic renal failure, intestinal parasitism, and exocrine pancreatic insufficiency) and diseases causing polyuria and polydipsia (diabetes mellitus, chronic renal failure, and hepatic disease).

Consequences of untreated hyperthyroidism include cardiac disease and hypertension. On occasion, treatment of hyperthyroidism can result in decompensation of chronic renal failure.

Untreated hyperthyroidism commonly results in a hypertrophic form of cardiomyopathy but also, in rare cases, it may result in a dilatative form of cardiomyopathy. Therefore, any older cat with cardiomyopathy of any form should be assessed for hyperthyroidism. Cardiomyopathy due to hyperthyroidism (thyrotoxic cardiomyopathy) very uncommonly causes CHF.

Up to 87% of hyperthyroid cats are hypertensive. Diagnosis and management of hypertension should be closely considered in hyperthyroid cats; however, hypertension generally resolves following successful treatment of hyperthyroidism and production of a euthyroid state.

Although hyperthyroidism does not directly induce renal pathology, decreased renal size and/or chronic renal failure are seen in many cats with hyperthyroidism because these findings are common in older cats. The importance of recognizing renal failure in hyperthyroid cats prior to treatment is based on the effects of thyroid hormone on glomerular blood flow (GBF) and glomerular filtration rate (GFR). Hyperthyroidism produces a hyperdynamic cardiac state, which increases both GBF and GFR. This results in improved renal function and delays the clinical and biochemical effects of renal failure in some cats with hyperthyroidism. When these cats are treated for hyperthyroidism, deterioration of renal function may occur, leading to clinical and biochemical signs of renal failure.

 D i a g n o s i s

Primary Diagnostics

- **Cervical palpation for thyroid enlargement:** This is a very sensitive and specific test for thyroid enlargement when the technique is performed properly. A thyroid lobe that is palpable should be considered abnormal.
- **Chemistry profile:** Around 90% of affected cats have an elevation of either ALT or ALP, but this is not thought to represent significant hepatic disease. Azotemia is present in some cats.
- **CBC:** Half of the affected cats may demonstrate a mildly elevated PCV. A normal CBC should be confirmed prior to beginning medical management of hyperthyroidism.

- **Urinalysis:** Poorly or nonconcentrated urine may be present as a result of hyperthyroidism or chronic renal failure.
- **Total T_4 (TT_4):** This value is elevated in 90–98% of affected cats. Some cats have normal TT_4 levels as a result of either fluctuation of TT_4 levels in and out of the normal range or suppression of elevated TT_4 levels into the normal range secondary to concurrent nonthyroidal illness.

Ancillary Diagnostics

- **T_3 suppression test:** This test is indicated when hyperthyroidism is suspected and T_4 levels are normal (2–10% of cases). Results are extremely accurate. The test procedure is described in Appendix F.
- **TRH response test:** This test is indicated when hyperthyroidism is suspected and T_4 levels are normal (2–10% of cases). It is described in Appendix F.
- **Thoracic imaging:** Radiography or ultrasonography may demonstrate cardiac changes, pleural effusion, or, rarely, metastatic or mediastinal disease.
- **Blood pressure:** Hypertension is present in up to 87% of affected cats.
- **ECG:** Tachycardia, left anterior fascicular bundle branch block, cardiac chamber enlargement, and arrhythmias may be present. However, many hyperthyroid cats have normal ECGs.
- **Pertechnetate thyroid scanning (⁹⁹ᵐTc):** Nuclear scanning accurately indicates overt and occult hyperthyroidism and can differentiate bilateral and unilateral disease. It can also determine if ectopic thyroid tissue is involved and whether metastasis is present.

Diagnostic Notes

- Serum T_3 levels are of limited usefulness in the diagnosis of feline hyperthyroidism. About 25% of affected cats with elevated serum T_4 levels have normal serum T_3 levels. Few, if any, hyperthyroid cats have normal levels of T_4 and elevated levels of T_3. Free T_4 (fT_4) levels, using proper techniques, are not more accurate than TT_4 levels in the diagnosis of overt hyperthyroidism but may be useful in the diagnosis of occult hyperthyroidism. Some hyperthyroid cats with normal or slightly high TT_4 values will have elevated fT_4 levels. However, some cats with nonthyroidal illness will have subnormal total T_4 levels and elevated fT_4 levels. Therefore, the fT_4 should not be used alone as a screening test. If fT_4 is to be measured, the equilibrium dialysis and direct dialysis assay methods are accurate and reliable. The radioimmunoassay or analogue method is not.
- The TSH stimulation test is an inaccurate test and is not useful in the diagnosis of hyperthyroidism.

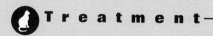

Treatment

Primary Therapeutics
Initial Phase

- **Methimazole:** This drug inhibits the synthesis of thyroid hormone. It is used during the initial phase of treatment to stabilize the cat and reverse the clinical signs, unless radioactive iodine therapy will be performed 2–3 weeks following diagnosis. Side effects are seen in about 15% of cats. Treatment varies with body weight and T_4 elevation. A common approach to a cat with mild hyperthyroidism begins with 2.5 mg BID PO for 2 weeks. Serum T_4 levels and a CBC should be assessed at the end of 2 weeks. If the T_4 level is still elevated, increase the dose by 2.5–5-mg/day increments, and recheck the serum T_4, serum creatinine, and CBC weekly until normal.

Definitive or Long-term Treatment

- **Radioactive Iodine (^{131}I):** This isotope destroys hyperfunctioning tissue without affecting normal thyroid tissue. It is reported to be effective 90% of the time (although this author [MAC] feels the success rate is much higher). It is a noninvasive, simple, safe procedure. The only stress involved is the travel to the facility and the 1–2-week posttreatment hospitalization required to allow the cat's surface radiation to fall to a safe level. Cats usually become euthyroid within 1 week of therapy. ^{131}I therapy is only available at approved facilities and is moderately expensive. Cats must be off all antithyroid medications for 1 week prior to therapy. It is preferable for the treatment to be performed without the cat having been on antithyroid medication.

- **Surgical excision:** Removal of one or both thyroid lobes or hyperfunctioning ectopic tissue is an effective, invasive, moderately difficult, and moderately expensive procedure for the treatment of hyperthyroidism. Because anesthesia is necessary, preoperative stabilization of the hyperthyroid state (medical management with methimazole) and associated conditions (cardiomyopathy, hypertension) is required. Some surgeons remove only the affected lobe(s), whereas others prefer to do bilateral thyroidectomy on all hyperthyroid cats. Original and modified intracapsular and extracapsular techniques have been used for many years. Recently, this author (GDN) reported a parathyroid transplant technique that is considerably less difficult to perform and has a very small chance for recurrence or for hypocalcemia.

- **Methimazole:** This drug can be continued as long-term therapy. It is an effective, inexpensive treatment for hyperthyroidism. It inhibits the synthesis of thyroid hormones but does nothing to prevent progression of thyroid enlargement. Therefore, the serum T_4 level (and a CBC) should be checked every 4–6 months. Side effects have occurred up to 6 months after therapy has begun. Anorexia and vomiting are most common, but several others are possible (see below).

Secondary Therapeutics

- **Propylthiouracil (PTU):** This drug inhibits the synthesis of thyroid hormones. It is an effective, inexpensive treatment for hyperthyroidism. Side effects are more frequent (20–25%) and potentially more severe compared with methimazole. Thus, this drug should only be used if methimazole is unavailable or if the cat reacts to methimazole. PTU is dosed at 11 mg/kg BID PO and adjusted to effect as per methimazole.

- **Hypertension:** Hypertension should be treated, if present, with amlodipine (0.625 mg/cat SID PO) or benazepril (2.5–5 mg/cat SID PO). Once hyperthyroidism has been corrected, hypertension therapy should be tapered while reassessing blood pressure. Effective treatment of hyperthyroidism will result in correction of hypertension in most cats.

- **Therapy for cardiac disease:** Treatment for cardiac disease should be instituted if indicated. Propranolol (5 mg/cat BID-TID PO), atenolol (6.25–12.5 mg/cat SID PO), or sustained-release diltiazem (30 mg/cat SID-BID PO) is most commonly used. Hyperthyroid-induced cardiomyopathy often improves with treatment of hyperthyroidism, allowing discontinuation or reduction of cardiac medications.

Therapeutic Notes

- Clinical side effects of medical antithyroid therapy include anorexia, vomiting, lethargy, facial pruritus, self-excoriation, icterus, and bleeding. Laboratory abnormalities associated with antithyroid therapy include eosinophilia, neutropenia, lymphocytosis, agranulocytosis, thrombocytopenia, positive antinuclear antibody titre and Coombs' tests, and increases in liver enzymes. Many side effects from methimazole are mild and resolve following cessation of therapy for a few days. Severe side effects or persistent mild side effects will usually resolve when the drug is discontinued. The side effects of PTU are often more severe. As a result of the side effects seen with medical management, a CBC should be monitored along with serum T_4 levels every 4–6 months, and sooner if mild changes are noted. If severe clinical or laboratory abnormalities occur (especially hepatotoxicity), antithyroid therapy should be discontinued, and ^{131}I therapy or surgery should be recommended.

- Because treatment of hyperthyroidism has the potential to worsen chronic renal disease, methimazole should be attempted first in animals with possible renal compromise. If worsening of renal failure occurs (this must be differentiated from side effects of therapy), hyperthyroidism should not be treated or should be treated to bring the T_4 into the range of 5.0 to 6.0 µg/dL.

- Serum calcium should be checked once daily for 3 days following surgery. Transient, clinical hypoparathyroidism is seen in 5–15% of cats undergoing bilateral thyroidectomy due to damage to the parathyroid glands or their blood supply. Transient, mild hypocalcemia without clinical signs is common but does not warrant therapy. Clinical signs usually occur within 1–3 days following surgery but may occur up to 7 days following surgery. They usually resolve by 3 weeks following surgery but may take up to 6 months to resolve. In rare cases, hypoparathyroidism may be permanent. Clinical signs of hypocalcemia include tetany, seizures, muscle twitching, and/or anorexia. Clinical or severe (< 7.5 mg/dL) hypocalcemia needs immediate therapy, as this is a life-threatening condition. Therapy includes 0.5–1.5 mL/kg IV of 10% calcium gluconate over a 10-minute period while monitoring the heart rate. Infusion should be stopped if bradycardia occurs. Following initial therapy, one to two mL of 10% calcium gluconate diluted 1:1 in 0.9% saline is administered TID SC to prevent recurrence of clinical hypocalcemia (alternatively, one could add 10 to 20 mL of 10% calcium gluconate to 500 mL of 0.9% saline, depending on the severity of the hypocalcemia, and infuse at standard maintenance rate). Calcium levels are monitored two to three times daily, and therapy is adjusted as needed. Maintenance therapy for hypocalcemia is often needed for 2–3 weeks following surgery and occasionally longer. Maintenance therapy consists of either active vitamin D_3 (calcitriol or 1,25 dihydroxycholecalciferol) at 2.5–10 ng/kg SID or synthetic vitamin D_3 (dihydrotachysterol) at 0.02–0.03 mg/kg SID for 3 days, followed by 0.01–0.02 mg/kg QOD to SID along with oral calcium at 25 mg/kg BID-TID. Serum calcium should be measured every 1–3 days and adjustments made as needed. Vitamin D and calcium therapy should be tapered and, if serum calcium remains normal, stopped 2–3 weeks following surgery. It should be noted that post-thyroidectomy hypocalcemia can usually be avoided by performing bilateral thyroidectomies in two stages, allowing 3–4 weeks between removal of each lobe.
- Laryngeal paralysis, voice change, or Horner's syndrome is seen in a rare number of cats following surgery. Voice changes and Horner's syndrome are usually temporary and are clinically insignificant. Laryngeal paralysis is also usually temporary but may require tracheostomy for management of laryngeal obstruction until the condition resolves.

Hyperthyroidism recurs in 5–10% of cats undergoing bilateral thyroidectomy and in 20% of cats undergoing unilateral thyroidectomy using standard intracapsular and extracapsular techniques. Recurrence may occur 8 to 63 months following surgery, but usually occurs within 2 years.

Thyroid levels are transiently low (usually 1–3 weeks) following ^{131}I therapy or bilateral surgery, but persistent hypothyroidism as a result of either is rare. Thyroid supplementation is not indicated following these procedures unless thyroid levels are persistently low 6 months following ^{131}I therapy or surgery.

- It is important to weigh the advantages and disadvantages of medical versus surgical versus ^{131}I therapy prior to making recommendations to the client. Items of concern include the age of the cat, how well the cat does away from home, the financial ability of the client, the presence or absence of renal failure, the willingness of owners to travel to the facility, and the availability of facilities that offer ^{131}I therapy.

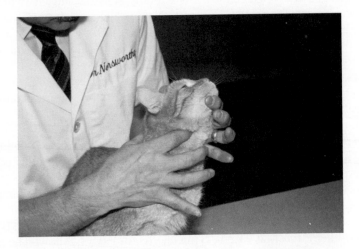

FIGURE 73.1. Hyperthyroidism: Proper palpation can reveal an enlarged thyroid lobe, often before the T_4 elevates.

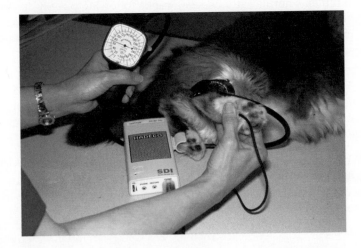

FIGURE 73.2. Over 20% of hyperthyroid cats have systemic hypertension. If possible, the cat's blood pressure should be determined before thyroidectomy. Doppler blood pressure units are the most accurate for cats. (Available from Pet Recovery Products, 1-800-484-6255 PIN 7778.)

Prognosis

Most cats with hyperthyroidism can be successfully treated. Cats with concurrent renal failure have the poorest prognosis.

Suggested Readings

Feldman EC, Nelson RW. Feline hyperthyroidism (thyrotoxicosis). In: Feldman EC, Nelson RW, eds. Canine and feline endocrinology and reproduction, 2nd ed. Philadelphia: WB Saunders, 1996;118–165.

Meric SM. Cats with overactive thyroid glands: the best tests and treatments. *Vet Med* 1989;10:954–981.

Norsworth GD. Feline thyroidectomy: a simplified technique that preserves parathyroid function. *Vet Med J* 1995;90(11):1055–1063.

Peterson ME. Hyperthyroid diseases. In: Ettinger SJ, Feldman EC, eds. Textbook of veterinary internal medicine, 4th ed. Philadelphia: WB Saunders, 1995;1466–1487.

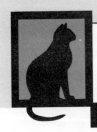

CHAPTER 74

Hypertrophic Cardiomyopathy

John-Karl Goodwin

Overview

Hypertrophic cardiomyopathy (HCM) is the most common cardiac disease of the cat and is characterized by unexplained and significant left ventricular hypertrophy. The left ventricle is nondilated and often hyperdynamic. There is no definable cause contrasting left ventricular hypertrophy that occurs secondary to hyperthyroidism, systemic hypertension, or subaortic stenosis.

Although the etiology is currently unknown, myocardial beta-myosin heavy chain mutations have been demonstrated in humans with HCM and may be responsible for the disease in cats as well. Other theories include altered myocardial calcium transport, enhanced myocardial sensitivity to catecholamines, and increased production of myocardial trophic factors.

Left ventricular hypertrophy results in a stiff, noncompliant chamber, causing diastolic (ventricular filling) dysfunction. This results in elevated left ventricular filling pressures and subsequent left atrial dilatation. As the disease progresses, pulmonary venous pressures increase and pulmonary edema develops. Left atrial enlargement predisposes affected cats to atrial arrhythmias. Stasis of blood within the dilated left atrium may result in thrombus formation and thromboembolic disease. Affected cats may also develop fatal ventricular arrhythmias secondary to myocardial ischemia.

The mean age of affected cats is 6 years with an age range from 8 months to 16 years. Approximately 75% are male. Reported breed incidences are: domestic shorthair (DSH) (89.1%), Persian (6.5%), domestic longhair (DLH) (2.2%), and Maine coon (2.2%).

Clinical signs are variable. Many cats have no clinical signs at the time HCM is documented. These cats are most often examined because a murmur, gallop rhythm, or other arrhythmia is detected during routine examination. On the other hand, cases may be first diagnosed only after severe clinical signs become apparent, such as fulminant pulmonary edema or systemic thromboembolism.

Physical examination abnormalities are dependent upon the stage of disease. Cats with congestive heart failure will exhibit tachypnea and labored breathing. Those with systemic thromboembolism will have characteristic signs (see Chapter 117). A heart murmur is present in approximately 65 to 95% of all cats with hypertrophic cardiomyopathy. Other auscultatory findings may include a gallop rhythm (40%) and other arrhythmia (25%).

 D i a g n o s i s

Primary Tests

- **Electrocardiography:** Evidence of left atrial enlargement (P-mitrale—widened P-waves) and left ventricular enlargement (increased R-wave amplitude and/or increased QRS duration) are present. Arrhythmias are frequent. Most cats with hypertrophic cardiomyopathy will have a sinus tachycardia. Atrial and ventricular arrhythmias may be present. Intraventricular conduction deficits, such as left anterior fascicular block, are occasionally present.

- **Radiography:** Variable enlargement of the cardiac silhouette is seen. Left atrial enlargement is often most prominent. Early in the course of the disease, the cardiac silhouette may be normal. Cats with congestive heart failure may demonstrate enlargement of the pulmonary veins, variable pulmonary edema, and pleural effusion.

- **Echocardiography:** Left ventricular hypertrophy involving the left ventricular free wall and, usually to a greater degree, the interventricular septum is present. The mean septal thickness of affected cats is reportedly 6.5 mm (normal 3.7 ± 0.7 mm).

Left ventricular hypertrophy is diffuse in approximately 67% of cats and regional in 33%. Affected cats tend to have greater hypertrophy of the basilar portion of the left ventricle than the apical portion (57%), whereas others have fairly equal hypertrophy in both regions (43%).

In several cats, a localized area of hypertrophy is often found at the proximal interventricular septum, which protrudes into the left ventricular outflow tract. This is often referred to as asymmetric septal hypertrophy, or ASH, and is thought to cause a variable degree of obstruction to left ventricular emptying. A stenotic lesion such as this results in compensatory ventricular hypertrophy, which may lead to further obstruction.

The diameter of the left ventricle in diastole is typically within normal limits, whereas the left ventricular diameter in systole is often decreased, resulting in an increased fractional shortening in some cats. Most cats with HCM will have a normal fractional shortening (30–60%). Left atrial enlargement is consistently present (mean of 18 mm; normal 11 mm) and if absent should cause one to question the diagnosis in cats with slight left ventricular hypertrophy. Other echocardiographic findings may include mitral valve leaflet thickening, occasionally a slight pericardial effusion, and intracardiac thrombi. Systolic anterior motion (SAM) of the mitral valve is observed in approximately 67% of affected cats.

Ancillary Diagnostics

- **Doppler echocardiography:** Mild to marked left ventricular outflow obstruction occurs in cats with SAM. Due to the malposition of the anterior leaflet in systole, mitral insufficiency is present in cats with SAM.

Diagnostic Notes

- Because systemic blood pressure is not routinely measured in cats, inevitably cats with hypertensive heart disease are included in descriptions of hypertrophic cardiomyopathy.
- Always rule out overt or occult hyperthyroidism as the cause of left ventricular hypertrophy in cats over 6 years of age.

 T r e a t m e n t

Primary Therapeutics

- **Reduce stress:** Take all measures to minimize any stress to cats exhibiting respiratory distress (e.g., delay radiographs and catheter placement).
- **Facilitate breathing:** Thoracocentesis should be performed in all dyspneic cats when pleural effusion is suspected (muffled lung sounds). With the cat sternal, place a 19–22 gauge butterfly catheter just into the pleural space (5th to 7th intercostal space, just cranial to adjacent rib) and aspirate. Use a closed system, and tap both sides of the chest. Give furosemide when pulmonary edema is present. In the crisis setting, give 2–4 mg/kg IV initially, then 1–2 mg/kg IV or IM every 4–6 hours until the edema has resolved. Furosemide is often continued as needed (6.25–12.5 mg SID-BID) to control edema formation. Apply ¼ inch of nitroglycerin to a hairless area every 4–6 hours until the edema has resolved.
- **Oxygen:** Administer via face mask if tolerated; otherwise use an oxygen cage or tent (50% oxygen).

Secondary Therapeutics

- **Diltiazem:** This may improve myocardial relaxation and control arrhythmias. Give 7.5 mg TID or 30 mg of a sustained release preparation SID-BID.
- **Other cardiac drugs:** Alternatively to diltiazem, a beta blocker such as atenolol (6.25 mg SID-BID) or propranolol (5 mg BID-TID) may be used.

- **Enalapril:** The use of 0.25 mg/kg SID may be beneficial. ACE inhibitors have been shown to reduce left ventricular hypertrophy in cats with HCM.
- **Aspirin:** This drug may reduce chance of thrombus formation; Give 81 mg every third day.
- **Periodic centesis:** Thoracocentesis or abdominocentesis may be needed periodically.

Therapeutic Notes

- There are relative advantages of either diltiazem (calcium channel blocker) or beta blockers (atenolol and propranolol), and no consensus has been reached on the most effective therapy. Cats with persistent tachycardia may benefit more from a beta blocker than a calcium channel blocker. Those with severe left ventricular hypertrophy may benefit more from a calcium channel blocker.
- Monitor renal function if enalapril is used.
- Warfarin (5 mg SID) may be used in lieu of aspirin but has a much greater chance of inducing a hemorrhagic crisis.
- The dose of a diuretic and the need for antiarrhythmic agents may change during the course of the disease. Frequent monitoring is recommended.

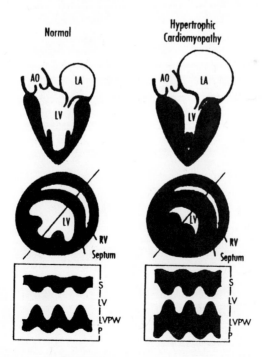

FIGURE 74.1. Hypertrophic CM: Two different M-mode echocardiograms identifying the left ventricle (LV), interventricular septum (S), left ventricular posterior wall (LVPW), and pericardium (P).

P r o g n o s i s

The prognosis of affected cats is dependent upon the severity of disease. Those with no clinical signs have a median survival of nearly 5 years. Cats presented with evidence of congestive heart failure reportedly have a median survival of 3 months, although this should be increased with advances in therapeutics. Systemic thromboembolism is a concern and often results in exacerbation of the congestive heart failure state. Recurrence is also likely.

S u g g e s t e d   R e a d i n g

Pion PD, Kienle RD. Feline cardiomyopathy. In: Miller MS, Tilley LP, eds. Manual of canine and feline cardiology, 2nd ed. Philadelphia: WB Saunders, 1995.

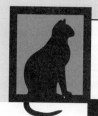

CHAPTER 75

Hypokalemia

Mitchell A. Crystal

Overview

Hypokalemia is the most common cause of ventral neck flexion and generalized muscle weakness in cats. Hypokalemia results from excessive urinary losses of potassium, which is usually concurrent with renal dysfunction. Decreased dietary intake of potassium and acidosis may also contribute to the development of hypokalemia, although the latter causes a shift of potassium from intracellular sites (the place of activity) to the blood, thus masking the severity of the potassium depression. Cats affected usually are middle aged to older (usually around 9 years of age). There does not appear to be any breed predilection, though a periodic muscle weakness due to hypokalemia has been recognized in Burmese kittens. There are two clinical syndromes: a subclinical form and a severe form. The subclinical form produces obscure signs often confused with aging. These include reduced appetite, gradual weight loss, low-grade anemia, and reduced activity. Clinical signs of the severe hypokalemic polymyopathy usually appear acutely and include ventral neck flexion and generalized muscle weakness. About 25% of cats will demonstrate a stiff or stilted gait and muscle pain. Cats may also be polyuric and polydipsic as a result of hypokalemia or underlying chronic renal failure. Rarely, cats with severe hypokalemia may demonstrate dyspnea due to respiratory muscle paralysis. The differential diagnosis for cats with ventral neck flexion and generalized muscle weakness should also include diabetes mellitus (distal neuropathy and/or hypokalemia), hypernatremia, hyperthyroidism, idiopathic polymyositis, myasthenia gravis, chronic organophosphate toxicity, portosystemic shunt, and thiamine deficiency.

 ## Diagnosis

Primary Diagnostics

- **Clinical signs:** The clinical signs of the subclinical form are listed above. Cervical ventroflexion due to muscle weakness is classic for the severe form.

- **Chemistry profile:** Serum potassium is decreased and creatine kinase is usually markedly increased. Abnormalities associated with chronic renal failure may also be present (azotemia, hyperphosphatemia, acidosis).
- **Therapeutic trial:** Serum potassium levels are usually normal in the subclinical form. A trial of 4 mEq/day of potassium gluconate for 4–6 weeks will result in a dramatic response for affected cats.

Ancillary Diagnostics

- **Urinary fractional excretion of potassium:** This is usually greater than 6% in affected cats.
- **Electromyography:** Generalized abnormalities are expected (excessive insertional activity, spontaneous sharp waves and fibrillation potentials, bizarre high-frequency discharges).

Diagnostic Notes

- Only 2% of the body's potassium is found in the blood. There is very poor correlation with blood levels and tissue levels. Therefore, the subclinical and early clinical forms should not be ruled out based on a low-normal or normal serum potassium level.
- Diagnostic tests for other differential diagnoses for ventral neck flexion and generalized muscle weakness should be performed if indicated by clinical signs or chemistry abnormalities.
- Other causes of hypokalemia should be considered and evaluated if suggested by clinical signs or history (gastrointestinal disease, loop diuretic therapy).
- Muscle biopsies are generally not needed but, if performed, are normal.

 T r e a t m e n t

Primary Therapeutics

- **Oral potassium therapy:** Potassium is given at 5 to 10 mEq per cat per day in divided doses until serum potassium is within the normal range (severe form) or until clinical response is achieved (subclinical form), followed by 2 to 4 mEq per cat per day in divided doses. Oral potassium therapy is more effective than parenteral potassium supplementation and should be used for all but the most severely affected cats. Potassium gluconate as a powder, gel, or tablet (Tumil-K) or elixir (several sources) provides the most available source of potassium; however, palatability can be a problem. The tablets are preferred so that administration is confirmed. The powder is generally more palatable than the elixir. Potassium chloride is also effective but is generally less palatable and may worsen pre-existing acidosis.

Secondary Therapeutics

- **Parenteral potassium therapy:** For the severe form, intravenous potassium is given at 0.25–0.5 mEq/kg/hour in parenteral fluids until normalization and stabilization of serum potassium are achieved. Fluids should be given at slow rates and contain a high concentration of potassium (e.g., 160 mEq/L administered at 2.0 mL/kg/hour). Fluids with low potassium concentrations administered at rapid rates may further lower serum potassium and worsen clinical signs, leading to respiratory muscle paralysis. Oral therapy should be started concurrently, if possible.

- **Continuous infusion of dopamine:** The infusion of this drug at 0.5 mg/kg/hr may induce transient elevation in serum potassium and thus help in treating severe cases.

Therapeutic Notes

- Administration rates of fluids containing high concentrations of potassium should be closely monitored to prevent cardiac arrhythmias.

- Cats with either form of hypokalemia should receive long-term potassium supplementation.

P r o g n o s i s

The prognosis for the subclinical form is excellent. In the severe form, response to therapy usually begins within 24 hours. Considerable improvement is seen in 2 to 3 days, although complete remission may take several weeks. With appropriate

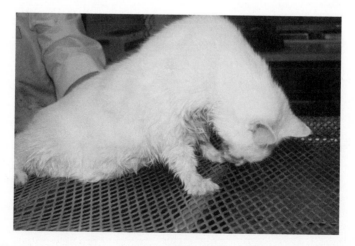

FIGURE 75.1. Hypokalemia: The severe form of hypokalemia results in profound muscle weakness. Affected cats experience cervical ventroflexion because they do not have enough muscle strength to raise their heads.

therapy and long-term potassium supplementation, the prognosis for recovery from hypokalemic polymyopathy is excellent, although the underlying renal dysfunction may carry a less favorable prognosis for long-term survival. Treatment failure usually results from administering fluids of low potassium concentration at a rapid rate.

Suggested Readings

Dow SW, LeCouteur RA. Hypokalemic polymyopathy of cats. In: Kirk RW, ed. Current veterinary therapy X: small animal practice. Philadelphia: WB Saunders, 1989;812–815.

Dow SW. Potassium depletion in cats: causes and consequences. In: Dow SW, DiBartola SP, Schaer M, eds. Hypokalemia: clinical manifestations and treatment. St. Petersburg, FL: Daniels Pharmaceuticals, 1993;3–6.

Taboada J. Ventroflexion of the neck in cats. Proceedings of the Twelfth Annual Veterinary Medical Forum, 1994;385–389.

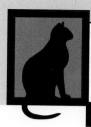

CHAPTER 76
Immune-Mediated Skin Diseases

Sharon K. Fooshee

Overview

Skin disease caused by autoimmune disorders is uncommon in the cat. Two main types are noted: pemphigus complex and systemic lupus erythematosus. In the pemphigus group of disorders, autoantibody is directed against the intercellular cement of the stratified squamous epithelium. Vesicles, and eventually pustules, form as cellular adhesions are destroyed. When these lesions dry, the characteristic crusting of pemphigus appears. Two types of pemphigus have been recognized in cats: pemphigus foliaceous (PF) and pemphigus erythematosus (PE). With systemic lupus erythematosis (SLE), autoimmunity is directed against a wide range of host antigens, rather than specifically against the skin. Clinically, PF and PE may appear quite similar. Lesion distribution is more generalized in PF; with PE, lesions are limited to the head and face. Crusting, scaling, and exudation are characteristic lesions. Vesicles and pustules will rarely be seen. Nasal crusting with associated periocular crusting is a hallmark for pemphigus. Paronychia may be noted in some cats. Pruritus is variable, and peripheral lymphadenopathy may be present. Affected cats oftentimes appear ill (fever, weight loss, anorexia). Lesions of SLE can be similar with additional findings of mucocutaneous ulceration, alopecia, erythema, and depigmentation.

Diagnosis

Primary Diagnostics

- **Clinical signs:** Crusting dermatitis or paronychia should raise one's index of suspicion.
- **Skin scraping and fungal culture:** These tests should be included in the initial diagnostic evaluation of most diseases of the skin. If intact pustules can be located, cytologic preparations can be helpful in identifying acantholytic cells of PE and PF. If necessary, submit the slide to a pathologist for interpretation.

- **Skin biopsy:** Histopathology provides the most effective means of diagnosing immune-mediated skin disease. Either punch or excisional biopsy may be performed, depending on size of the lesion, and the sample placed in 10% formalin.
- **Minimum data base:** A CBC, chemistry profile, urinalysis, FeLV and FIV tests are all important as part of the minimum data base. These tests are useful in evaluating the overall health of the cat and in identifying complicating factors in treatment. Hematologic disturbances and proteinuria are found with SLE.
- **ANA:** Cats with SLE have not typically produced high ANA titers; also, false-positive and false-negative results can occur. The LE cell test is more specific than the ANA but is less sensitive.

Ancillary Diagnostics

- **Immunofluorescence testing:** If routine histopathology is diagnostic, there may be no need for direct tissue immunofluorescence. If the latter is desired, a small tissue sample should be placed in Michel's medium. This is best done at the time of initial biopsy. If the sample is not needed, it may be discarded. With each IFA, the pathologist should be consulted for potential causes of false-negative and false-positive test results.

Diagnostic Notes

- The skin *should not* be scrubbed or prepped prior to biopsy. This may destroy the architecture of the surface lesions.
- A dermatopathologist or veterinary pathologist with an interest in dermatology should be used for histopathologic evaluation of submitted samples.
- Diagnosis of SLE is based on the presence of major and minor signs. Even with this, the diagnosis is often not straightforward. A detailed internal medicine text should be consulted for further information related to diagnosis of feline SLE.

 T r e a t m e n t

Primary Therapeutics

- **Steroids:** Glucocorticoids are the first choice for treatment of pemphigus and SLE. Oral prednisone or prednisolone at 4–6 mg/kg/day (may be divided into two doses) can be used initially. With response to therapy, the dose can be tapered to alternate day therapy at 1–2 mg/kg every 48 hours.

Secondary Therapeutics

- **Other immune suppressants:** If glucocorticoids alone are not sufficient to provide remission for pemphigus, aurothioglucose (1–2

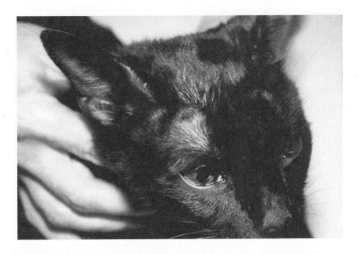

FIGURE 76.1. Immune-mediated skin diseases: The lesions of systemic lupus erythematosis are limited to the head and face and are characterized by crusting, scaling, and exudation.

mg/kg IM weekly) or chlorambucil (0.1–0.2 mg/kg PO q 24 hr) can be added to the protocol. For refractory cases of SLE, chlorambucil may be administered at 0.25–0.5 mg/kg q 48–72 hr. Detailed information related to monitoring and side effects should be obtained prior to institution of these drugs.

- **Therapeutic shampoo:** Cleansing shampoos are useful in removing excess scales and crusts from the skin of cats with PF and PE.

Therapeutic Notes

- Clipping of the hair, especially in long-haired cats, may make it easier to monitor response to therapy, because development of new lesions (and healing of older lesions) can be determined.

- For refractory cases of PE, PF, and SLE, it is recommended to *avoid* azathioprine due to the cat's extreme sensitivity for myelosuppression.

P r o g n o s i s

The prognosis is good for a reasonable quality of life for cats with PE and PF. However, in many cases, treatment is long-term, and relapses are common. For cats with SLE, the prognosis must remain guarded because of the potential for multi-organ failure.

Suggested Readings

Moriello KA. Diseases of the skin. In: Sherding RG, ed. The cat: diseases and clinical management. Philadelphia: WB Saunders, 1994;1999–2009.

Scott DW, Walton DK, Slater MR, Smith CA, Lewis RM. Immune-mediated dermatoses in domestic animals: Ten years after—Part I. *Compend Contin Educ Pract Vet* 1985;9:424–437.

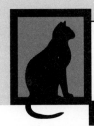

CHAPTER 77

Inflammatory Bowel Disease

Mitchell A. Crystal

Overview

I diopathic inflammatory bowel disease (IBD) is a group of gastrointestinal disorders caused by infiltration of normal inflammatory cells into the mucosa of the gastrointestinal tract. IBD may present with a variety of clinical signs, the most common being chronic intermittent vomiting (compared with the dog, in which the most common clinical sign is diarrhea). Other signs seen with this disorder include diarrhea, weight loss, anorexia, and, rarely, intermittent episodes of increased appetite. Physical examination is often normal or may demonstrate weight loss, palpably thickened intestinal bowel loops, or rarely evidence of diarrhea.

The IBDs are classified according to the type of inflammatory cell infiltrating the gastrointestinal wall. The most common type is lymphocytic-plasmacytic gastroenteritis or colitis. Other less common forms of IBD include eosinophilic, granulomatous, suppurative (neutrophilic), and histiocytic gastroenteritis or colitis. The etiology of IBD is unknown, although several theories have been presented to explain the cause, including immune-mediated disease, gastrointestinal permeability defects, dietary allergy or intolerance, genetic influence, psychologic influence, and infectious disease.

IBD is most commonly seen in middle-aged to older cats with the mean age (in 128 cats from eight studies) around 8 years and a range of 5 months to 20 years. There is no reported breed or sex predilection, although two reports suggest that males are more commonly affected. Many other diseases clinically resemble IBD, and because the gastrointestinal tract responds to insults of any cause with inflammatory cells, a biopsy without diagnostically excluding other differential diagnoses does not constitute a diagnosis of IBD. To make a diagnosis of IBD, all differential diagnoses must be excluded, and inflammatory cells within the mucosa of the gastrointestinal tract must be demonstrated upon histopathologic examination of biopsies. Differential diagnoses to consider include parasites (nematodes, *Giardia*, *Cryptosporidium*), neoplasia (alimentary lymphoma and other neoplastic diseases), endocrinopathies (hyperthyroidism, diabetes mellitus), infectious gastrointestinal diseases (*Helicobacter* gastritis, FeLV/FIV-associated diseases, salmonellosis, campylobacteriosis), metabolic diseases (chronic renal failure, hepatic disease, chronic pancreatitis), and exocrine pancreatic insufficiency (EPI).

D i a g n o s i s

Primary Diagnostics

- **Database (CBC, chemistry profile, and urinalysis):** A database should be submitted to evaluate for diabetes mellitus (hyperglycemia, glucosuria, a low urine specific gravity), liver disease (hyperbilirubinemia, decreased BUN, increased ALT, ALP, and GGT, bilirubinuria), renal disease (elevated BUN and creatinine with a decreased urine specific gravity), signs of hyperthyroidism (increased ALT and/or ALP, a mild increase in PCV, a low urine specific gravity), and signs of lymphoma (occasional cats demonstrate circulating lymphoblasts and anemia). Protein-losing enteropathy from a variety of causes is an uncommon finding in cats with diarrhea (hypoalbuminemia, hypoglobulinemia).

- **Fecal:** A zinc sulfate flotation should be performed to evaluate for nematodes and *Giardia*.

- **Total T_4 (TT_4):** This test should be performed on all cats over 10 years of age with signs of chronic gastrointestinal disease to evaluate for hyperthyroidism.

- **FeLV/FIV Test:** These tests are not confirmatory for disease but may suggest that secondary diseases are present.

Ancillary Diagnostics

- **Feline-specific trypsin-like immunoreactivity (TLI):** A 12-hour fasting serum sample can be submitted for cats with diarrhea to evaluate for EPI and for cats with vomiting to evaluate for pancreatitis. Decreased pancreatic function (i.e., EPI) leads to decreased leakage of trypsinogen into the vascular space, resulting in a subnormal TLI. Some cases of pancreatitis have elevations in TLI, although many are normal (see Chapter 96).

- **Fecal culture for *Salmonella* and *Campylobacter*:** Fecal samples can be submitted for *Salmonella* and *Campylobacter* culture and sensitivity in cats with diarrhea. Samples are best submitted in special media (selenite or tetrathionate media for *Salmonella*; *Campylobacter* media for *Campylobacter*), as high numbers of normal enteric bacteria present in feces tend to overgrow and mask *Salmonella* and *Campylobacter* growth. A positive culture without evidence of other disease processes supports a diagnosis. A negative culture does not necessarily eliminate the possibility of infection (see Chapter 109).

- **Fecal evaluation for *Cryptosporidium*:** Feces and fecal smears can be submitted in cats with diarrhea for concentration techniques and special staining. Fecal ELISA and IFA assays are also available at many laboratories.

- **Intestinal biopsy/histopathology:** This procedure should be performed to investigate for primary intestinal diseases after other differentials have been excluded. Biopsies may be collected via endoscopy, exploratory laparotomy, or, in the case of diffuse or focal intestinal thickening greater than 2–3 cm, by ultrasound-guidance. Histopathology may reveal IBD, alimentary lymphoma, *Cryptosporidium*, and/or *Helicobacter* gastritis.

- **Urea test** (*Campylobacter*-like organism [CLOtest—Delta West PTY LTD, Perth, Australia; distributed in the USA by Tri-Med Specialists Inc., Overland Park, KS.]) **on gastric biopsies:** This test can be performed to evaluate for indirect evidence of *Helicobacter* (see Chapter 65).

Diagnostic Notes

- All differential diagnoses must be excluded prior to making a diagnosis of IBD.

- Many cases of IBD have mild to moderate elevations in liver enzymes. This is believed to be a result of periportal inflammation due to inflammatory efflux from the gastrointestinal tract.

- Alimentary lymphoma can only be differentiated from IBD via biopsy and histopathology, as clinical signs are identical and most cats with gastrointestinal lymphoma are FeLV negative (see Chapter 82.)

- Contrast gastrointestinal radiographs are usually not helpful in the diagnosis of chronic gastrointestinal diseases. They are time consuming, difficult to perform and interpret, and seldom reveal a diagnosis. Even when lesions are present, gastrointestinal biopsy and histopathology are required for a diagnosis.

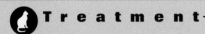 **T r e a t m e n t**

Primary Therapeutics

- **Corticosteroids:** Prednisolone is the drug of choice (along with dietary therapy) for all types of IBD except lymphocytic-plasmacytic colitis. Begin at 1 mg/kg PO BID for 4 weeks, then taper the dosage as follows: 1.5 mg/kg PO SID for 4 weeks, 1.0 mg/kg PO SID for 4 weeks, 0.75 mg/kg PO SID for 4 weeks, 0.5 mg/kg PO SID for 4 weeks, 0.5 mg/kg PO QOD for 4 weeks. After this, discontinue therapy if clinical remission is present. If clinical signs recur during the taper, maintain the cat on the lowest effective dose for 4–6 months and attempt to taper again.

- **Sulfasalazine:** This is the drug of choice (along with dietary therapy) if drug therapy is needed (see following diet bullet) for lymphocytic-plasmacytic colitis. Begin at 15 mg/kg PO SID for 3 weeks, then decrease the dosage to 7.5 mg/kg PO SID for 1 month, then discontinue medication if clinical remission is present. If clinical signs recur after discontinuing therapy, maintain the cat on the lowest effective dose for 2 months and attempt to discontinue therapy again.
- **Diet:** Diet is a critical part of therapy in all forms of IBD. A highly digestible, easily assimilated low-fat diet should be instituted. Diets of a novel protein source may also provide benefit in some cats. In cats with lymphocytic-plasmacytic colitis, clinical remission may be achieved with diet alone. Cats with colonic IBD often benefit either from maintaining a high-fiber diet or from supplementing a highly digestible, easily assimilated low-fat diet with a fiber source such as psyllium (Metamucil) at 1/2–1 teaspoons (about 1.7–3.4 g) PO with food SID-BID or canned pumpkin at 1–2 teaspoons PO with food SID-BID (see Appendix E).
- **Omega-3 fatty acids:** These fatty acids have been shown to have anti-inflammatory effects on the gastrointestinal tract and may prove helpful in the management of IBD. Omega-3 fatty acid supplementation can be found as part of some balanced commercial cat foods (see Appendix E).

Secondary Therapeutics

- **Metronidazole:** Therapy with metronidazole along with the protocols described above may help manage IBD as a result of its antimicrobial effects. Metronidazole has also been reported to inhibit cell-mediated immunity, although this has not been demonstrated in the cat. The dose is 10–20 mg/kg PO BID for 2–3 weeks. Single-agent therapy with metronidazole may be effective in mild cases of IBD.
- **Other immunosuppressive therapy:** Along with the above therapy, azathioprine (0.3 mg/kg PO QOD), chlorambucil (2 mg/m² QOD), or cyclophosphamide (50 mg/m² 4 days on, then 3 days off) are immunosuppressive agents that might be useful in refractive cases of IBD. Drugs should be used for 3 weeks, then tapered by 25–50% for an additional 3–4 months. Neutrophil counts should be monitored weekly for the first month of therapy, then every 2–3 weeks while the cat is on therapy. Drug therapy should be stopped or tapered if the neutrophil count drops below 3000/mL. Cyclosporine is a cell-mediated immunity modulator that has shown promise in cases of human IBD. The dose for cats is 10 mg/kg PO BID. Therapeutic blood levels should be measured 2–4 times monthly at first, then less frequently later, and the dose is adjusted to maintain a whole-blood cyclosporine trough level of 250 ng/mL.

Therapeutic Notes

- No good controlled studies exist on the effectiveness of therapeutics once diet, corticosteroids, or sulfasalazine have proven ineffective. Most information is based on limited cases or extrapolated from human medicine.

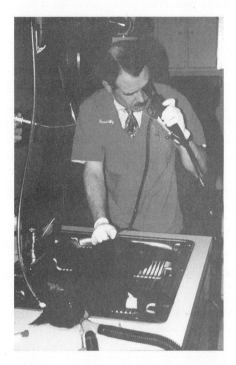

FIGURE 77.1. Inflammatory bowel disease: The diagnosis of IBD is confirmed with biopsies of the stomach or intestinal tract. The stomach and colon can be biopsied with an endoscope.

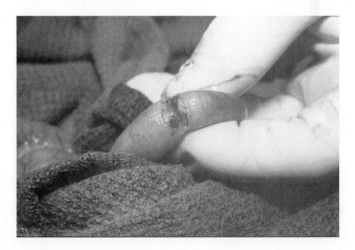

FIGURE 77.2. Small-intestinal biopsies (except in the duodenum) require surgical techniques. At surgery, the intestinal wall is often found to be thickened and/or friable.

> Most cats with responsive IBD show signs of clinical improvement within a week of beginning therapy.

Prognosis

With appropriate dietary therapy and intermittent drug therapy, lymphocytic-plasmacytic IBD is often controllable but rarely curable. Lymphocytic-plasmacytic colitis is usually manageable with dietary therapy alone. Other forms of IBD do not usually respond to therapy. Unlike that of the dog, eosinophilic enterocolitis in the cat is usually aggressive and almost neoplastic in nature, often infiltrating other organs, including the bone marrow (hypereosinophilic syndrome).

Suggested Readings

Guilford WG. Idiopathic inflammatory bowel diseases. In: Strombeck's small animal gastroenterology, 3rd ed. Philadelphia: WB Saunders, 1996:451–486.

Tams TR. Chronic feline inflammatory bowel disorders, part I. Idiopathic inflammatory bowel disease. *Compend Contin Educ Pract Vet* 1986;8(6):371–376.

Tams TR. Chronic feline inflammatory bowel disorders, part II. Feline eosinophilic enteritis and lymphosarcoma. *Compend Contin Educ Pract Vet* 1986;8(7):464–471.

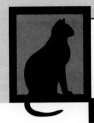

CHAPTER 78

Ischemic Encephalopathy

Sharon K. Fooshee

Overview

Feline ischemic encephalopathy (FIE) is an idiopathic neurologic disorder that develops secondary to infarction of a major blood vessel (usually the middle cerebral artery). The cause is unknown, although sometimes there is a history of recent illness—upper respiratory infection in particular. Some circumstantial evidence exists linking FIE with migration of *Cuterebra* larvae. Cardiomyopathy is not associated with this disorder, and the FeLV and FIV status is unrelated. No breed or sex predilection is reported, although the disorder usually involves adult cats and is most common in the summer months and in the eastern/northeastern United States.

 Diagnosis

Primary Diagnostics

- **Clinical signs:** Neurologic signs are peracute in onset and often lateralizing. Seizures are commonly reported. Other reported findings include circling (toward the affected side), motor deficits, blindness, and behavior changes such as aggression or depression. When blindness occurs, pupillary light reflexes will be normal on the side opposite the lesion (cortical blindness). Other than the neurologic disturbance(s), the physical examination is usually unremarkable.

Ancillary Diagnostics

- Other diagnostic tests are normal: thoracic, abdominal, and skull radiographs; clinicopathological examination; cerebrospinal fluid analysis.

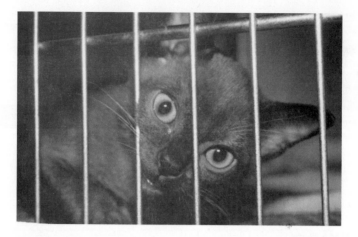

FIGURE 78.1. Ischemic encephalopathy: Like vestibular disease, ischemic encephalopathy can cause a head tilt and circling.

Diagnostic Notes

The main differential diagnosis of trauma should be ruled out with the history and physical examination. Vestibular disease also can mimic FIE.

T r e a t m e n t

Primary Therapeutics

- Treatment does not appear to alter the course of the disease, although glucocorticoid therapy may be useful in decreasing cerebral edema. Rapid-acting formulations would be preferred (i.e., prednisolone sodium succinate).
- Supportive care, such as oxygen, anticonvulsant therapy, and nutritional support, should be provided as needed.

Therapeutic Notes

- Acepromazine should be avoided because of the potential to lower the seizure threshold. Ketamine may increase intracranial pressure.
- Fluid therapy should be used with caution to avoid worsening of the cerebral edema.
- Most cats begin to improve within 3–7 days. Long-term seizure control may require diazepam or phenobarbital.

Prognosis

The prognosis is usually favorable. Signs can disappear with time, although residual signs, such as behavior changes and seizures, often remain. In some cats, aggressive behavior requires euthanasia.

Suggested Reading

Meric SM. Seizures. In: Nelson RW, Couto CG, eds. Essentials of small animal internal medicine. St. Louis: Mosby Year Book, 1992;752–763.

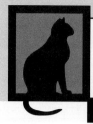

CHAPTER 79

Linear Foreign Body

Gary D. Norsworthy

Overview

A linear foreign body is a gastrointestinal (GI) foreign body that is linear in shape. It may lodge in the GI tract due to its diameter or composition, or it may lodge because it exceeds the length of a peristaltic wave, i.e., about 30 centimeters. Most linear foreign bodies are string, sewing thread, or ribbon. Materials of this type often lacerate the intestinal wall, resulting in bacterial peritonitis. Clinical signs include anorexia, retching, vomiting, lethargy, and fever. Rapid weight loss will occur if the foreign body is present for several days.

 Diagnosis

Primary Diagnostics

- **Clinical signs:** Cats with repeated vomiting or retching for several days should be suspected of ingesting a linear foreign body. Abdominal pain occurs in many cats, especially if bowel perforation and peritonitis occur.
- **Oral examination:** Some linear foreign bodies, especially sewing thread, are wrapped around the base of the tongue. They may be visualized by lifting the tongue by pressing in the intermandibular space with one's finger.
- **Imaging:** Linear foreign bodies often cause loops of small bowel to become bunched or accordion pleated. These may be suspected on survey radiographs or ultrasound, but they are much more easily detected by using positive contrast material.

Diagnostic Notes

If bowel perforation is suspected, barium is contraindicated; an iodine-based contrast material or iohexol should be used.

⬤ T r e a t m e n t

Primary Therapeutics

- **Surgery:** Surgery is required to remove a linear foreign body. Surgery may require a gastrotomy and multiple enterotomies. However, a technique can be used in many cats that requires only one enterotomy incision (see Suggested Reading). Aggressive treatment of bacterial peritonitis should be part of the surgical procedure.
- **Antibiotics:** Because many of these cats have bowel perforation, antibiotics should be given before and after surgery.

Therapeutic Notes

- Symptomatic treatment for vomiting will only prolong and worsen this condition.
- Some cats have a propensity to playing with sewing thread, string, and ribbons. These items should be removed from their environment to prevent future ingestion.

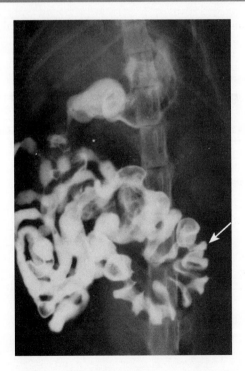

FIGURE 79.1. Linear foreign body: The classic radiographic sign of a linear foreign body is accordion pleating of the intestinal tract.

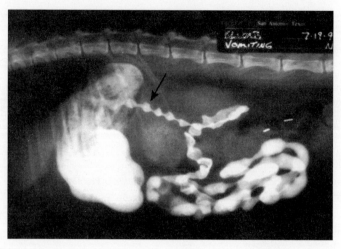

FIGURE 79.2. The "string of pearls" sign is a normal finding that can be mistaken for a linear foreign body.

Prognosis

The prognosis is good if surgery is performed before bacterial peritonitis occurs. The prognosis is guarded if bacterial peritonitis is present.

Suggested Reading

Sherding RG. Diseases of the intestines. In: Sherding RG, ed. The cat: diseases and clinical management, 2nd ed. Philadelphia: Churchill Livingstone, 1994;1211–1285.

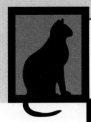

CHAPTER 80

Liver, Biliary, and Pancreatic Flukes

Gary D. Norsworthy

Overview

The cat may be infected with several species of flukes, including *Amphimerus pseudofelineus*, *Opisthorcus tenuicollis*, *Metorchus conjunctus*, and *Platynosomum concinnum*. The latter, *P. concinnum*, is the most common. Infections are limited to cats living in semitropical climates (especially Hawaii, south Florida, and Puerto Rico) and exposed to two intermediate hosts. *P. concinnum* is about 2 mm × 5 mm and lives in the bile ducts and gall bladder; it is occasionally found in the small intestine and pancreas. The first intermediate host is the land snail. The second intermediate host is most commonly a lizard (thus the term "lizard poisoning"), but it may be the Bufo toad, skink, or gecko. Adult flukes develop about 1 week after ingestion of the second intermediate host, and ova can be detected in the cat's feces about 2–3 months later. Many infected cats are asymptomatic, and others have nonspecific signs including vomiting, diarrhea, inappetence, weight loss, eosinophilia, and icterus. Because these signs are common in many other diseases, the detection of fluke ova does not necessarily mean that flukes are the causative agent.

Diagnosis

Primary Diagnostics

- **History and clinical signs:** Icteric cats in appropriate geographic locations should be suspected of flukes; however, there are many causes of icterus (See Chapter 15).

- **Fecal examination:** This is a specific but not extremely sensitive test because egg production is limited in number. Ova may be found on fecal floatation, but the most sensitive method is formalin-ether sedimentation (see Appendix F).

- **Ultrasound:** The findings include dilated hepatic ducts and bile duct and an enlarged gall bladder with echogenic (thickened) bile.

Ancillary Diagnostics

- **Laparotomy:** This is indicated when evidence of biliary obstruction is found. It permits liver biopsy and manual expression of the gallbladder to relieve biliary obstruction. If manual expression is not successful, the gallbladder should be explored and the bile duct cannulated and flushed. Sometimes, flukes and ova can be seen in the bile, grossly or microscopically.

Diagnostic Notes

Fecal floatation is not indicated. Direct fecal-saline preparations may reveal ova, but sedimentation techniques are best.

 T r e a t m e n t

Primary Therapeutics

- **Praziquantel:** Administer at 20 mg/kg SC SID for 3–5 days.
- **Supportive care:** Because some affected cats have profound anorexia, orogastric tube feeding or surgically-implanted tube feeding may be needed for several days. Dehydration should be corrected with a balanced electrolyte solution.

Secondary Therapeutics

- **Prednisolone:** This drug is indicated if the histopathology reveals significant eosinophilic pericholangitis. Begin at 1.1 mg/kg PO and taper after 1 week. Some cats require long-term treatment for chronic cholangiohepatitis.
- **Fenbendazole:** This drug is thought to be less efficacious than praziquantel. It has been given at 50 mg/kg PO BID for 5 days.
- **Ursodeoxycholic acid:** This drug is a choleretic agent that is dosed at 10–15 mg/kg PO SID. It is contraindicated in extrahepatic biliary obstruction.

Therapeutic Notes

Drugs that appear to be nonefficacious include thiabendazole, levamisole, and mebendazole.

P r o g n o s i s

The prognosis is good as long as appropriate supportive care is given. Limiting access to the intermediate hosts is important in preventing reinfection.

S u g g e s t e d   R e a d i n g s

Hitt ME. Liver fluke infection in South Florida cats. *Feline Pract* 1981;11:26.

Tams TR. Hepatobiliary parasites. In: Sherding RG, ed. The cat: diseases and clinical management, 2nd ed. Philadelphia: WB Saunders, 1994;607–611.

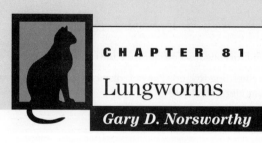

CHAPTER 81

Lungworms

Gary D. Norsworthy

Overview

L ungworms are helminths that live in the alveoli, bronchioles, bronchi, and trachea of cats. Many affected cats are asymptomatic, whereas many others develop a dry cough. This is one of the few causes of chronic coughing of cats and should be considered if the geographic area is endemic for feline lungworms.

There are two lungworms of the cat: *Capillaria aerophila* and *Aelurostrongylus abstrusus*. **Capillaria** has a direct life cycle and may be transmitted through earthworms and rodents. Cats are infected by ingestion of the embryonated ova or one of the paratenic hosts. Adult worms live within the epithelium of the trachea, bronchi, and bronchioles and produce ova about 40 days after infection. The ova are coughed up, swallowed, and passed in the feces. They become embryonated in 1–2 months but can survive in the environment for over a year. The cat becomes infected with **Aelurostrongylus** when it eats the intermediate hosts (snails or slugs) or paratenic hosts (birds, rodents, amphibians, or reptiles). The adults live in the alveoli and are capable of producing ova about 25 days after ingestion. The ova hatch and become larvae, which migrate up the bronchi and trachea into the pharynx. They are swallowed and passed in the feces, where they can survive for several months. An intense immune response, causing focal interstitial pneumonia, is responsible for elimination of the worms in most cats.

 Diagnosis

Primary Diagnostics

- **Clinical signs:** Many cats are asymptomatic. Others have a nonproductive cough, which can be elicited by tracheal palpation, or dyspnea due to secondary bacterial pneumonia.
- **Baermann fecal examination:** Larvae may be found, sometimes in large numbers.

- **Radiography:** Many cats have normal thoracic radiographs. Others have peribronchial infiltrates, bronchial thickening, or a diffuse interstitial pattern.
- **CBC:** Absolute and relative eosinophilia may occur.

Ancillary Diagnostics

- **Transtracheal wash, bronchial wash, or bronchoalveolar lavage:** Larvae may be recovered.
- **Tracheal endoscopy:** This examination may reveal inflamed bronchial or tracheal epithelium or large numbers of larvae.

Diagnostic Notes

A fecal examination using a Baermann apparatus should be performed on any coughing cat in a lungworm-endemic area.

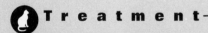Treatment

Primary Therapeutics

- **Fenbendazole:** Give 50 mg/kg/day for 10 days for capillariasis and for 21 days for aelurostrongylosis.

Secondary Therapeutics

- **Ivermectin:** Give 400 µg/kg subcutaneously or orally; repeat in 2 weeks.

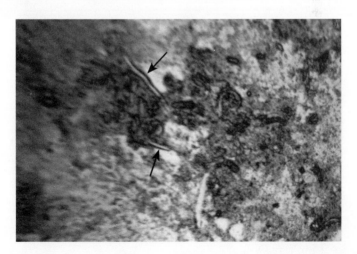

FIGURE 81.1. Lungworms: Lungworm larvae may be found using the Baermann technique in a fecal sample. This should be part of the diagnostic workup for coughing cats in lungworm-endemic areas.

Therapeutic Notes

Treatment is often unnecessary for capillariasis, and most cases of aelurostrongylosis will resolve spontaneously.

P r o g n o s i s

Feline lungworm infections may be self-limiting but also respond well to the listed anthelminthics. The prognosis is generally good.

S u g g e s t e d   R e a d i n g

Pechman RD. Respiratory parasites. In: Sherding RG, ed. The cat: diseases and clinical management, 2nd ed. Philadelphia: WB Saunders, 1994;613–622.

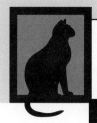

CHAPTER 82
Lymphoma
Mitchell A. Crystal

Overview

L ymphoma (also known as malignant lymphoma or lymphosarcoma) is the most common neoplasia in the cat, accounting for one-third of all feline neoplasms. It arises form lymphoid tissue and may involve any organ or tissue. Lymphoma is believed to be caused by the feline leukemia virus (FeLV), although alimentary and cutaneous lymphoma are usually FeLV negative and renal lymphoma is negative in about half of the cases. Other forms of lymphoma are usually positive but can be negative. Cats with feline immunodeficiency virus (FIV) infections are also at an increased risk of developing lymphoma.

The average age of cats with lymphoma is 3 years for those that are FeLV positive and 7 years for those that are FeLV negative. There is no sex or breed predilection. The most common anatomic form of lymphoma is alimentary lymphoma, followed by mediastinal and multicentric lymphoma (hepatosplenomegaly and generalized lymphadenopathy). Extralymphoid tissue sites are less common and include renal, ocular, bone marrow, central nervous system (CNS) (usually spinal leading to posterior paresis), cutaneous, pulmonary, and nasal lymphoma. Peripheral lymphadenopathy alone is rare and is more likely to be due to hyperplasia than lymphoma. Renal lymphoma may have a tendency to later involve the CNS. Clinical signs and differential diagnoses are variable depending on the organ/tissues involved.

Diagnosis

Primary Diagnostics

- **CBC:** Circulating lymphoblasts are occasionally found. Some cats may demonstrate cytopenias due to bone marrow involvement.
- **FeLV/FIV test:** About 70% of cats are FeLV positive.
- **Fine-needle aspiration/cytology or biopsy/histopathology of liver, spleen, mediastinal mass, kidney, or lymph node:** This is necessary to

cytologically or histopathologically confirm lymphoma involving these tissues.

- **Intestinal biopsy:** Intestinal biopsy by endoscopy, exploratory laparotomy, or ultrasound-guidance is necessary to confirm a diagnosis of alimentary lymphoma.

Ancillary Diagnostics

- **Chemistry profile and urinalysis:** Abnormalities may be found in renal (azotemia, decreased urine specific gravity) and multicentric (liver enzyme elevation) lymphoma. Hypercalcemia is rarely present; it is more common in the mediastinal form but still is rare. Hyperglobulinemia (monoclonal gammopathy) is uncommon.

- **Abdominal imaging:** Abnormalities may be found in renal, multicentric, and alimentary lymphoma.

- **Thoracic radiographs:** A mediastinal mass is present in mediastinal lymphoma.

- **Bone marrow aspirate/cytology:** This is necessary to confirm a diagnosis of bone marrow lymphoma and document bone marrow involvement with other forms of lymphoma. It also is helpful in confirming a diagnosis of spinal lymphoma; spinal lymphoma usually has bone marrow involvement and is more easily diagnosed with a bone marrow aspirate than a cerebrospinal fluid (CSF) tap.

- **CSF tap/cytology:** This can confirm CNS lymphoma but is less definitive than bone marrow aspiration; only 30–50% will demonstrate lymphoblasts in the CSF.

- **Skin biopsies/histopathology:** These are needed to confirm a diagnosis of cutaneous lymphoma.

Diagnostic Notes

- A negative FeLV test and/or lack of CBC changes does not exclude lymphoma.
- A positive FeLV test (without cytologic or histologic evidence of lymphoma in involved tissue) does not confirm or indicate a diagnosis of lymphoma.

T r e a t m e n t

Primary Therapeutics

- **Combination chemotherapy:** See Appendix B.

Secondary Therapeutics

- **Supportive care:** Fluids, nutritional supplementation, or other supportive measures may be needed depending on the location and severity of the lymphoma.

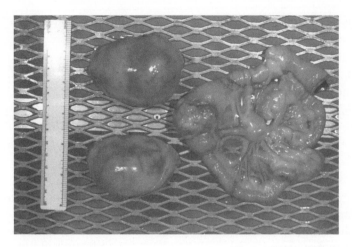

FIGURE 82.1. Lymphoma: Lymphoma can affect almost any organ in the body. The multicentric form affects several organs simultaneously, as seen in this cat with intestinal and renal disease.

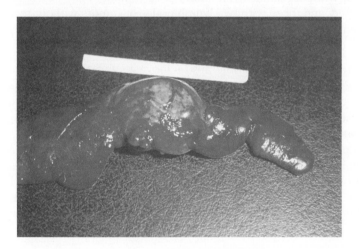

FIGURE 82.2. The spleen was the only organ involved with this cat.

Therapeutic Notes

- Chemotherapy generally is well tolerated. Most cats experience self-limiting side effects (anorexia, lethargy) at some point in the protocol. Serious side effects are infrequent and include vomiting, diarrhea, protracted anorexia, and sepsis (due to neutropenia) (see Appendix B).
- Prednisone alone will achieve remission in many cats; however, response rates and survival times are less than those achieved with combination chemotherapy.

- For more information on recognizing and managing chemotherapy reactions, see Appendix B.
- Radiation therapy is effective for localized lymphoma (e.g., single node, nasal).
- Cats that test positive for FeLV antigens will remain positive after successful chemotherapy and are contagious to other cats.

P r o g n o s i s

The prognosis for cats with lymphoma varies depending on several factors. Factors that improve survival times include: a negative FeLV test; a positive response to chemotherapy (cats that achieve complete remission have 5–7-month survival times, cats that achieve partial remission have 2-month survival times, and cats that do not respond to chemotherapy have 1–2-month survival times); a lack of significant clinical illness; and a less severe stage of disease (cats with a single tumor with or without regional lymph-node involvement, those with a single lymph node affected, and those with two lymph nodes or tumors without regional node involvement on the same side of the diaphragm have significantly better survival times than cats with more extensive disease).

Response rates to initial chemotherapy (achievement of complete remission) generally range from 60–80%, with the duration of initial remission ranging from 5–7 months. Second-time remission rates (rescue) and duration of remission are much reduced. About 30% of cats with lymphoma undergoing chemotherapy survive greater than 1 year. A positive FeLV status does not affect response to therapy but is associated with decreased survival times when compared with FeLV negative cats. Little information is available for cutaneous lymphoma. The prognosis with alimentary lymphoma varies. On the average, remission of alimentary lymphoma can be sustained with cyclical combination chemotherapy for about 50 to 200 days, although some cats will be less responsive, and some will have response rates in excess of 1 to 2 years.

S u g g e s t e d   R e a d i n g s

MacEwen GE. Feline lymphoma and leukemias. In: Withrow SJ, MacEwen EG, eds. Small animal clinical oncology, 2nd ed. Philadelphia: WB Saunders, 1996;479–495.

Mauldin GE, Mooney SC, Maleo KA, Matus RE, Mauldin GN. Chemotherapy in 132 cats with lymphoma: 1988–1994. Proceedings of the Veterinary Cancer Society 15th Annual Conference 1995;35–36.

Moore AS, Mahony OM. Treatment of feline malignant lymphoma. In: Bonagura JD, ed. Kirk's current veterinary therapy XII: small animal practice. Philadelphia: WB Saunders, 1995;498–502.

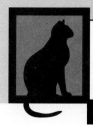

CHAPTER 83

Mast Cell Tumors

Mitchell A. Crystal

Overview

Mast cell tumors are the second most common feline skin tumor (following basal cell tumors). There are two forms: a mastocytic form that histologically resembles normal mast cells and a histiocytic form that histologically has features of histiocytic mast cells. Cats with an average age of 10 years are most commonly affected by the mastocytic form, and Siamese cats may be predisposed; however, tumors have been reported in all breeds of all ages. Young Siamese cats are predisposed to the histiocytic cutaneous form. Mast cell tumors may be cutaneous or visceral.

Cutaneous mast cell tumors are often benign but can metastasize to the regional lymph nodes, spleen, liver, bone marrow, and, rarely, the lung. Reports of rates of metastasis vary from 0 to 22%. Cutaneous tumors occur more commonly on the head and neck, may be pruritic or nonpruritic, and have a variety of appearances (solitary or multiple, soft or firm, raised or plaque-like, papules or nodules, well-circumscribed or poorly demarcated, pink, red, white, or yellow, ulcerated or nonulcerated, alopecic or nonalopecic). The histiocytic cutaneous form seen in 6-week-old to 4-year-old Siamese cats appear as multiple, firm, pinkish papules on the head and pinnae that spontaneously regress over 4 to 24 months. Clinical signs in cats without metastasis are limited to the presence of the tumor. Differential diagnoses for cutaneous mast cell tumor include squamous cell carcinoma, melanoma, basal cell tumor, fibrosarcoma, cutaneous hemangioma or hemangiosarcoma, hair follicle tumors, and sebaceous gland tumors.

Visceral mast cell tumors occur most commonly in the spleen and less commonly in the liver and intestine. Visceral mast cell tumors are much more likely to metastasize than the cutaneous form. Common presenting signs include lethargy, anorexia, vomiting (secondary to histamine-induced gastric erosions or ulcers) and weight loss. Splenomegaly, hepatomegaly, abdominal effusion, or an abdominal mass may be found on physical examination. Differential diagnoses for systemic mast cell tumor include lymphoma and neoplasia of abdominal organs/structures.

Diagnosis

Primary Diagnostics

- **Fine-needle aspiration/cytology:** This simple test may be performed on cutaneous and visceral (spleen, liver, lymph nodes, intestine) lesions. Effusions, if present (abdominal or thoracic), are often diagnostic. The histiocytic form is more difficult to diagnose with fine-needle aspiration.
- **Surgical removal or biopsy and histopathology:** This is definitive.
- **CBC:** Anemia may be present from splenic sequestration, gastrointestinal hemorrhage, or bone marrow involvement. Mastocytemia may be present in cats with metastatic disease.

Ancillary Diagnostics

- **Buffy coat preparation:** This may reveal mastocytemia in cats with metastatic disease. A negative result does not exclude metastatic disease.
- **Bone marrow aspiration:** This may reveal infiltration with malignant mast cells.
- **Abdominal imaging:** Radiographs and ultrasound may reveal hepatomegaly, splenomegaly, abdominal lymphadenopathy, abdominal effusion, or intestinal masses.
- **Thoracic imaging:** Mast cell tumors rarely metastasize to intrathoracic locations, although pleural effusions have been reported.
- **Coagulation profile:** Abnormalities have been reported in a significant number of cats with splenic mast cell tumors. These abnormalities are rarely clinically significant.

Diagnostic Notes

- Histologic appearance may help predict metastatic potential. Tumors with a high mitotic index and an anaplastic appearance may be more likely to metastasize.
- A complete systemic evaluation (CBC, buffy coat preparation, bone marrow aspiration, abdominal and/or thoracic imaging) will define the extent of the disease and assist in selection of the most appropriate therapeutic approach. This should be performed in all visceral mast cell tumors and in cutaneous mast cell tumors with lymphadenopathy or an aggressive histologic appearance.
- Up to 50% of cats with splenic mast cell tumors have buffy coat and/or bone marrow involvement.
- Mast cell granules occasionally do not stain well with quick-staining methods.

⬤ T r e a t m e n t

Primary Therapeutics

- **Surgical excision:** Complete removal is curative in most cases of cutaneous mast cell tumor. Splenectomy in cats with splenic mast cell tumors (with or without effusions or involvement of other organs) will prolong survival time. Median survival times are: without splenectomy, 6 months; with splenectomy, 19 months.

Secondary Therapeutics

- **Laser ablation, cryotherapy, electrosurgery for cutaneous lesions:** These may be used to remove lesions on the skin.
- **Antihistamines:** Both H_1 (diphenhydramine [2.2 mg/kg BID-TID PO, IM, slowly IV] or chlorpheniramine [2.2 mg/kg BID-TID PO]) and H_2 blockers (ranitidine [3.5 mg/kg BID PO, IV], cimetidine [10 mg/kg TID-QID PO, IV], or famotidine [0.5 mg/kg SID-BID PO]), may help control systemic effects in cats with disseminated or extensive disease.

Therapeutic Notes

- Wide surgical margins (3 cm) should be attempted. Reported recurrence rates are from 0 to 24% and usually occur within 6 months.
- Intestinal mast cell tumors require removal of 5 to 10 cm of bowel on either side of the lesion. Microscopic extension usually exceeds visible gross disease.

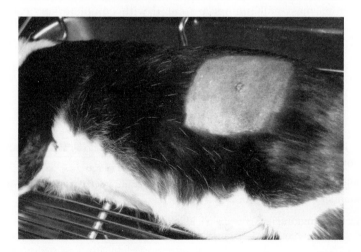

FIGURE 83.1. Mast cell tumor: Mast cell tumors may appear to be small, insignificant masses, or have the look and feel of a lipoma.

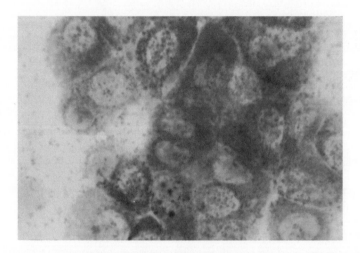

FIGURE 83.2. The characteristic cells can be aspirated and identified easily with a modified Wright's stain. The granules are deep purple and may be found extracellularly, because the cells rupture easily.

- The effectiveness of chemotherapy (including corticosteroids) and radiation therapy have not been evaluated in the cat. Chemotherapy (including corticosteroids) has been used in a limited number of cases without apparent improvement in survival times.

Prognosis

Most cutaneous mast cell tumors are cured with complete surgical excision. Splenic mast cell tumors have a median survival time of 19 months with splenectomy and 6 months without splenectomy. Nonsplenic visceral and metastatic mast cell tumors carry a poor prognosis.

Suggested Readings

Elmslie RE. Basal cell tumor. In: Smith FWK, Tilley LP, eds. The 5-minute veterinary consult. Baltimore: Williams & Wilkins, 1996; 387.

Scott DW, Miller WH, Griffin CE. Miller & Kirk's small animal dermatology, 5th ed. Philadelphia: WB Saunders, 1995;1056–1064.

Vail DM. Mast cell tumors. In: Withrow SJ, MacEwen EG, eds. Small animal clinical oncology, 2nd ed. Philadelphia: WB Saunders, 1996;202–210.

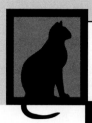

CHAPTER 84

Mammary Gland Neoplasia

Mitchell A. Crystal

Overview

Mammary gland neoplasia is the third most common neoplasia in the cat (following hematopoietic and skin neoplasia), accounting for 17% of all neoplasms in the female cat. Mammary gland neoplasia occurs at an average age of 10 to 12 years but has a reported age range of 9 months to 23 years. Siamese cats may be at an increased risk of developing mammary gland neoplasia and may acquire tumors at a younger age. Intact female cats are most commonly affected, suggesting that an hormonal influence may be involved. Reports have shown that some mammary tumors contain progesterone receptors, and that some cats have developed mammary neoplasia following prior progesterone administration. In the dog, early ovariohysterectomy has a sparing effect on the incidence of mammary neoplasia.

Feline mammary tumors are malignant 80–90% of the time (in contrast to 42% of the time in dogs). The most common tumor type is the adenocarcinoma (tubular, papillary, or solid), which presents as singular or multiple nodules or as a diffuse swelling. Tumors may be present in one or more glands and are often ulcerated. In addition, they may incite a marked inflammatory response or produce secretions that resemble lactation. Metastasis is common and often involves regional lymph nodes, lungs, pleura, and/or liver. Regional lymph node metastasis typically occurs in the inguinal lymph nodes for tumors involving the caudal four mammae and in the axillary lymph nodes for tumors involving the cranial four mammae.

Benign mammary gland adenoma is uncommon and presents as a small, single, firm nodule. This is a differential diagnosis for malignant mammary neoplasia. Other differential diagnoses include malignant and benign skin tumors, mastitis, and mammary gland hyperplasia. Mammary gland hyperplasia can present as massive enlargement of the mammary glands soon after pregnancy or pseudopregnancy or within a year of ovariohysterectomy. This hyperplasia occurs as a result of rapidly decreasing progesterone levels, stimulating prolactin secretion and growth of mammary tissue (see Chapter 85).

Diagnosis

Primary Diagnostics

- **Surgical excision/histopathology:** This is the procedure of choice for diagnosis and treatment (see below). Because 80–90% of mammary gland tumors are malignant, a diagnosis should be based on histopathology rather than cytology.

Ancillary Diagnostics

- **Lymph node aspiration/cytology:** This may reveal evidence of regional metastasis. Lymph node aspiration/cytology should be performed whenever lymphadenopathy is seen in combination with mammary tumors.
- **Thoracic radiographs:** These may reveal evidence of metastasis to the lungs, pleura, or intrathoracic lymph nodes. Thoracic radiographs should be performed prior to anesthesia and surgery in all cats with mammary tumors.
- **Pleurocentesis/cytology:** This is indicated if pleural effusion is present. Cytologic evaluation of fluid collected may reveal evidence of metastasis.
- **Fine-needle aspiration/cytology:** This may suggest whether a tumor is malignant or benign.

Diagnostic Notes

Mammary tumor fine-needle aspiration/cytology alone should not be used to determine a definitive diagnosis, as a geographical miss during aspiration of a tumor may delay a diagnosis of malignancy and rapid surgical intervention. If fine-needle aspiration suggests a benign or non-neoplastic lesion, a less aggressive surgery (i.e., local removal instead of radical mastectomy) may be initially planned to confirm the diagnosis.

Treatment

Primary Therapeutics

- **Surgical excision:** This is the treatment of choice for mammary gland neoplasia. Current recommendations include unilateral radical mastectomy for mammary tumors confined to one side. Bilateral radical mastectomy (simultaneous bilateral radical mastectomy or unilateral radical mastectomy staged 2–3 weeks apart) is indicated if there is disease in both left and right mammary chains. The inguinal lymph nodes should always be removed at the time of surgery, whereas the axillary lymph nodes should only be removed if they are palpably enlarged.

Secondary Therapeutics

- **Chemotherapy:** Doxorubicin (20–30 mg/m^2 IV, slowly [over 10 to 15 minutes], on day 0) followed by cyclophosphamide (50 mg/m^2 PO on days 3,4,5, and 6) can be used once every 3 weeks for three to six treatments in cats with metastatic and/or nonresectable disease. This protocol has been shown to significantly increase survival time. Complete or partial responses can be seen in 50% of cats (one study reported survival times of 283 days in cats receiving therapy versus 57 days in cats without therapy). Dose-limiting side effects include profound anorexia and moderate myelosuppression. Side effects are decreased by either dosing doxorubicin at 20 mg/m^2 or substituting mitoxantrone at 5 mg/m^2 for doxorubicin in the above protocol.

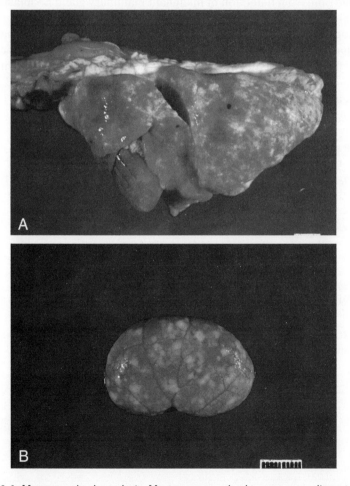

FIGURE 84.1. Mammary gland neoplasia: Most mammary gland tumors are malignant and metastasize early, often before the mammary mass is detected. Metastasis may occur to the lungs (*A*), kidneys (*B*), or other organs.

- **Pleurocentesis:** Therapeutic pleurocentesis should be considered for cats that are dyspneic as a result of pleural metastasis/pleural effusion.

Therapeutic Notes

- Radiation, immune therapy, and endocrine therapy have not been shown to improve survival times in cats with mammary gland neoplasia.
- Controlled studies evaluating mastectomy with or without chemotherapy and chemotherapy with or without mastectomy have not been published.

Prognosis

The average time from detection of malignant mammary gland neoplasia to death is 1 year. Significant factors affecting survival include the size (most important) and histologic grade of the tumor. Cats with tumors that are greater than 3 cm in diameter have a median survival time of 4 to 6 months; cats with tumors that are 2–3 cm in diameter have a median survival time of 2 years; and cats with tumors that are less than 2 cm in diameter have a median survival time of over 3 years. Tumors with a high histologic grade (poor cellular differentiation, high mitotic index) have a worse prognosis than those of low histologic grade. About 10% of cats with a high-grade histologic tumor type will survive 1 year compared with 50% of cats with a low-grade histologic tumor type. The extent of the surgical procedure affects the recurrence rate of the tumor but does not affect the cat's survival time. Cats undergoing radical mastectomy had a reduced rate of local recurrence (i.e., improved disease-free survival time) than did cats undergoing local surgical removal.

Suggested Readings

Hahn KA. Adjuvant chemotherapy in feline mammary carcinoma. Proceedings of the Thirteenth Annual Veterinary Medical Forum 1995;885–889.

MacEwen EG, Withrow SJ. Tumors of the mammary gland. In: Withrow SJ, MacEwen EG, eds. Small animal clinical oncology, 2nd ed. Philadelphia: WB Saunders, 1996;356–372.

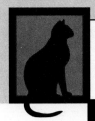

CHAPTER 85

Mammary Hyperplasia

Gary D. Norsworthy

Overview

Mammary hyperplasia, or rapid growth of mammary tissue, involves both epithelial and mesenchymal tissue. Its typical presentation is in young, cycling females. However, it also has been associated with exogenous progestin administration in neutered male and female cats. It is considered a benign condition, but it must be differentiated from mammary neoplasia.

D i a g n o s i s

Primary Diagnostics

- **Clinical findings:** Rapid growth of mammary glands is typical. This may occur in cycling female cats and in cats of both genders receiving progesterone compounds.

Ancillary Diagnostics

- **Biopsy and histopathology:** These are important as means of differentiating this condition from mammary neoplasia.

Diagnostic Notes

Serum progesterone concentrations are increased in about one-third of affected cats, so this is not a sensitive diagnostic tool.

T r e a t m e n t

Primary Therapeutics

- **Progesterone withdrawal:** If the source of progesterone can be withdrawn, the condition will correct itself. Unspayed females should be spayed.

- **Spontaneous remission:** Cats not receiving progesterone compounds usually have remission within a few weeks.

Secondary Therapeutics

- **Analgesics:** Pain-relieving medication can make the cat more comfortable.
- **Mastectomy:** This surgical procedure should be considered if the abnormal tissue outgrows its blood supply or if progesterone withdrawal does not produce a cure.

P r o g n o s i s

The prognosis for mammary hyperplasia is good. Spontaneous remission occurs in some cats, and progesterone withdrawal cures most others.

S u g g e s t e d   R e a d i n g

Johnson CA. Female reproduction and disorders of the female reproductive tract. In: Sherding RG, ed. The cat: diseases and clinical management, 2nd ed. Philadelphia: WB Saunders, 1994;1855–1876.

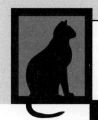

CHAPTER 86

Megacolon

Mitchell A. Crystal

Overview

I diopathic megacolon is an acquired condition of colonic dilation and decreased motility that usually is associated with constipation or obstipation due to colonic dysfunction from unknown etiology. Muscular dysfunction is thought to be the cause of this disease. Cats of a wide age range are affected (1–15 years of age), with 1 study of 38 cats reporting a mean age of 4.9 years. There is no breed or sex predilection. Obese, less-active cats may be at an increased risk. Clinical signs of megacolon include chronic constipation/obstipation with poor responses to treatment with laxatives and enemas. Clinical signs may be present for weeks to years. Physical examination reveals a distended colon and no other abnormal findings.

The differential diagnosis for idiopathic megacolon should include causes of acquired colonic distention and constipation such as extralumenal constriction (pelvic fractures, neoplasia), intralumenal constriction (foreign bodies, impacted ingesta, neoplasia), pseudocoprostasis (matting of hair and debris in the perineal area, obstructing passage of feces), colonic or rectal stricture, perineal hernia, dyschezia (such as that due to inflammatory disease of the rectoanal area), lumbosacral disease (trauma, stenosis, deformities like those of the manx cat), hypokalemia, drug therapy (vincristine, antacids, sucralfate, phosphate binders, anticholinergics, narcotic analgesics), and dysautonomia. Environmental stress or changes as well as an inability to posture and use the litter box (e.g., due to hindlimb fractures, hip dysplasia, bilateral luxating patallae) may also lead to decreased bowel movements and subsequent constipation and colonic distention.

Diagnosis

Primary Diagnostics

- **History:** The client should be questioned about any changes in the environment, the household or diet, whether the cat's defecation is painful, and if any current drug therapy is in use.

- **Neurologic examination:** A complete neurologic examination should be performed with close attention paid to the perineal area. Signs of lumbosacral disease, such as poor anal tone, easily expressible bladder, hind-limb weakness, or pain on lifting the tail or palpating the caudal spinal area, may be evident. If these signs are found, lumbosacral spinal radiographs with or without an epidurogram should be performed. Signs of diffuse autonomic dysfunction indicating the need for further evaluation of the autonomic nervous system may be seen in the rare event of dysautonomia.

- **Chemistry profile and urinalysis:** These may reveal abnormalities in serum potassium, hydration status, and renal function.

- **Abdominal/pelvic radiographs:** These are indicated to confirm diffuse colonic distention, look for masses and foreign bodies, search for evidence of stricture (colonic fecal distention in the cranial but not the caudal portion of colon), evaluate the pelvis for fractures, and examine the lumbosacral area for obvious abnormalities.

- **Rectal examination:** This is best performed under anesthesia in conjunction with initial therapy (enema administration/manual colonic evacuation). The rectoanal area should be evaluated for rectal strictures, masses, and perineal hernias.

Ancillary Diagnostics

- **Colonoscopy with biopsy/histopathology:** This is indicated if the cat has a history of painful defecation or if radiography or rectal examination reveals the possibility of a mass, stricture, or foreign body. Colonic evacuation and preparation with oral cathartic solutions (polyethylene-glycol solutions at 30 mL/kg PO via orogastric or nasogastric tube 18–24 and 8–12 hours prior to colonoscopy) are needed prior to performing colonoscopy.

Diagnostic Notes

- Barium enemas may be helpful in identifying colonic strictures or masses but are usually less helpful than colonoscopy.

- Other differential diagnoses for colonic distention/constipation must be excluded prior to making a diagnosis of idiopathic megacolon.

T r e a t m e n t

Primary Therapeutics

- **Treat any underlying causes:** The idiopathic form of this disease has no underlying cause, but many cases are secondary to another disease.

- **Enema administration/manual colonic evacuation:** This is indicated as the initial step in the medical management of megacolon. This is best performed with the cat under anesthesia. The enema should utilize 15–20 mL/kg of warm water without soap or other additives (to minimize mucosal irritation and damage). The volume delivered should be repeated several times to completely empty the colon. Manual evacuation via abdominal palpation and rectal digital manipulation should be performed in conjunction with enema administration for maximal colonic evacuation. A small amount of water-soluble lubrication will help in removing feces.

- **Cisapride:** This is a prokinetic motility enhancer that has proven effective and is the drug of choice in combination with stool softeners in the medical management of megacolon. The dose is 5–7.5 mg/cat PO TID.

- **Diet:** Fiber creates a soft stool with some increased bulk, which might be helpful in managing megacolon. However, diets high in fiber may create excessive fecal bulk and complicate or worsen colonic distention. Easily digestible, low-bulk diets (see Appendix E) with or without fiber supplementation (e.g., psyllium (Vetasyl, Metamucil) at 1/2–1 teaspoons (about 1.7–3.4 g) PO with food SID-BID or canned pumpkin at 1–2 teaspoons PO with food SID-BID) are indicated in megacolon treatment.

Secondary Therapeutics

- **Lactulose:** This is an osmotic stool softener that may help in managing megacolon when used in combination with cisapride. The dose is 0.5–1.0 mL/kg PO BID-TID.

- **Subtotal colectomy:** This is an effective therapy for megacolon and should be recommended if medical management has failed on more than two or three attempts.

Therapeutic Notes

- Assuring proper hydration by administering IV fluids at one-and-a-half times the maintenance dose (70–80 mL/kg/day) for 12-24 hours prior to anesthesia and enema will facilitate more complete, faster, and easier colonic evacuation.

- A large number of stool softeners, available commercially, can be used in combination with cisapride to attempt to medically manage megacolon.

- Stool softeners, laxatives, and diet change, in combination or alone (without cisapride), are rarely effective in the management of idiopathic megacolon.

- Most surgeons prefer to perform a subtotal colectomy without prior colonic evacuation.

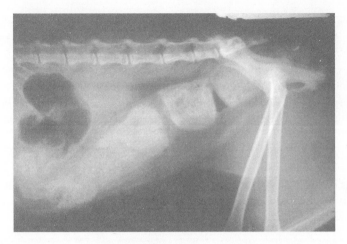

FIGURE 86.1. Megacolon: The colon of an obstipated cat is easily palpable. Its diameter should be at least two times the diameter of the body of L7.

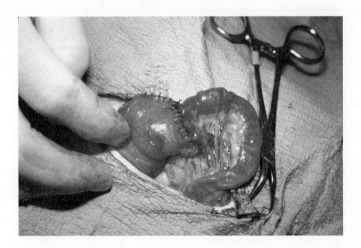

FIGURE 86.2. Most cats ultimately need a subtotal colectomy, because conservative therapy usually fails after weeks or months.

Prognosis

Megacolon can often be controlled with prolonged doses of therapy with cisapride, stool softener, and dietary therapy, although a large number of cats will require subtotal colectomy to prevent frequent recurrences of constipation/obstipation. Cats that respond to medical management may still have infrequent episodes of constipation/obstipation that require enema therapy.

Significant postoperative complications occur in only 2% of cats that undergo subtotal colectomy and may include stricture at the surgical site and anastamosis dehiscence/peritonitis. Common, transient postoperative problems include tenesmus and diarrhea. Tenesmus usually resolves within a few days of surgery. Diarrhea usually resolves within 6 weeks of surgery (80% of the cats in one study), although it has been documented to persist for as long as 6 months. A small number of cats may develop constipation weeks to months following surgery, but this usually responds to medical management.

S u g g e s t e d   R e a d i n g s

DeNovo RC, Bright RM. Chronic feline constipation/obstipation. In: Bonagura JD, Kirk RW, eds. Current veterinary therapy XI: small animal practice. Philadelphia: WB Saunders, 1992;619–626.

Dimski DS. Pathophysiology and treatment of constipation. Proceedings of the Ninth Annual Veterinary Medical Forum 1991;153–155.

Rosin E. Megacolon in cats: the role of colectomy. In: Lieb MS, ed. Small animal practice. Philadelphia: WB Saunders, *Vet Clin North Am* 1993;23(3):587–594.

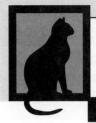

CHAPTER 87

Meningioma

Sharon K. Fooshee

Overview

Meningioma, the most common primary brain tumor of the cat, arises from connective tissue elements of the meninges. Intracranial meningiomas are more common than intraspinal ones, and the tumor is most often found in the meningeal covering of the cerebral hemispheres. Growth is by expansion or excavation of nearby brain tissue, rather than by infiltration of the tissue, thus explaining the typical slow onset of clinical signs. The cause of this benign brain tumor is unknown. There is no known breed disposition; old cats are more frequently affected than young cats. Some reports have suggested that male cats may have a slightly greater incidence of meningiomas than female cats. Frequently, multiple tumors are present.

 D i a g n o s i s

Primary Diagnostics

- **Clinical signs:** Signs of neurologic disturbance may be acute or chronic in onset; usually, they are slowly progressive in nature. A change in mentation is commonly noted—for example, aggression, depression, or stupor. Physical examination is suggestive of a focal cerebral lesion. If circling occurs, it is toward the side of the lesion. Visual, postural, and proprioceptive deficits are contralateral to the tumor. Occasionally, the fifth and seventh cranial nerves are affected. Seizures are not consistently a feature of this tumor but can occur.

- **Radiography:** Skull radiographs can demonstrate a calcified meningioma. Hyperostosis of the adjacent calvarium (or erosion of the calvarium) may be recognized.

- **Magnetic resonance imaging and computed tomography scans:** These diagnostic imaging techniques are very helpful in detecting the presence of an intracranial mass.

- **Electroencephalography (EEG):** The EEG will not establish a definitive diagnosis of meningioma but can be useful in localizing a cerebral lesion.

Ancillary Diagnostics

- **Cerebral spinal fluid (CSF) collection and analysis:** CSF analysis is unlikely to establish the diagnosis of meningioma. Nonspecific findings of increased CSF protein and normal cell counts (albuminocytologic dissociation) may be reported. Occasionally, cell counts are increased. Cytology usually is normal. Collection of CSF may lead to herniation when intracranial pressure (ICP) is increased; therefore, this procedure is generally not recommended when meningioma is strongly suspected.

Diagnostic Notes

Other types of primary brain tumors and tumors that metastasize to the brain are usually more rapidly progressive than meningiomas.

 T r e a t m e n t

Primary Therapeutics

- **Surgical excision:** Surgical excision of all visible tumor gives a good prognosis. This tumor grows so slowly that, even if microscopic tumor remains, most cats will do well for a long period following surgery. One retrospective study suggested that adjunctive radiation therapy is only indicated when surgery does not remove all visible tumor or there is recurrence of the tumor.

Secondary Therapeutics

- **Corticosteroids:** Tumor-related edema may be managed with glucocorticoids.
- **Anticonvulsant therapy:** Phenobarbital is the anticonvulsant of choice for cats with meningioma. Side effects of anticonvulsant therapy may appear similar to tumor-related signs.

Therapeutic Notes

- Only those experienced with cranial surgery should attempt to remove this tumor.
- The anesthetic protocol should strive to minimize increases in ICP. Ketamine should be avoided for this reason. An ultra-short-acting barbiturate is preferred for induction because of the effect on ICP. Mildly hyperventilating the patient is also beneficial, as it causes vasoconstriction and a decrease in ICP.

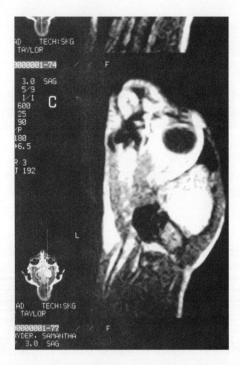

Figure 87.1. The large mass caudal to the eye is an extradural meningioma that was causing circling and a head tilt. It was removed surgically, and the signs resolved.

- Preoperative CT scans can be helpful in identifying the correct location for craniotomy.
- Brain herniation is a risk during the immediate postoperative period; the patient should be monitored carefully for signs of this complication.

Prognosis

The prognosis is improved significantly when surgical intervention succeeds in localizing and excising the tumor. Otherwise, the long-term prognosis is poor.

Suggested Readings

Braund KG, Ribas JL. Central nervous system meningiomas. *Compend Contin Educ Pract Vet* 1986;8:241–249.

Gallagher JG, Berg J, Knowles KE, Williams LL, Bronson RT. Prognosis after surgical excision of cerebral meningiomas in cats: 17 cases (1986–1992). *J Am Vet Med Assoc* 1993;203: 1437–1440.

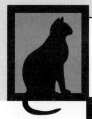

CHAPTER 88
Methemoglobinemia and Heinz-Body Hemolytic Anemia
Sharon K. Fooshee

Overview

Oxidative agents cause two major types of injury to feline erythrocytes. The first, Heinz body (HB) formation, occurs when feline hemoglobin is denatured and precipitates on the erythrocyte membrane. Feline hemoglobin is an easy target for oxidative injury since it contains more sulfhydryl groups per molecule than other species; conformational changes in the sulfhydryl molecule lead to formation of the HB. Additionally, the feline spleen is relatively inefficient at removing HB aggregates from the erythrocyte. As a consequence of these distinctions, even clinically normal cats have greater numbers of HB in circulation compared with other species. The irreversible cellular damage caused by HB formation leads to a primarily extravascular Heinz-body hemolytic anemia (HBHA) when the erythrocyte reaches a critical level of fragility and must be cleared from circulation. The second type of oxidative injury, methemoglobinemia, is reversible; it develops when the ferrous ($+2$) iron of hemoglobin is oxidized to the ferric ($+3$) state, rendering hemoglobin incapable of carrying oxygen. With HBHA, mucous membranes will be pale and perhaps icteric. Weakness, depression, and tachypnea are other significant clinical signs. When methemoglobinemia is present, the membranes will be cyanotic or brownish.

 D i a g n o s i s

Primary Diagnostics

- **Clinical signs:** When methemoglobinemia is present, the membranes will be cyanotic or brownish. This is an important sign.
- **CBC:** HB are visible with routine blood stains and wet mounts of new methylene-blue stain (the stain commonly used to identify reticulocytes). HB appears as large single inclusions that may bulge from the cell surface. Within a few days of HBHA onset, a regenerative response is reflected with increasing numbers of circulating reticulocytes.

Ancillary Diagnostics

As a screening test for methemoglobinemia, a spot of the patient's blood can be placed on a piece of white absorbent paper and compared with a spot of a control patient's blood. Methemoglobinemia makes the patient's blood noticeably brown compared to that of the control. Also, larger commercial laboratories may be able to assay blood for methemoglobin levels. Send a feline control sample along with the patient's blood and contact the lab for details on proper submission.

Diagnostic Notes

The presence of large numbers of HBs in a cat does not necessarily indicate an impending hemolytic crisis, as the HBs may be present in a variety of diseases. Because a wide variety of chemical agents may cause oxidant injury to feline erythrocytes, a detailed history is important. Potential causes of HBHA and methemoglobinemia include methylene blue, acetaminophen, benzocaine, phenazopyridine, and methionine. Propylene glycol, now discontinued as a humectant in semimoist cat foods, was previously a significant cause of HB formation.

 T r e a t m e n t

Primary Therapeutics

- Generally, supportive care is the only requirement for treating HBHA. With appropriate bone marrow stimulation, reticulocytes will replace damaged erythrocytes within a few days. Rarely, a transfusion of whole blood is needed. The kidneys should be protected against hemoglobin-induced injury with fluid therapy.
- For details on treatment of methemoglobinemia, refer to Chapter 25.

Therapeutic Notes

Be sure that all potential causes of ongoing oxidative injury to erythrocytes are avoided.

P r o g n o s i s

Although HBHA is nonreversible, the prognosis for recovery from it is better than for the cat with methemoglobinemia. Methemoglobinemia will result in the death of the cat if its oxygen-carrying potential drops below a critical level. The cat with methemoglobinemia is less likely to survive without intervention than is the cat with HBHA.

S u g g e s t e d   R e a d i n g s

Harvey JW. Methemoglobinemia and Heinz-body hemolytic anemia. In: Kirk RW, Bonagura J, eds. Current veterinary therapy XII. Philadelphia: WB Saunders, 1995;443–446.

Norsworthy GD. Heinz-body hemolytic anemia and methemoglobinemia. In: Norsworthy GD, ed. Feline practice. Philadelphia: JB Lippincott, 1993;384–387.

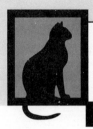

CHAPTER 89

Mitral Valve Dysplasia

John-Karl Goodwin

Overview

Mitral valve dysplasia (MVD) is a common congenital cardiac anomaly of the cat. A wide spectrum of lesions has been observed including abnormal papillary muscle structure and dysplasia of chordae tendineae and mitral valve leaflets. MVD may be seen in conjunction with other congenital abnormalities such as ventricular septal defects. The typical lesion is one of valvular incompetence that results in mitral regurgitation of blood into the left atrium. There may also be a component of valvular stenosis.

Physical examination typically reveals a prominent (grade IV to VI) holosystolic regurgitant murmur over the mitral valve area. The cardiac impulse may also be displaced due to significant cardiomegaly in association with ventricular volume overload.

Cats may be presented for evaluation of a murmur heard during routine examination or may have developed signs of left-sided congestive heart failure (tachypnea, dyspnea). Weight loss may occur. Most affected cats exhibit a degree of fatigue during exertion.

 D i a g n o s i s

Primary Tests

- **Radiography:** Prominent left atrial enlargement occurs with variable left ventricular enlargement. There may be enlargement of the pulmonary veins, venous congestions, and pulmonary edema. Pleural effusion is uncommon.

- **Echocardiography:** Severe left atrial enlargement is typically present. Dysplasia of the mitral valve leaflets (shortened, malformed leaflets) and chordae tendineae are evident. There is variable left ventricular enlargement. Contractility is usually within normal limits or slightly increased.

- **Electrocardiography:** Evidence of left ventricular enlargement (tall and wide R waves) and left atrial enlargement (widened P waves) may be seen. Atrial arrhythmias (atrial premature complexes) may also occur.

Ancillary Diagnostics

- **Doppler echocardiography:** This will demonstrate significant mitral regurgitation. The extent of the regurgitant jet, rather than the velocity, correlates well with severity.

Diagnostic Notes

Many cats present within the first 2 years of life, although it is not unusual for cats to survive for years without clinical signs when the lesion is mild.

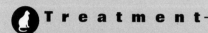 T r e a t m e n t

Primary Therapeutics: Congestive Heart Failure

- **Stress:** Take all measures to minimize any stress to cats exhibiting respiratory distress (e.g., delay radiographs and catheter placement).
- **Facilitate breathing:** Thoracocentesis should be performed when pleural effusion is suspected (muffled lung sounds). Furosemide should be administered when pulmonary edema is present. In the crisis setting, give 2–4 mg/kg IV initially, then 1–2 mg/kg IV or IM every 4–6 hours until the edema has resolved. Furosemide is often continued as needed (6.25–12.5 mg SID-BID) to control edema formation. One-fourth inch of nitroglycerin should be applied to a hairless area every 4–6 hours until the edema has resolved.
- **Oxygen:** Administer by face mask, if tolerated, or by oxygen cage or tent (50% oxygen).

Secondary Therapeutics

- **Enalapril:** Give 0.25 mg/kg SID.
- **Digoxin:** Give if contractility is reduced. Administer one-quarter of a 0.125-mg tablet every 24 to 48 hours.
- **Aspirin:** This may reduce the chance of thrombus formation. Give 81 mg every third day.
- **Periodic centesis:** Thoracocentesis or abdominocentesis may be needed periodically.

Therapeutic Notes

- Monitor renal function if enalapril or digoxin is used.

- Warfarin (5 mg SID) may be used in lieu of aspirin but has a much greater chance of inducing hemorrhagic crisis.
- Surgical correction of the defect has been of limited success and is associated with high morbidity and cost.

Prognosis

The prognosis for cats with MVD depends on the severity of the valvular incompetence and degree of ventricular volume overloading. Cats with mild lesions usually remain asymptomatic and have a good prognosis. Cats with significant lesions and evidence of moderate-to-severe volume overload early in life have a guarded-to-poor prognosis and usually develop congestive heart failure.

Suggested Reading

Fox PR. Congenital feline heart disease. In: Fox PR, ed. Canine and feline cardiology. New York: Churchill Livingstone, 1988;391–408.

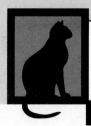

CHAPTER 90

Nasal and Frontal Sinus Infections

Gary D. Norsworthy

Overview

There are three common categories of infection in the nasal cavity and frontal sinuses: bacterial, viral, and fungal. All three are likely to be chronic and produce a nasal discharge. Several theories are related to the pathophysiology of these disorders. One author feels that most disorders are idiopathic, whereas others feel that most begin as a chronic infection with the feline herpesvirus or the feline calicivirus. The latter theory states that a chronic viral infection predisposes the cat to secondary bacterial or even fungal infections. The bacteria most commonly cultured include *Pseudomonas aeruginosa*, *Proteus mirabilis*, and *Staphylococcus aureus*. The most common fungal infections are due to *Cryptococcus neoformans* or *Histoplasma capsulatum*. Underlying immunosuppression due to the FeLV or the FIV has not been found to be a factor. The typical clinical signs are recurrent episodes of sneezing and a chronic purulent nasal discharge. Cats with fungal infections may progress to systemic signs of weight loss, inappetence, and lethargy.

D i a g n o s i s

Primary Diagnostics

- **Radiographs:** Lateral, open-mouth, and skyline views should be taken to localize the infection. It is important to know whether the frontal sinuses are involved. Infectious, instead of neoplastic, diseases tend to produce bilateral lesions.

- **Culture and cytology:** After the site of the lesion is identified by radiographs, a 20 or 22 gauge needle is drilled through the hard palate into the lesion. Material is aspirated for culture and cytology. If the site is chosen properly, a diagnostic quality sample may be obtained. If this is not feasible or successful, a 3.5 Fr. catheter is passed 1–2 cm into the nasal cavity. Marks should be placed so it can be determined how far the catheter is passed. Five to 10 mL of saline are flushed through the nasal cavity. The material is caught on a 2×2 gauze square in the pharynx. It is important that a cuffed endotracheal tube be in place. This method is not as likely to recover a diagnostic sample as the aspiration technique.

- **Histopathology:** Material is recovered via a rhinotomy incision through the nasal bones.

Ancillary Diagnostics

- **Traumatic nasal flush:** This procedure is used to recover material for histopathology. The catheter should not be advanced past the medial canthus of the eye to prevent damaging the brain.
- **Viral culture:** This procedure is useful if it can be performed properly. Contact your laboratory for specific instructions.
- **Fungal serology:** False negatives are common, but high or increasing titers are diagnostic.

Diagnostic Notes

- The presence of blood in the nasal discharge does not strongly correlate with neoplasia as it does in the dog.
- It is unusual for a primary bacterial infection to cause chronic rhinitis or rhinosinusitis. An underlying viral (or fungal) infection should be suspected.

 T r e a t m e n t

Primary Therapeutics

- **Antibiotics:** The choice of antibiotic should be made based on culture and sensitivity. If this is not feasible, antibiotics should be chosen that are likely to be effective against *P. aeruginosa*. The most practical is high-dose enrofloxacin (4 mg/kg BID PO for 30 days).
- **Interferon:** Low-dose oral interferon is used to slow viral replication and contain (not eliminate) viral infections. It is dosed at 6–12 units/kg SID PO. If effective, it is used as a long-term treatment.
- **Itraconazole:** This drug is used at a dose of 5 mg/kg BID PO for at least 6 months when a fungal infection is present.

Secondary Therapeutics

- **Frontal sinus obliteration:** If infection is present in the frontal sinuses, medical therapy will not be effective. The purpose of this procedure is to remove the frontal sinuses as a site of infection.

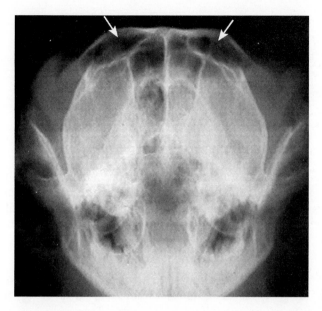

Figure 90.1. Nasal and frontal sinus infections: It is important to localize the infection. The frontal sinuses can be visualized with the skyline view. Both frontal sinuses of this cat are normal.

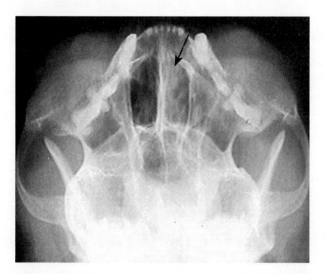

Figure 90.2. The nasal cavity can be seen with an open-mouth ventrodorsal (VD) view. The left nasal cavity is abnormally radiopaque.

Therapeutic Notes

- Cats with viral and bacterial infections that are controlled may have periodic relapses requiring the use of antibiotics.
- Cats with viral and bacterial infections usually do not have systemic signs. If they are not treated, they can be expected to live many years with their nasal discharge.

Prognosis

The prognosis is guarded for cats with chronic viral and bacterial infections. Aggressive, long-term treatment is usually required. The prognosis for cats with fungal infections is variable. Some recover completely after several months of treatment, whereas others succumb to their infections if the infections become systemic.

Suggested Readings

Cape L. Feline idiopathic chronic rhinosinusitis: A retrospective study of 30 cases. *J Am Anim Hosp Assoc* 1992;28:149–155.

Norsworthy GD. Finding the cause of chronic nasal discharge in cats. *Vet Med* 1995;90(11):1038–1047.

Norsworthy GD. Treating chronic nasal discharge in cats. *Vet Med* 1995;90(11):1048–1054.

Norsworthy GD. Chronic nasal discharge. In: Norsworthy GD, ed. Feline practice. Philadelphia: JB Lippincott, 1993;266–273.

O'Brien RT, Evans SM, Wortman JA, Hendrick MJ. Radiographic findings in cats with intranasal neoplasia or chronic rhinitis: 29 cases (1982–1988). *J Am Vet Med Assoc* 1996;208(3):385–389.

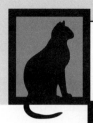

CHAPTER 91

Nasal and Nasopharyngeal Polyps

Gary D. Norsworthy

Overview

Inflammatory polyps are polypoid benign growths that arise from mucous membranes of the nose (nasal polyps) or the base of the eustachian tube (nasopharyngeal polyps). The latter can extend into the middle ear, external ear, pharynx, and nasal cavity. The primary clinical sign is a chronic, purulent nasal discharge that may be unilateral or bilateral. Frequently, the cat will have a draining, fistulous tract over the nasal bone, a head tilt, or chronic otitis externa. Other signs include dyspnea, Horner's syndrome, and otitis externa. The majority of cats reported had onset of signs at less than 1 year of age.

 Diagnosis

Primary Diagnostics

- **Clinical signs:** Chronic nasal discharge is present and is usually in a young cat. Inconsistently found are draining tracts over the nasal bone, head tilt, chronic otitis, dyspnea, Horner's syndrome, and otitis externa.
- **Examination:** Nasopharyngeal masses can often be visualized if the soft palate is retracted rostrally while the cat is anesthetized.
- **Radiography:** Radiographs usually reveal increased density in the nasal cavity with turbinate destruction. The bullae are often thickened if otitis media is present.
- **Histopathology:** This test is confirmatory. Biopsy material may be recovered from the pharynx or nasal cavity.

Ancillary Diagnostics

- **Rhinotomy:** This will reveal the masses and permit biopsy for histopathology.

- **Rhinoscopy:** This will also permit visualization of the mass if appropriate instrumentation is available.

Diagnostic Notes

The presence of a draining tract over the nasal bone in a young cat with a chronic nasal discharge should raise the index of suspicion for nasal or nasopharyngeal polyps.

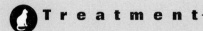 Treatment

Primary Therapeutics

- **Oral surgery:** Initially, the mass should be approached orally with rostral retraction of the soft palate. The mass should be grasped at its base so it avulses from its point of attachment. Failure to remove all of the mass will often result in regrowth.
- **Nasal surgery:** Nasal polyps and parts of nasopharyngeal polyps can be removed via a rhinotomy incision.
- **Bulla osteotomy:** If there is evidence of otitis media, this procedure is necessary to remove the polyp within the bulla.

Secondary Therapeutics

- **Antibiotics:** Appropriate antibiotics should be used for concurrent bacterial otitis.

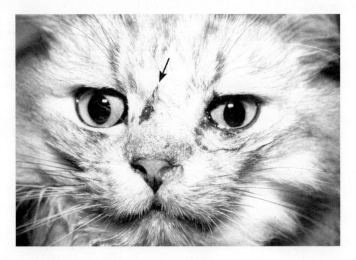

Figure 91.1. Nasal and nasopharyngeal polyps: Inflammatory polyps often cause pressure necrosis. This polyp created a draining tract through the right side of the nasal bone.

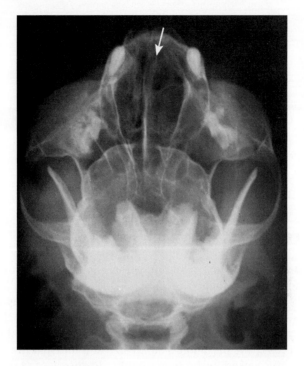

Figure 91.2. The bony destruction can be seen on the radiograph of the nasal cavity.

Therapeutic Notes

Horner's syndrome or facial paralysis are possible complications following bulla osteotomy. Most cases resolve spontaneously.

Prognosis

The prognosis is good if all of the polyp can be removed. However, because of the location, this is not always possible.

Suggested Readings

Levy JK, Ford RB. Diseases of the upper respiratory tract. In: Sherding RG, ed. The cat: diseases and clinical management, 2nd ed. Philadelphia: WB Saunders, 1994;947–978.

Norsworthy GD. Finding the cause of chronic nasal discharge in cats. *Vet Med* 1995;90(11): 1038–1047.

Rosychuk RAW, Luttgen P. Diseases of the ear. In: Ettinger SJ, Feldman EC, eds. Textbook of veterinary internal medicine, 4th ed. Philadelphia: WB Saunders, 1995;533–567.

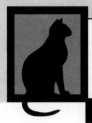

CHAPTER 92

Ollulanis Infection

Mitchell A. Crystal

Overview

*O*llulanis tricuspis is a gastric nematode parasite that causes gastric erosions and chronic fibrosing gastritis. *O. tricuspis* is acquired via ingestion of infected vomitus. There is no extragastric migration; transplacental and transmammary infection do not occur. Clinical signs include vomiting, anorexia, and weight loss. Physical examination may be normal or reveal evidence of weight loss. The organism's small size and unusual life cycle (neither eggs nor larvae are passed in the feces) make diagnosis of *O. tricuspis* difficult.

D i a g n o s i s

Primary Diagnostics

- **Direct microscopic examination of vomitus:** Adults and/or larvae may be seen. An emetic agent such as xylazine (0.2 mg/kg IV or SC) can be given to provide vomitus for examination.
- **Baermann's apparatus on vomitus for concentrating adults and larva:** Adults or larvae may be seen.

Ancillary Diagnostics

- **Gastric biopsy and histopathology:** Adults or larvae may be seen on histologic sections.

Diagnostic Notes

Histopathologic examination of three gastric mucosal sections reveals *O. tricuspis* in only half of the cats infected with the parasite.

Treatment

Primary Therapeutics

- **Fenbendazole:** Give 12.5 mg/kg BID PO for 5 days.
- **Oxfendazole:** Give 10 mg/kg BID PO for 5 days.

Therapeutic Notes

The difficulty in identifying an effective therapeutic agent results from the uncommon incidence of the disease, the difficulty in initially identifying the parasite, and the difficulty in identifying whether the parasite is still present following therapy.

Optimal therapy for naturally-occurring *O. tricuspis* infection has not been definitively identified.

Prognosis

The prognosis is uncertain as a result of the problems listed above. If significant gastric fibrosis has occurred, clinical signs may persist despite effective therapy.

Suggested Readings

Guilford WG, Strombeck DR. Chronic gastric diseases. In Strombeck's small animal gastroenterology, 3rd ed. Philadelphia: WB Saunders, 1996;275–302.

Willard MD. Diseases of the stomach. In: Ettinger SJ, Feldman EC, eds. Textbook of veterinary internal medicine, 4th ed. Philadelphia: WB Saunders, 1995;1159.

Wilson RB, Presnell JC. Chronic gastritis due to *Ollulanus tricuspis* infection in a cat. *J Am Anim Hosp Assoc* 1990;26:137–139.

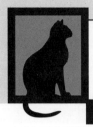

Organophosphate and Carbamate Toxicosis

Gary D. Norsworthy

Overview

C ats are commonly exposed to organophosphates (OP) and carbamates found in topical, systemic, and environmental pest control products. Common OPs include fenthion, malathion, chlorpyrifos, diazinon, dichlorovos, phosmet, and propetamphos. Common carbamates include fenoxy-carb, methomyl, bendiocarb, aldicarb, carbaryl, carbofuran, and propoxur. All of these products affect the nervous system by inhibiting acetylcholinesterase (AChE). This permits acetylcholine accumulation at the postsynaptic receptor, causing stimulation of effector organs. Spontaneous reactivation of AChE is very slow in young cats and almost nonexistent in older cats; it occurs more easily in carbamate toxicosis. The clinical signs occur from parasympathetic stimulation and, to some degree, sympathetic stimulation. There is a progression of signs that begins with restlessness and progresses to hyperexcitability or hypoexcitability. Salivation and muscle twitching are commonly observed. Vomiting, diarrhea, abdominal pain, and frequent urination follow. Cyanosis and generalized tetany signal that advanced toxicosis is present. These signs shortly precede seizures, respiratory failure, and death. Two notable exceptions are fenthion and chlorpyrifos toxicosis. The former may be tolerated by the cat for several weeks before toxicosis begins, and prolonged anorexia may be the predominant clinical sign. The latter also may cause onset of clinical signs after several days of exposure and may cause the clinical signs of anorexia, ataxia, posterior paralysis, and cervical ventroflexion. Both may require several weeks of antidotal therapy and nutritional support.

OP-impregnated flea collars have been associated with two syndromes. Spinal disease can occur, resulting in posterior ataxia, which progresses cranially. It generally occurs 10–14 days after application of the collar. Typically, clinical signs resolve after the collar is removed. Flea collars may cause a local dermatitis if the collar is applied too tightly and gets wet or if more than one collar is applied. Collar removal usually results in healing, but some cats need aggressive treatment with oral and locally applied corticosteroids.

Chlorpyrifos toxicosis usually occurs several days after exposure, resulting in posterior ataxia or paralysis or cervical ventroflexion. Tremors and fasciculations are common. Anorexia of several weeks' duration may also occur.

 D i a g n o s i s

Primary Diagnostics

- **History:** Recent application of a topical or systemic OP or carbamate should raise the index of suspicion.
- **Clinical signs:** Salivation, muscle twitching, vomiting, diarrhea, abdominal pain, and frequent urination are the common early signs. Cyanosis, generalized tetany, respiratory distress, coma, and death may follow. Prolonged anorexia without other cause and local irritation to the skin near the collar are also possible.
- **Whole-blood AChE:** A level below 25% of normal (Normal > 1000 IU/L) is indicative of exposure, but this value is highly variable in normal cats. This is the only means of determining depressed cholinesterase activity in living cats.

Ancillary Diagnostics

- **Tissue AChE:** Tissue levels can be confirmatory. The best tissues for analysis include the brain (include samples of cerebellum, cerebrum, and brain stem), liver, body fat, stomach and intestinal contents, and skin and subcutaneous tissue.
- **Tissue toxins:** Tissue levels of OPs and carbamates can be confirmatory.

Diagnostic Notes

- It is important to correlate the whole-blood AChE level with exposure and clinical signs because there is considerable variation in AChE levels in normal cats.
- Tissue samples for toxin analysis must be taken and frozen quickly because tissue levels of the toxins decrease rapidly.

 T r e a t m e n t

Primary Therapeutics

- **Respiratory support:** A patent airway should be secured and oxygen support administered if needed.
- **Seizure control:** If seizures occur, administer diazepam (0.05–0.1 mg/kg IV) or phenobarbital (3.0–30 mg/kg IV) **to effect.**

- **Atropine:** This drug should be given initially IV at 0.2–0.5 mg/kg. (NOTE: This is 5–10 times the preanesthetic dose.) The drug's effects may last only 10–15 minutes, so it may be necessary to repeat it frequently. When the cat is stable, it may be given subcutaneously.

- **Pralidoxime chloride (2-PAM):** This drug is dosed at 10–20 mg/kg IM, SC, or IV slowly over 30 minutes BID-TID. Each dose lasts 6–8 hours. It is indicated for OP toxicosis only; it is not beneficial for carbamate toxicosis.

Secondary Therapeutics

- **Bathing:** If dermal exposure has occurred, the cat should be bathed in a mild detergent soap to remove any remaining toxin. If this is not done, the cat may ingest more toxin by grooming.

- **Activated charcoal and cathartic:** Activated charcoal is given at the rate of 2.0 g/kg (10 mL/kg) PO. Sodium sulfate is given at 1 g/kg. These drugs are combined in some antidotal products (Actidose with Sorbitol, Paddock Laboratories).

- **Gastric lavage/through-and-through enema:** These may be used to remove remaining toxins from the GI tract. Note that gastric lavage should not be done if the cat is unconscious because of the potential for aspiration.

- **Diphenhydramine:** This drug may be helpful in controlling muscle fasciculations. It is dosed at 2–4 mg/kg PO q8h.

Therapeutic Notes

- Chlorpyrifos toxicosis often requires several weeks of therapy with 2-PAM. Relapse is common and often requires reinstitution of 2-PAM therapy.

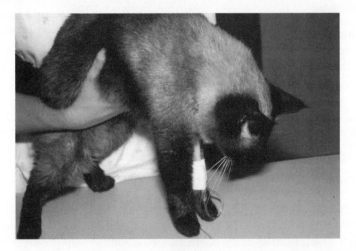

Figure 93.1. Organophosphate and carbamate toxicosis: There are a variety of clinical signs produced by organophosphate and carbamate toxicosis. Chlorpyrifos may result in cervical ventroflexion that is clinically identical to hypokalemia and thiamine deficiency.

Because of the prolonged anorexia that may occur, nutritional support in the form of an implanted feeding tube may be needed.

- 2-PAM has a 2-week shelf life if it is refrigerated in the dark, i.e., wrap the bottle in aluminum foil.

- Although control of seizures is imperative, it is important that CNS depression not be induced except for that purpose.

Prognosis

The prognosis for OP and carbamate toxicoses is good if diagnosed and treated quickly. However, the clinician should note that treatment may require intensive care for several days and continued treatment for several weeks. Long-term effects are not likely.

Suggested Readings

Groff RM, Miller JM, Stair EL, et al. Toxicoses and toxins. In: Norsworthy GD, ed. Feline practice. Philadelphia: JB Lippincott, 1993;551–569.

Rumbeiha WK, Oehme FW, Reid FM. Toxicoses. In: Sherding RG, ed. The cat: diseases and clinical management, 2nd ed. Philadelphia: WB Saunders, 1994;215–249.

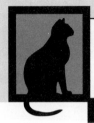

CHAPTER 94

Otitis Externa

Gary D. Norsworthy

Overview

O titis externa refers to any inflammatory disease of the external ear canal. The most common pathogens include *Staphylococcus spp.*, *Proteus mirabilis*, *Pseudomonas aeruginosa*, *Escherichia coli*, and *Malassezia pachydermatitis*. Ear mites, *Otodectes cynotis*, are also commonly found when the other pathogens are present. Clinical signs include head shaking, ear scratching, and an otic discharge.

 D i a g n o s i s

Primary Diagnostics

- **Clinical signs:** A discharge from the external ear canal is highly suspicious for otitis externa. The discharge is often fetid.

- **Cytology:** A modified Wright's stained smear can be used to classify the infection as cocci (*Staphylococcus spp.*), small rods (usually *P. mirabilis* or *P. aeruginosa*), large rods (usually *E. coli*) or yeast (*M. pachydermatitis*). This information is important in selecting appropriate medication.

- **Otoscopic examination:** This should be performed to identify ear mites, the degree of debris buildup, foreign bodies, and whether or not the ear drum is intact. This may require sedation in some cats.

Ancillary Diagnostics

- **Bacterial culture:** This is generally not necessary when cytology is performed. Because yeasts usually do not grow on aerobic cultures, culture should not be performed without cytology.

- **Viral testing:** The FeLV and FIV may predispose the cat to bacterial otitis. If a bacterial infection is present and ear mites are not present, or if the cat does not respond to initial therapy, these tests should be performed.

Diagnostic Notes

Primary ear infections are uncommon in cats, so an underlying disease should be sought.

 T r e a t m e n t

Primary Therapeutics

- **Antibiotics:** Topical antibiotics are indicated when bacterial infections are present. Their choice should be based on culture and sensitivity. The use of systemic antibiotics should be considered in severe or resistant infections.
- **Antifungals:** Topical antifungals (clotrimazole or miconazole) are indicated when fungal infections are present. Resistant infections can be

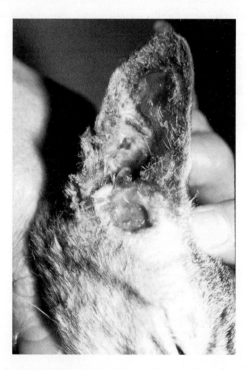

Figure 94.1. Otitis externa: Purulent otitis externa may be caused by a variety of micro-organisms. However, it is often secondary to an underlying disease or immunosuppressive agent.

treated with ketoconazole (10 mg/kg PO SID) or itraconazole (5 mg/kg PO BID).

- **Insecticide:** This is indicated when ear mites are present. See Chapter 48.

Secondary Therapeutics

- **Ear flushing:** Some practitioners are aggressive in flushing the ears of sedated cats. However, wax solvents or solvent-containing antibiotic products are usually effective in dissolving the debris and permitting the cat to shake it out of the ear canal. Excessive force in flushing should be avoided, as a fragile tympanum may rupture. Although it will usually heal, it may predispose the cat to otitis media and interna.

Therapeutic Notes

The use of cotton-tipped swabs by owners is contraindicated, as they tend to push debris deeper into the ear canal.

Prognosis

The prognosis is good with proper diagnostics and appropriate therapy unless the FeLV or FIV are present. These viruses warrant a guarded prognosis.

Suggested Reading

Haagen A.J. Venker-van. Diseases and surgery of the ear. In: Sherding RG, ed. The cat: diseases and clinical management, 2nd ed. Philadelphia: WB Saunders, 1994;1999–2009.

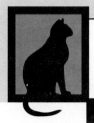

CHAPTER 95

Otitis Media and Interna

Sharon K. Fooshee

Overview

Otitis media and interna are defined as inflammation of the middle and inner ear, respectively. Middle ear structures include the tympanic membrane and air-filled tympanic cavity, the tympanic nerve (a branch of the facial nerve), the eustachian tube, and three auditory ossicles (the malleus, stapes, and incus). Sympathetic and parasympathetic nerves pass through the middle ear. Inner ear structures include the cochlea, vestibule, and semicircular canals; these are housed within a membranous labyrinth contained within a bony labyrinth. Otitis media may be difficult to diagnose, as it may be clinically silent or overshadowed by concurrent otitis externa. Signs of otitis interna usually allow a more straightforward diagnosis. Otitis media may be a primary or secondary disease and may also occur iatrogenically. In some cases, it develops secondary to extension of otitis externa through a ruptured tympanic membrane. In cats, it occasionally occurs by extension up the eustachian tube following upper respiratory infection. Other possible causes include polyps, tumors, trauma, and bacterial infection. Many cases of otitis interna have an associated otitis media; thus, the middle ear may serve as the most common route of infection for the inner ear.

A complete physical examination should be performed. The oral cavity should be examined for evidence of inflammation or polyps protruding from the eustachian tube. When examining the external ear canal, it is important to document the patency of the tympanic membrane, if possible. Bulging or rupture of the membrane and changes in opacity or color indicate middle ear pathology. Signs of otitis media include shaking the head or pawing at the ear and, occasionally, a head tilt (associated with pain). When the facial nerve is involved, paralysis or drooping of the lip or ear, diminished or absent palpebral reflexes, and widened palpebral fissures may be seen. Sympathetic nerve involvement may produce Horner's syndrome: enophthalmos, protrusion of the membrana nictitans, ptosis, and miosis. Signs of otitis interna include head tilt toward the affected side, asymmetric ataxia, and spontaneous horizontal or rotary nystagmus. Nausea and vomiting may occur due to disturbance of vestibular connections to the emetic center in the brain stem.

Diagnosis

Primary Diagnostics

- **Clinical signs:** Otitis media and/or interna should be suspected in cats with head tilt or signs of facial nerve abnormalities.
- **Radiography:** Radiographic changes of otitis media include the presence of a fluid density in the tympanic bulla or thickening of the bulla. Radiographic changes may not always be apparent, even when otitis media is present. Where available, CT or MRI scans are useful. Rarely does otitis interna produce any radiographic signs.

Ancillary Diagnostics

- **Myringotomy:** If the membrane is bulging but intact, an exudate may be present in the middle ear. Myringotomy may be helpful for draining the fluid, obtaining a sample for culture and sensitivity, and flushing the middle ear.

Diagnostic Notes

Unilateral otitis media may be more suggestive of neoplasia, polyps, or a foreign body.

Treatment

Primary Therapeutics

- **Antibiotics:** Treatment depends upon the underlying cause. In many cases, it is prudent to administer systemic antimicrobials for 3 to 6 weeks. When possible, the antibiotic should be selected based on culture and sensitivity.

Secondary Therapeutics

- **Otitis externa:** If otitis externa is also present, it should be appropriately managed. Patency of the tympanum should be considered before placing medication into the external canal. See Chapter 94.
- **Flushing the middle ear:** A 20 gauge spinal needle is usually used for myringotomy. Once the eardrum has been punctured, the middle ear may be gently flushed with warm sterile saline. A reference text should be consulted for details, because this procedure poses risk for delicate structures within the middle and inner ear.
- **Antiemetics:** These may be used to control vestibular signs and associated nausea.

Therapeutic Notes

- The only safe solution for flushing the middle ear is sterile saline. All disinfectants should be avoided.
- Known ototoxic agents should not be placed into the ear canal when the eardrum is ruptured. These include aminoglycosides, iodinated compounds, chlorhexidine, and chloramphenicol.

Prognosis

Prognosis for otitis media or interna is dependent upon the underlying cause.

Suggested Readings

Rosychuk RAW. Diagnosis and management of otitis media in the dog and cat. In: Proceedings of the American College of Veterinary Internal Medicine, 13th Annual Meeting. 1995;838–841.

Shell L. Otitis media and otitis interna. In: August JR, ed. Diseases of the ear canal. *Vet Clin North Am*, Philadelphia: WB Saunders, 1988;885–899.

Venker-van Haagen AJ. Diseases and surgery of the ear. In: Sherding RG, ed. The cat: diseases and clinical management. Philadelphia: WB Saunders, 1994;1999–2009.

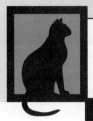

CHAPTER 96

Pancreatitis

Gary D. Norsworthy

Overview

P ancreatitis has been reported in the cat as a chronic disease accompanied by cholangiohepatitis or inflammatory bowel disease. Histologically, the acute forms are classified as necrotizing or suppurative. The etiology of pancreatitis is usually not determined, but cases have been reported associated with trauma, toxoplasmosis, feline Herpesvirus I, feline infectious peritonitis, hepatic lipidosis, organophosphate intoxication, hepatobiliary infections, drugs (acemannan), pancreatic flukes (*Amphimerus pseudofelineus* and *Eurytrema procyonis*) and feline parvovirus infection. Because the feline pancreatic duct and bile duct converge, surgical expression of a distended gall bladder can force bile into the pancreas, causing necrotizing pancreatitis. High-fat meals and glucocorticoid administration do not seem to be associated with feline pancreatitis. Cats with pancreatitis exhibit nonspecific signs. Fever and abdominal pain are much less common than in dogs; cats with the chronic form often have a history of weight loss, depression, and anorexia. The acute necrotizing form may present as an acute onset of lethargy, anorexia, icterus, marked hyperglycemia, and dehydration. Cats with suppurative pancreatitis are often hypoglycemic.

Diagnosis

Primary Diagnostics

- **Clinical signs:** The clinician should suspect necrotizing pancreatitis in a cat presented with an acute onset of depression, icterus, and hyperglycemia. Vomiting is an inconsistent finding. The clinical signs of the other forms are similar to other gastrointestinal and metabolic diseases.
- **Feline trypsin-like immunoreactivity (TLI):** This test is the most reliable biochemical test available at this time. The cat with pancreatitis will have a TLI value significantly above the normal range. It is important that the cat be fasted for 12 hours prior to blood sampling.

358

Ancillary Diagnostics

- **Radiography:** Abdominal radiographs may reveal peritonitis in the right anterior quadrant of the abdomen, ascites, and displacement of the duodenum.

- **Ultrasound:** Cats with pancreatitis often reveal a nonhomogenous mass and loss of echogenicity in the right anterior abdominal quadrant. Dilated bile ducts are often found.

- **Liver aspiration:** This test should be utilized because of the concurrence of pancreatitis and hepatic lipidosis and the resulting treatment implications.

- **Laparotomy and pancreatic biopsy:** Many cases are diagnosed during exploratory laparotomy performed for nonspecific signs of abdominal disease. Many other cases are diagnosed by necropsy. Pancreatic biopsy is advised in an attempt to find an underlying cause and when vague signs are present but the diagnosis is uncertain.

Diagnostic Notes

- Serum amylase and lipase levels have virtually no value in diagnosing feline pancreatitis.

- Feline TLI is performed by GI Lab, Texas A & M University, College Station, TX 77843 (Ph: 409-862-2861).

- Plasma or urine trypsinogen activation peptides (TAP) have shown promise of being specific and sensitive for diagnosing feline pancreatitis.

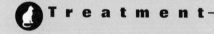

T r e a t m e n t

Primary Therapeutics

- **Supportive care:** Intravenous fluids, such as lactated Ringer's solution supplemented with 30–40 mEq of KCl per liter, are important in correcting and preventing dehydration. A balanced electrolyte fluid should be used, but KCl administration should not exceed 0.5 mEq/kg/hr.

- **Jejunostomy tube:** If concurrent hepatic lipidosis is present, nutritional support is essential and can be safely performed in this manner. Otherwise, food should be withheld.

- **Analgesics:** These should be employed if abdominal pain is present.

- **Antemetics:** If vomiting is present, chlorpromazine (8–10 mg/kg BID IM or IV) is usually the most effective drug. Metoclopramide (0.1–0.3 mg/kg BID IM) may also be beneficial.

Secondary Therapeutics

- **Insulin:** Cats that have marked hyperglycemia benefit from a short and well-monitored course of regular insulin IM.
- **Plasma:** Plasma administration can be beneficial because it contains albumin and protease inhibitor.
- **Hetastarch:** This colloid should be used if hypoproteinemia is present. It helps maintain normal fluid mechanics at the capillary level.
- **Dopamine:** This drug is gaining popularity when given at a constant rate infusion of 5 μg/kg/min. It is thought to decrease permeability in the pancreas and decrease inflammation by limiting release of proteases.
- **Antibiotics:** The concurrence of cholangiohepatitis warrants the use of antibiotics according to culture and sensitivity or, if unavailable, drugs likely to be effective against anaerobes (amoxicillin, ampicillin, metronidazole).
- **Relief of biliary obstruction:** Surgery for this purpose is necessary when it occurs.
- **Fenbendazole:** This drug is indicated when liver flukes are present. It is dosed at 30 mg/kg SID for 6 or more days.

Therapeutic Notes

- Antibiotics and antisecretory drugs have not proven to be of value in pancreatitis not accompanied by infection.
- Corticosteroids seem to be helpful in selected patients.
- When feeding is resumed, small, frequent meals should be offered.

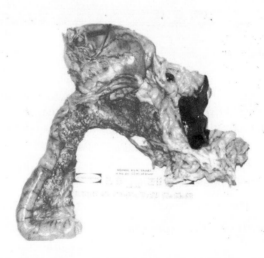

Figure 96.1. Pancreatitis: Necrotizing pancreatitis is less common than the chronic recurrent form. However, it does occur in the cat and is often fatal.

P r o g n o s i s

The prognosis is variable. The acute forms are often fatal. The chronic forms usually have a good prognosis, especially if an underlying cause can be determined and corrected. Concurrent pancreatitis and hepatic lipidosis can be very difficult to manage as a result of conflicting nutritional strategies unless a jejunostomy tube is used.

S u g g e s t e d   R e a d i n g s

Akol KG, Washabau RJ, Saunders HM, et al. Acute pancreatitis in cats with hepatic lipidosis. *J Vet Int Med* 1993;7:205–209.

Hardy RM. Diseases of the exocrine pancreas. In: Sherding RG, ed. The cat: diseases and clinical management, 2nd ed. Philadelphia: WB Saunders, 1994;1287–1296.

Hill RC, Van Winkle TJ. Acute necrotizing pancreatitis and acute suppurative pancreatitis in the cat. A retrospective study of 40 cases (1976–1989). *J Vet Int Med* 1993;7:25–33.

Williams DA. Feline exocrine pancreatic disease. *Fel Health Topics* 1995;10(4):1–8.

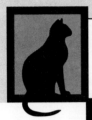

CHAPTER 97

Patent Ductus Arteriosus

John-Karl Goodwin

Overview

P atent ductus arteriosus (PDA), although not as common in the feline as in the canine, is important because it represents one of the few cardiovascular anomalies that may be corrected surgically.

In the fetus, the ductus arteriosus allows shunting (right-to-left) of blood away from the pulmonary vascular bed through the pulmonary artery to the descending aorta. Following birth, the ductus arteriosus normally constricts and eventually closes in response to increases in local partial pressure of oxygen and inhibition of prostaglandins. If the ductus remains patent, a left-to-right shunt occurs, which eventually causes severe left ventricular volume overload and left-sided heart failure. Changes in the pulmonary vascular resistance may cause reversal of the shunt, which results in right-sided heart failure.

The magnitude of left-to-right shunting is dependent on the luminal diameter and resistance within the ductus and on the pulmonary vascular resistance. The clinical features of PDA depend on the direction and degree of the shunting.

A left-to-right shunt typically causes a continuous left basilar cardiac murmur, bounding femoral pulses, and left atrial and ventricular enlargement suggested by a caudally displaced cardiac impulse. In right-to-left shunts, a murmur usually is not present, the femoral pulses are not bounding, and signs of right-sided (i.e., ascites and jugular pulses and/or distention) or biventricular heart failure (i.e., pleural effusion) predominate.

Diagnosis

Primary Tests

- **Echocardiogram:** This reveals left atrial and ventricular dilatation; enlargement of the pulmonary artery and ascending aorta; normal systolic function in most cases (decreased function in cases with cardiomyopathy of overload); continuous turbulent flow in the distal main pulmonary artery; and mitral and sometimes aortic regurgitation (secondary to aortic root dilation), as demonstrated by spectral or color-flow Doppler.

Ancillary Diagnostics

- **Electrocardiography:** Increased R-wave amplitude suggestive of left ventricular enlargement; wide P wave suggestive of left atrial enlargement; right-axis shift in cases with reversed shunting; premature atrial complexes; and ventricular arrhythmias may be present.
- **Thoracic radiography:** left atrial and ventricular enlargement; pulmonary artery and aortic dilation; pulmonary vascular overcirculation; evidence of congestive heart failure (pulmonary venous congestion, mixed interstitial-alveolar pattern consistent with pulmonary edema).

Diagnostic Notes

- Reverse PDA probably occurs less frequently in the cat than in the dog.
- Cardiac catheterization is rarely required for the diagnosis.
- PDA may occur in the presence of other congenital cardiac defects.

 Treatment

Primary Therapeutics

Surgical ligation of the patent ductus arteriosus is the treatment of choice.

Secondary Therapeutics

Preoperative stabilization of patients in congestive heart failure is essential and usually requires only diuretic therapy (furosemide 1–4 mg/kg IV, IM, or PO SID-QID depending on the severity of the clinical signs).

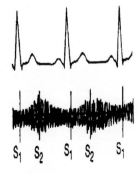

S_1 S_2 S_1 S_2 S_1

Figure 97.1. Patent ductus arteriosis: A machinery murmur is typical of a cat with PDA.

Therapeutic Notes

Surgical intervention is recommended as soon as possible in most cases.

Small shunts are less likely than large shunts to cause significant volume overloading of the left ventricle and potentially may not require surgical intervention. However, the size of the ductus may only be determined accurately by cardiac catheterization and angiocardiography.

Prognosis

In general, a good prognosis is given to patients that undergo surgical ligation of the ductus (a 5–10% complication rate is commonly quoted, with most of the complications occurring in the perioperative period). Cats with evidence of myocardial dysfunction may have irreversible pathology and, therefore, a more guarded prognosis.

Suggested Readings

Fox PR. Congenital feline heart disease. In: Fox PR, ed. Canine and feline Cardiology. New York: Churchill Livingstone, 1988;391–408.

Liska W, Tilley LP. Patent ductus arteriosus. *Vet Clin North Am, Small Anim Pract* 1979;9:195–206.

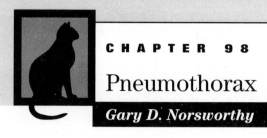

CHAPTER 98

Pneumothorax

Gary D. Norsworthy

Overview

Pneumothorax is an accumulation of air in the pleural space. It occurs in three forms: 1) **open,** in which there is an opening in the chest wall; 2) **closed,** in which there is an opening in the lungs, bronchi, trachea, or esophagus; and 3) **tension,** in which a tear in the pleura permits air to enter the pleural space during inspiration but not to exit during expiration. Pneumothorax occurs **spontaneously** or due to **trauma.** The former may be idiopathic, but it is most commonly associated with lung disease that results in necrosis of the visceral pleura, permitting air leakage. The clinical signs are an acute onset of dyspnea and tachypnea (due to anoxia) and cyanosis (due to decreased venous return). Many affected cats are anxious or panicked. Frothy blood may exit the nose and mouth. If the trachea or esophagus is lacerated, cervical subcutaneous emphysema may occur.

 D i a g n o s i s

Primary Diagnostics

- **Physical examination:** External signs of trauma may be present.
- **Clinical signs:** These include an acute onset of dyspnea and tachypnea. Cyanosis may be present.
- **Auscultation:** Lung sounds are decreased dorsally; heart sounds are usually muffled.
- **Thoracentesis:** This is the diagnostic test of choice if asthma, diaphragmatic hernia, and bleeding disorders are unlikely. A needle is inserted in the dorsal two-thirds of the thorax in the seventh to ninth intercostal spaces; it is inserted just deeply enough to enter the pleural space. Free aspiration of air is confirmatory.
- **Radiography:** On the lateral view, the heart appears elevated off the sternum due to lateral displacement that occurs when the cat is placed in

lateral recumbency. Other findings include an identifiable, air-filled pleural space, partial lung collapse, and lung margins that are retracted from the thoracic wall.

Ancillary Diagnostics

- **Bronchoscopy:** This may be used to identify tears in the trachea or main-stem bronchi.

Diagnostic Notes

Dyspneic cats should be handled very carefully because increased stress may be fatal. Extreme care should be taken when doing the physical examination, radiographs, and thoracentesis. It may be necessary to place the cat in an oxygen cage for several minutes prior to diagnostics and between diagnostic procedures. The least stressful radiographic view is the dorsoventral (DV); it may be the only view that is practical in some cases. However, the lateral view is needed to confirm pneumothorax.

 T r e a t m e n t

Primary Therapeutics

- **Thoracentesis:** The least amount of sedation should be employed. If sedation is needed, the use of 2 mg/kg of ketamine IV is generally safe. Aspirate both sides of the chest, and remove as much air as possible. A needle or catheter is inserted in the dorsal two-thirds of the thorax in the seventh to ninth intercostal spaces; it is inserted just deeply enough to enter the pleural space.

Secondary Therapeutics

- **Thoracostomy tube:** This permits continuous or intermittent chest drainage without further stress to the cat. Generally, one tube will drain both sides of the chest; however, some cases require bilateral tube placement. A thoracostomy tube is recommended if more than two thoracenteses are needed within 24 hours. If tension pneumothorax is present, a trocar should be used prior to tube placement to relieve pressure within the pleural space. The chest should be aspirated one to two times per day until less than 10 mL of air are removed in 12 hours.
- **Thoracotomy:** Cats that do not respond to 2–5 days of thoracentesis, have more than two episodes that recur after proper treatment, have tension pneumothorax, or appear to have pulmonary leakage are candidates for surgery. Lacerations, neoplastic lesions, and pulmonary blebs should be sought.

Therapeutic Notes

- Minor lacerations of the visceral pleura or the lung may heal within 48 hours. Therefore, a thoracostomy tube is generally not placed on the first

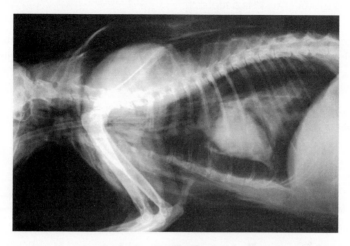

Figure 98.1. Pneumothorax: Tension pneumothorax occurs when a tear in the pleura permits air to enter the pleural space during inspiration but not to exit during expiration.

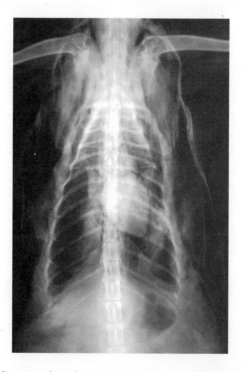

Figure 98.2. Air may dissect to the subcutaneous tissues, causing subcutaneous emphysema.

day of treatment unless there are signs of tension pneumothorax or repeated thoracentesis is needed.

- Repeated thoracentesis over several days may be used in place of thoracostomy tube placement. However, the former can be a painful procedure that may be too stressful for many cats that are fragile patients. The use of a chest drain is strongly recommended for patients that fit the above criteria.

- If anesthesia is administered, the use of anesthetic agents (ketamine plus diazepam) that permit rapid control of the airway is advised. Face-mask induction is generally not advised.

- Heimlich valves are generally not recommended in cats because cats are usually unable to produce enough intrathoracic pressure to activate the flutter valve.

P r o g n o s i s

Traumatic pneumothorax generally has a good prognosis if the source of the air leak is located and successfully controlled. The spontaneous form's prognosis depends on the underlying cause.

S u g g e s t e d   R e a d i n g s

Dramek BA, Caywood DD. Pneumothorax. *Vet Clin North Am, Small Anim Pract* 1987;17:285–300.

Sherding RG. Diseases of the pleural cavity. In: Sherding RG, ed. The cat: diseases and clinical management, 2nd ed. New York: Churchill Livingstone, 1994;1053–1091.

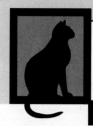

CHAPTER 99

Polycystic Kidney Disease

Gary D. Norsworthy

Overview

Polycystic kidneys contain multiple fluid-filled cysts 1 mm to 1 cm in diameter within the renal parenchyma. Although they may form due to intraluminal or extraluminal obstruction of renal tubules, the typical form seen is a genetic disease most commonly involving Persian and other long-haired breeds. In the Persian, it is an autosomal-dominant disease. The disease may be unilateral or bilateral, and concurrent hepatic cysts may be present. Severely affected kittens may die of renal failure by 8 weeks of age; however, the disease is usually subclinical until the cat is several years old. Clinical signs are those of renal failure: polydipsia, polyuria, weight loss, inappetence, and lethargy.

Diagnosis

Primary Diagnostics

- **Ultrasound:** This is the most specific, noninvasive test available. It reveals multiple, fluid-filled cysts throughout the kidney. The liver should also be imaged.

Ancillary Diagnostics

- **Plain radiographs:** Enlarged, irregular kidneys can be visualized, but this finding is not specific for polycystic kidney disease.
- **Excretory urogram:** The cysts may be seen as multiple radiolucent areas within the renal parenchyma.

Diagnostic Notes

Litter mates and parents of affected cats should have sonograms, because there may be many months or years of asymptomatic disease present. Early detection permits early therapy to support renal function.

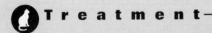

Treatment

Primary Therapeutics

- **Treatment for renal failure:** Renal failure is what makes this disease clinical. An aggressive approach should be taken to stabilize and maintain an affected cat. See Chapter 37.

Secondary Therapeutics

- **Nephrectomy:** This is indicated when unilateral disease is present and when renal failure is not present. An excretory urogram should be performed first to document function in the other kidney. This is not recommended in a Persian cat due to the genetic nature of the disease.

Therapeutic Notes

- Affected cats should not be bred.

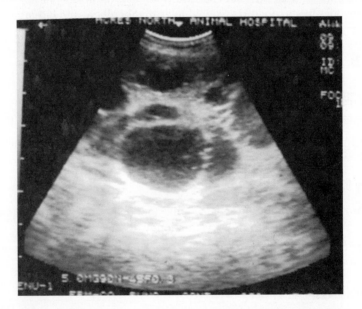

Figure 99.1. Polycystic kidney disease: The most sensitive diagnostic tool is ultrasound. The cysts can be easily visualized.

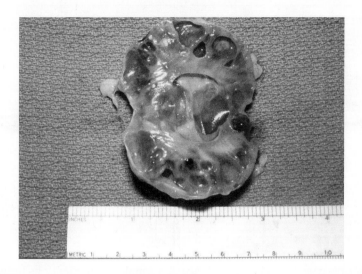

Figure 99.2. The cysts can be seen throughout this kidney of a 3-year-old Persian that presented in renal failure.

Prognosis

The prognosis depends upon the degree of renal failure, the cat's response to initial treatment for renal failure, and the owner's willingness to continue aggressive management for renal failure.

Suggested Reading

DiBartola SP, Rutgers HC. Diseases of the kidney. In: Sherding RG, ed. The cat: diseases and clinical management, 2nd ed. New York: Churchill Livingstone, 1994;1711–1767.

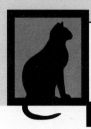

CHAPTER 100

Portosystemic Shunt

Mitchell A. Crystal

Overview

Portosystemic shunts (PSS) are abnormal communications between the portal and systemic venous system that allow intestinal blood to be delivered to the systemic circulation prior to hepatic detoxification. PSS may be singular or multiple, extrahepatic or intrahepatic, and congenital or acquired. Single, extrahepatic, congenital shunts are most common. Acquired multiple extrahepatic PSS may occur secondary to prolonged portal hypertension, such as that due to chronic hepatic disease or congenital shunt ligation in cats with hepatic vascular atresia.

Most cats with PSS demonstrate clinical signs within 1 year of age, although some cats have been as old as 4 years of age. Mixed-breed cats are most commonly affected, although Himalayan and Persian cats are over-represented in the affected population. Male cats develop PSS slightly more frequently than females. Many cats with PSS are reported to have copper-colored irises. Common clinical signs include ptyalism, seizures, ataxia, depression, and tremors. Other signs include intermittent blindness, aggression, mydriasis, stunted growth, anorexia and recurrent vomiting, diarrhea, and polyuria/polydipsia. Signs may wax and wane. Worsening of clinical signs with feeding is not a consistent finding. Some cats present for lower urinary tract signs that result from ammonium biurate calculi. Cats may have a history of prolonged/difficult anesthetic recovery. Differential diagnoses to consider include neurologic diseases, other hepatic diseases, and lower urinary tract disease.

Diagnosis

Primary Diagnostics

- **Database (CBC, chemistry profile, and urinalysis):** Cats with PSS will commonly demonstrate a mildly to moderately increased level of alanine aminotranferase (ALT) or alkaline phosphatase (ALP),

372

hypocholesterolemia, and red-cell microcytosis and poikilocytosis. Less common changes include hypoalbuminemia, hypoglobulinemia, decreased BUN, mildly to moderately decreased urine specific gravity, and ammonium biurate crystalluria. Some cats will have a normal database.

- **Bile acids:** Serum bile acids (fasting and 2-hour postprandial) are diagnostic of PSS. Most fasting samples and all postprandial samples will be elevated. Postprandial samples are typically greater than 100 mol/L.
- **Portography:** An intraoperative portogram can be performed to help locate the PSS if it is not visible upon exploration.

Ancillary Diagnostics

- **Ammonia tolerance test:** Serum ammonia levels taken fasted and after an oral ammonium chloride challenge are diagnostic of PSS; however, this test requires special sample handling and may create or exacerbate hepatoencephalopathy.
- **Abdominal imaging:** Survey abdominal radiographs may demonstrate microhepatica, and abdominal ultrasonography may demonstrate the shunting vessel.
- **Scintigraphy:** Rectal nuclear scintigraphy can confirm PSS but does not indicate the type or location of shunt present.

Diagnostic Notes

- Hyperbilirubinemia is not a feature of PSS.
- Left gastric-caval and porto-caval are the most frequent shunt locations. Porto-azygous shunts are rarely seen.
- Liver biopsies should be collected at the time of surgery to examine for fibrosis or primary hepatobiliary disease.

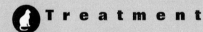 **T r e a t m e n t**

Primary Therapeutics

- **Surgical ligation:** This is the treatment of choice for single, extrahepatic shunts. Portal pressures should be monitored during ligation. If pressures rise over 20 cm of water or increase by more than 10 cm of water, the shunt should only be partially ligated so that these criteria are not exceeded. The use of an ameroid constrictor is strongly recommended.

Secondary Therapeutics

- **Medical management:** Several drugs are useful in the management of PSS-induced hepatoencephalopathy. Those commonly used include lactulose (1 mL given PO TID or as an enema [30% lactulose, 70% warm water] at 20 mL/kg per rectum and left in for 20–30 minutes), metronidazole (10 mg/kg PO BID), and neomycin (20 mg/kg PO TID). These agents are useful for preoperative patient stabilization and will temporarily help cats with inoperable PSS or those cats whose owners decline surgery.

- **Diet:** A diet of low quantity/high quality protein is indicated to help decrease signs of hepatoencephalopathy (see Appendix E).

Therapeutic Notes

- Use caution with pre-anesthetic and anesthetic agents. Cats should be masked or tanked down and maintained with isofluorane.
- Hypothermia due to prolonged anesthetic duration is common and should be prevented/addressed by using warm-water blankets intraoperatively and postoperatively.

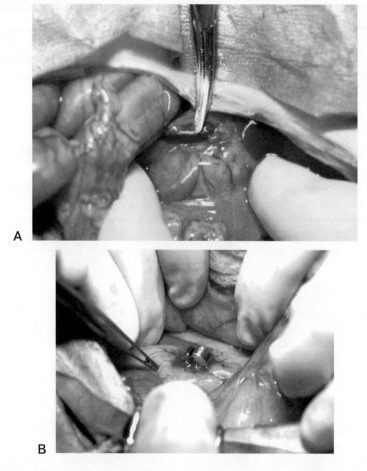

A

B

Figure 100.1. Portosystemic shunt. The most common shunt in the cat is the single extrahepatic form (*A*). The shunt should be ligated with an ameroid constrictor (*B*).

P r o g n o s i s

Cats with congenital, single, extrahepatic shunts without significant hepatic vascular atresia that undergo complete shunt ligation will likely be cured. Some cats with partial ligation may experience a recurrence and require a second surgery. Multiple and intrahepatic shunts are usually inoperable. Medical management can be attempted, but it is usually only temporarily successful in managing clinical signs. Some cats with partial or complete ligation will still demonstrate clinical signs and require continued temporary or permanent medical management.

S u g g e s t e d   R e a d i n g s

Birchard SJ, Sherding RG. Feline portosystemic shunts. *Compend Contin Educ Pract Vet* 1992;14(10):1295–1301.

Levy JK, Bunch SE, Komtebedde J. Feline portosystemic vascular shunts. In: Bonagura JD, ed. Kirk's current veterinary therapy XII: small animal practice. Philadelphia: WB Saunders, 1995;743–749.

VanGundy TE, Boothe HW, Wolf A. Results of surgical management of feline portosystemic shunts. *J Am Anim Hosp Assoc* 1990;26:55–62.

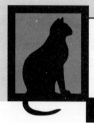

CHAPTER 101

Pulmonic Stenosis

John-Karl Goodwin

Overview

C ongenital obstruction of the right ventricular outflow tract is less common in the cat than in the dog. Isolated pulmonic stenosis (PS) has been reported infrequently in the cat. Right ventricular outflow obstruction secondary to valvular or infundibular stenosis causes right ventricular pressure overload and subsequent right ventricular concentric hypertrophy.

Physical examination findings suggestive of pulmonic stenosis include a left basilar systolic ejection-type murmur, jugular pulses and/or distention, and sometimes evidence of right-sided heart failure such as ascites. Affected cats may be asymptomatic, may experience weakness associated with exercise, or may develop right-sided congestive heart failure.

Cats with other congenital malformations may also have left basilar systolic ejection murmurs. Left-to-right shunting ventricular septal defects with significant shunting volumes demonstrate a murmur of relative pulmonic stenosis in association with the increased blood volume being ejected through the normal right ventricular outflow tract. Additionally, pulmonic stenosis is part of the tetralogy of Fallot, which is a relatively common congenital defect in the feline.

 D i a g n o s i s

Primary Diagnostics

- **Echocardiography:** right ventricular concentric hypertrophy, right atrial enlargement, and high-velocity (>2 m/sec) systolic turbulent flow across the obstruction as demonstrated by spectral or color-flow Doppler. Tricuspid valve regurgitation may also be present.

Ancillary Diagnostics

- **Electrocardiography:** Right-axis deviation may be present, with occasional atrial and ventricular premature complexes.
- **Thoracic radiography:** Right atrial and ventricular enlargement, poststenotic dilation of the pulmonary artery, diminutive pulmonary vasculature, and a distended caudal vena cava may be present depending on the severity of the outflow obstruction.

Diagnostic Notes

Electrocardiographic findings are variable. PS often occurs with other congenital defects.

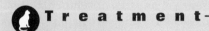 T r e a t m e n t

Primary Therapeutics

- Cardiac surgery may be palliative in cases with severe outflow obstruction.
- Balloon valvuloplasty of the obstruction may also be considered.

Secondary Therapeutics

- Beta blockers: Atenolol 6.25–12.5 mg PO SID or propranolol 2.5–5 mg PO BID-TID may be helpful.
- Therapy for right-sided congestive heart failure may be indicated in some patients.

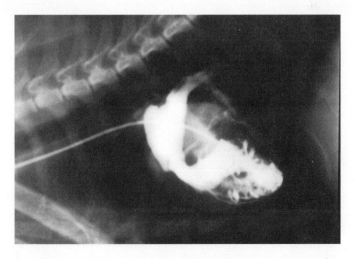

Figure 101.1. Pulmonic stenosis: An angiocardiogram showing pulmonic stenosis.

Therapeutic Notes

- The primary therapeutics noted above usually require referral of the patient to a specialist.
- Beta blockade may be cardioprotective by reducing myocardial oxygen consumption and slowing the heart rate.
- Interventional procedures such as balloon valvuloplasty and cardiac surgical procedures are performed infrequently in the feline.

P r o g n o s i s

The prognosis of pulmonic stenosis depends on the severity of the obstruction and the presence of concurrent lesions. The presence of an atrial or ventricular septal defect may allow right-to-left shunting to occur, leading to hypoxemia and cyanosis and chronic incapacitation. A severe lesion is likely if the Doppler gradient exceeds 70–100 mmHg.

Mild cases of pulmonic stenosis are unlikely to cause clinical disease.

S u g g e s t e d   R e a d i n g s

Loyer C. Pulmonic stenosis. In: Miller MS, Tilley LP, eds. Manual of canine and feline cardiology, 2nd ed. Philadelphia: WB Saunders, 1995.

Fox PR. Congenital feline heart disease. In: Fox PR, ed. Canine and feline cardiology. New York: Churchill Livingstone, 1998;391–408.

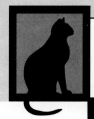

CHAPTER 102

Pyelonephritis

Gary D. Norsworthy

Overview

Pyelonephritis is inflammation of the renal interstitium, especially in the renal pelvis and adjacent medullary tissue. The etiology is typically bacterial, but urine cultures often do not recover the organism. Usually, the affected cat is presented for renal failure after many months or years of subclinical pyelonephritis; by this time, it is abacteriuric. The infection may arise hematogenously (bacterial endocarditis, abscesses, dental disease) or ascend from pre-existing cystitis. During the time of active infection, the cat may be febrile, anorectic, and lethargic. The kidneys may be painful to palpation, and polyuria and polydipsia may be present. However, some cats are asymptomatic or, at least, their disease is not recognized by their owners. Many cats showing non-specific signs of infection are treated empirically with antibiotics without a definitive diagnosis and subsequently recover. Evidence of the disease may be found years later following the onset of chronic renal failure or at necropsy, especially if it occurs unilaterally.

Diagnosis

Primary Diagnostics

- **Clinical signs:** If the cat is presented during active bacterial infection, it will have the systemic signs above. Pain in the kidneys is strongly suggestive.
- **Chemistry profile:** The typical findings during active infection are azotemia, hyperphosphatemia, nonregenerative anemia, and metabolic acidosis.
- **Urinalysis:** The typical findings during active infection are low specific gravity, proteinuria, bactiuria, pyuria, and hematuria.
- **Urine culture:** This should be performed to document the presence of bacteria and to provide data on which to base antibiotic selection.

Ancillary Diagnostics

- **Radiology:** An excretory urogram will reveal a dilated renal pelvis and blunting of the pelvic diverticula.
- **Ultrasound:** Active pyelonephritis produces an area of marked hyperechogenicity in the renal pelvis. The intensity of this finding will diminish, but it may persist for months or years following resolution of the active infection.

Diagnostic Notes

Experimentally, it has been shown that bacteria may impair renal concentrating ability. A positive urine culture in a cat with dilute urine is strongly suggestive of pyelonephritis, even in the absence of azotemia.

 Treatment

Primary Therapeutics

- **Antibiotics:** Specific antibiotic therapy should be given for at least 4 weeks.

Secondary Therapeutics

- **Renal support:** If azotemia is present, intravenous fluids should be given until the BUN and creatinine levels return to normal. Forty to 60 mEq of potassium chloride should be added to each liter of fluid, but the rate of administration should not exceed 0.5 mEq/kg/hour.

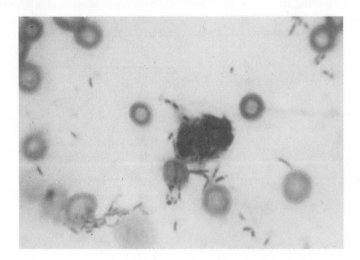

Figure 101.2. Pyelonephritis: Cats suspected with pyelonephritis should have a urinalysis and urine culture. Bacteruria is consistent with pyelonephritis; however, it can also be present in bacterial cystitis.

Therapeutic Notes

- One week following completion of antibiotic therapy, the urine should be recultured. If it is positive, antibiotics should be reinstituted for another 4–6 weeks.
- Pyelonephritis generally causes some permanent renal damage. The cat should be monitored periodically for early onset of renal failure.
- Some cases may require antibiotic therapy for life. One effective management program is to alternate nonnephrotoxic drugs each month.

Prognosis

The prognosis varies with the form of the disease. Cats diagnosed during the early acute phase that are treated aggressively have a good prognosis. Cats that are not treated early usually have some resulting permanent renal damage, which eventually leads to chronic renal failure. However, the ensuing renal failure may not occur for many years.

Suggested Reading

DiBartola S, Rutgers HC. Diseases of the kidney. In: Sherding RG, ed. The cat: diseases and clinical management, 2nd Ed. New York: Churchill Livingstone, 1994;1711–1767.

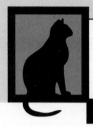

CHAPTER 103

Pyometra

Gary D. Norsworthy

Overview

Pyometra is a collection of purulent, usually septic, material within the lumen of the uterus. It is the result of a prolonged process, beginning with multiple estrogen-secreting estrous cycles without ovulation. This process results in endometrial hyperplasia and creates a uterine environment that supports bacterial growth; *Escherichia coli* and *Streptococcus* spp. are the most common isolates. Most queens that develop pyometra are at least 4 years of age. Clinical signs include abdominal distention, purulent vaginal discharge, anorexia, and lethargy. Unlike dogs, most cats do not have a history of polydipsia and polyuria. The history often includes an estrous cycle within 8 weeks prior to the onset of clinical signs.

 D i a g n o s i s

Primary Diagnostics

- **Clinical Signs:** The typical clinical signs, especially abdominal distention and vaginal discharge, in an intact female that cycled recently should raise one's index of suspicion for pyometra.
- **Imaging:** Radiography can detect uterine enlargement. Ultrasonography reveals an anechoic to hypoechoic tubular structure and can differentiate intrauterine fluid from noncalcified feti.

Ancillary Diagnostics

- **CBC:** Most cats have a marked neutrophilic leukocytosis with a regenerative left shift. Some have a mild anemia.

Diagnostic Notes

Because of the meticulous nature of cats, a vaginal discharge may go undetected.

❶ T r e a t m e n t

Primary Therapeutics

- **Antibiotics and fluids:** Regardless of the form of therapy chosen, many of these cats are septic and azotemic. Antibiotics should be chosen based on culture and sensitivity, if possible. If not possible or pending culture results, the following antibiotics are recommended: ampicillin, clavulanate-amoxicillin, cephalosporins, or enrofloxacin. One of the first two antibiotics can be combined with enrofloxacin.
- **Ovariohysterectomy:** This is the treatment of choice for most situations.
- **Prostaglandin $F_{2\alpha}$ therapy:** This drug can be used in queens that are to be used for future breeding. It is dosed at 200 µg/kg/day IM for 2 days, followed by 500 µg/kg/day IM for 3 days. See Therapeutic Notes.

Secondary Therapeutics

- **Hysterotomy and lavage:** This procedure produces mixed results but can be helpful in resolving infections so that future breeding is possible. It is indicated for closed-cervix pyometra.

Therapeutic Notes

- Prostaglandin therapy should be restricted to queens that meet all of the following conditions: a) have significant breeding value; b) are in stable condition; and c) have an open cervix.
- Prostaglandin therapy may produce vomiting, vocalizing, panting, salivation, urination, and defecation. These resolve within 1–2 hours after treatment and tend to diminish with subsequent injections.

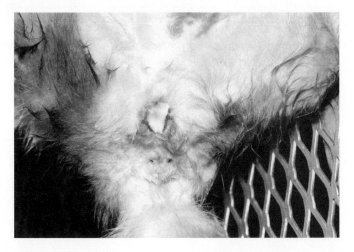

Figure 103.1. Pyometra: A purulent vaginal discharge is usually not noted in a cat with pyometra because of the fastidious nature of the cat.

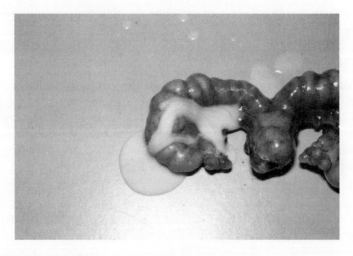

Figure 103.2. In cats with pyometra, the uterus is enlarged and filled with pus.

Prognosis

The prognosis is generally good if advanced sepsis has not occurred prior to treatment. However, about 20% of cats subjected to ovariohysterectomy die during or within a few days following surgery.

Suggested Readings

Eilts BE, Paccamonti DL, Causey R. Reproductive disorders. In: Norsworthy GD, ed. Feline practice. Philadelphia: JB Lippincott, 1993;458–476.

Johnson CA. Female reproduction and disorders of the female reproductive tract. In: Sherding RG, ed. The cat: diseases and clinical management, 2nd ed. New York: Churchill Livingstone, 1994;1855–1876.

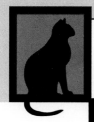

Pyothorax

Gary D. Norsworthy

Overview

Pyothorax is an accumulation of pus within the pleural cavity. It is almost always caused by a bacterial infection, but fungi may be causative; bacterial infections are usually due to anaerobic organisms. The causative organism generally gains entry into the pleural space through penetrating bite wounds from other cats, but foreign bodies, such as migrating plant awns, have been found within the pleural space and presumed to be causative. In addition, infections may arise from abscesses in adjacent organs, including the trachea and esophagus, and may originate hematogenously. The presence of the organisms and their toxins leads to the systemic effects of fever, inappetence, weight loss, and dehydration. Pulmonary compression results in dyspnea and tachypnea. As with most cases of dyspnea, the owner usually reports an acute onset.

 D i a g n o s i s

Primary Diagnostics

- **Clinical signs:** Clinical signs include dyspnea and tachypnea; some cats may have systemic signs of illness.
- **Auscultation:** Heart sounds are muffled; lung sounds are decreased ventrally and increased dorsally.
- **Radiography:** Pleural effusion with pleural fissures and scalloped lung borders are typical.
- **Thoracentesis:** A few milliliters of fluid may be removed to confirm the presence of pleural effusion and for subsequent analysis.
- **Pleural fluid analysis:** The protein content is greater than 5 g/dL, and the specific gravity is greater than 1.020. The nucleated cell count is greater than 15,000 cells/μL and often greater than 50,000 cells/μL.

- **Pleural fluid cytology:** Degenerative neutrophils, macrophages, and the causative organism are usually found.
- **Culture and sensitivity of pleural fluid:** Aerobic and anaerobic cultures are essential. More than 50% of pathogens are anaerobic. Some organisms take 2–4 weeks to grow.

Ancillary Diagnostics

- **Hemogram:** Marked neutrophilic leukocytosis and anemia of chronic disease are typical.
- **Serum chemistries:** These are often normal, but there may be increased total protein with a decreased A:G ratio.
- **Urinalysis:** This is usually normal. Proteinuria is present if glomerulopathy has developed.

Diagnostic Notes

Dyspneic cats should be handled very carefully, because increased stress may be fatal. Extreme care should be taken when doing the physical examination, radiographs, and thoracentesis. It may be necessary to place the cat in an oxygen cage for several minutes prior to diagnostics and between diagnostic procedures. The least stressful radiographic view is the dorsoventral (DV); it may be the only view that is practical in some cases and is usually sufficient to diagnose the presence of pleural effusion.

 T r e a t m e n t

Primary Therapeutics

- **Thoracentesis:** The least amount of sedation should be employed. If sedation is needed, the use of 2 mg/kg of ketamine IV is generally safe. Aspirate both sides of the chest, and remove as much fluid as possible. Aspirate below the costochondral junction in multiple locations beginning at the 4th to 6th IC space with the cat in sternal recumbency.
- **Antibiotics:** The initial choice should include drugs likely to be effective against anaerobic bacteria. Amoxicillin (high dose = 40 mg/kg TID IM, SC) plus metronidazole is the initial drug combination of choice. Antibiotics should be given for at least 1 month past apparent recovery based on clinical signs and radiographs. The choice of antibiotics should be based on culture and sensitivity.

Secondary Therapeutics

- **Thoracostomy tube:** This permits continuous or intermittent chest drainage without further stress to the cat. Generally, one tube will drain both sides of the chest; however, some cases require bilateral tube placement. The chest should be aspirated one to two times per day. Many clinicians flush the pleural space with warm saline solution with or without antibiotics. Most feel that parenteral antibiotics are sufficient, and overzealous use of certain antibiotics, especially aminoglycosides, may result in toxicity. The pleural space should be aspirated until less than 4 mL/kg of fluid is removed. (This amount is usually due to the presence of the tube.)

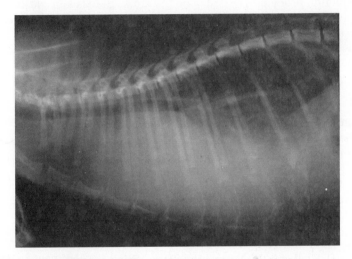

Figure 104.1. Pyothorax is the presence of pus in the pleural space. It cannot be distinguished radiographically from other causes of pleural effusion.

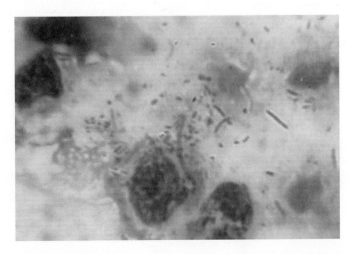

Figure 104.2. Cytology reveals copious numbers of bacteria and degenerative neutrophils.

- **Intravenous fluids:** Placement of an intravenous catheter and fluid administration should be delayed until thoracentesis has been performed due to the stress involved.
- **Thoracotomy:** Cats that do not respond to 5–10 days of chest drainage and appropriate systemic antibiotics are candidates for this surgery. The pleural space should be probed for foreign bodies.

Therapeutic Notes

Repeated thoracentesis may be used in place of thoracotomy. However, this can be a painful procedure that may be too stressful for many cats that are fragile patients. The use of a chest drain is strongly recommended for all but the most debilitated patients.

P r o g n o s i s

This is a serious and potentially fatal disease. However, with aggressive diagnostics and therapeutics, including a thoracotomy tube, most of these cats will recover. Recurrence is likely if antibiotic therapy is discontinued too soon; otherwise, the prognosis is good.

S u g g e s t e d   R e a d i n g s

Norsworthy GD. Pyothorax. In: Norsworthy GD, ed. Feline practice. Philadelphia: JB Lippincott, 1993;454–457.

Roudebush P. Bacterial infections of the respiratory system. In: Green C, ed. Infectious diseases of the dog and cat. Philadelphia: WB Saunders, 1990.

Sherding RG. Diseases of the pleural cavity. In: Sherding RG, ed. The cat: diseases and clinical management, 2nd ed. New York: Churchill Livingstone, 1994;1053–1091.

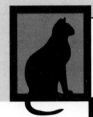

CHAPTER 105

Pyrethrin Toxicosis

Gary D. Norsworthy

Overview

Pyrethrins are insecticides commonly used on cats. The most popular ones are permethrin, allethrin, resmethrin, and tetramethrin. Fenvalerate plus diethyltoluamide (DEET) is used on dogs but is very toxic to cats. Pyrethrins are nontoxic to most mammals, but cats have less ability to degrade these products. Toxicity occurs in an occasional cat, but it is usually not fatal with the exception of DEET toxicity. Pyrethrins may be more toxic if combined with synergistic insecticides. Their toxicity is based on their ability to permit excessive amounts of sodium into cells, resulting in excessive nerve stimulation. Lethargy and salivation are the mildest clinical signs. The toxicity may progress to ataxia, tremors, and seizures.

 Diagnosis

Primary Diagnostics

- **History and clinical signs:** A combination of known exposure and clinical signs is the basis for diagnosis in most cases.

 Treatment

Primary Therapeutics

- **Atropine:** This drug is given (0.5 mg/kg SC or IM) to control salivation.
- **Diazepam:** This drug is given (in 0.5–1.25-mg increments IV) to control seizures. The dosage should not exceed 20 mg/cat.
- **Bathing:** It is important to remove remaining toxin from the skin with a noninsecticide-containing shampoo.

Therapeutic Notes

Full recovery is expected in 1–2 days.

Prognosis

The prognosis is good with the exception of DEET toxicity or toxicity due to pyrethrin-containing insecticide combinations. In the latter case, the prognosis will vary depending upon the other insecticide involved.

Suggested Reading

Rumbeiha WK, Oehme FW, Reid FM. Toxicoses. In: Sherding RG, ed. The cat: diseases and clinical management, 2nd ed. Philadelphia: WB Saunders, 1994;215–249.

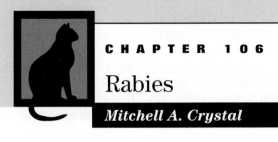

CHAPTER 106

Rabies

Mitchell A. Crystal

Overview

R abies is caused by the rabies virus, a labile, single-stranded RNA virus in the family Rhabdoviridae. Rabies is acquired via a bite from an infected animal, typically a raccoon or skunk or, uncommonly, a bat or other mammal. Other rare sources of infection acquisition include inhalation or ingestion. Younger cats are more susceptible to infection. Rabies virus has a predilection for nervous and salivary gland tissue. After being bitten by an infected animal, cats will undergo an incubation period without clinical signs, during which time the virus spreads to the central nervous system (CNS) by retrograde flow-up axons. The incubation period is of variable length depending on the site of the bite (shorter when closer to the CNS and in highly innervated tissue), age (shorter in younger cats), and the amount of virus introduced. Incubation periods may vary from 9 days to over a year, although the vast majority of cats will develop clinical signs within 4–6 weeks.

Clinical signs of rabies include increased vocalization with or without a change in voice; restlessness; a wild, anxious, or blank look to the eyes; anorexia; depression; flaccid hind-limb paresis or paralysis (reported by owners as ataxia); erratic and/or vicious/striking behavior; and weakness and/or incoordination. Signs may or may not progress from a less to a more severe clinical illness (sometimes referred to as progressing from a prodromal to a furious phase). A paralytic form of rabies also exists (dumb rabies), in which cats present for generalized paralysis, coma, and death. This form may follow a period of clinical signs as described above or may be the presenting complaint. Death typically occurs within 8–10 days of clinical signs, although a few experimental cases have had prolonged survival after development of clinical signs. Vaccine-induced rabies has been reported secondary to the use of modified live-virus rabies vaccines. Clinical signs begin 2 weeks after vaccination and include hind-limb weakness progressing to posterior, then generalized, paralysis. No modified live-virus rabies vaccines are currently available for use in cats.

Since 1981, cases of feline rabies have outnumbered cases of canine rabies. An increase in rabies in cats could result in an increase in exposure of humans to rabies. This is potentially due to the free-roaming/predatory nature and more limited vaccination of cats as well as to the recent rabies outbreak in the mid-Atlantic states. Rabies is a public health concern. Although the incidence of human rabies in developed countries is low, infection is nearly 100% fatal. Therefore, early recognition and prevention are essential. Any human potentially exposed to a rabid animal is advised to consult his or her physician to discuss therapy with human rabies immune globulin and rabies vaccination. Individuals who are at an increased risk of exposure should receive pre-exposure rabies prophylaxis.

 Diagnosis

Primary Diagnostics

- **Direct immunofluorescent antibody test:** This test performed on brain tissue will demonstrate virus in all cats excreting virus in their saliva. The entire head, chilled but not frozen, should be submitted to the proper testing facility.

- **Quarantine and observation:** Any vaccinated cat that bites a human should be confined for observation for 10 days. Rabies vaccination should not be administered during this time. If neurologic signs develop, the cat should be euthanized and the head submitted to the proper authorities for rabies testing. The individual receiving the bite should be contacted and referred to a physician immediately.

Diagnostic Notes

- There are no rapid, definitive antemortem tests for rabies.
- Any unvaccinated cat that bites a human should be euthanized and the head submitted to the proper authorities for rabies testing.
- Freezing of a brain to be examined for rabies will interfere with and delay the diagnostic testing.
- Gloves and masks should be used when handling tissue that is potentially infected with rabies.
- Containers used to ship or transport tissue that is potentially infected with rabies should be clearly marked as a biologic hazard.

 Treatment

Primary Therapeutics

- **Euthanasia:** No therapy is effective once clinical signs of rabies are present. Because rabies is a human health concern, euthanasia is indicated followed by submission of the head to the proper authorities for rabies testing.

- **Vaccination:** All cats should be vaccinated with a killed vaccine given intramuscularly at one location in the thigh at 3 to 4 months of age, at one year of age, then at the appropriate interval determined by duration of product immunity and local public health regulations.
- **Nonvaccination preventive measures:** Any wound from a possible animal bite should be thoroughly cleansed. Owners should be discouraged from allowing their cats to roam free in areas endemic for rabies. Owners should be advised to immediately report any free-roaming wild or domestic animal demonstrating neurologic signs to the appropriate animal or wildlife control officials.

Secondary Therapeutics

- **Quarantine:** Any vaccinated cat that is bitten by a known or suspected rabies-infected animal should be revaccinated, kept under owner control, and observed for 45 days. An unvaccinated cat that is bitten by a known or suspected rabies-infected animal should be euthanized. If the owner is unwilling to have this done, the cat should be isolated for 6 months and vaccinated 1 month prior to being released.

Therapeutic Notes

Any humans potentially exposed to rabies should be referred to their physician to discuss appropriate preventative therapy.

Prognosis

Rabies is nearly 100% fatal in animals and people. Due to public health concerns, cats suspected of having rabies should not be treated. Immediate euthanasia is indicated followed by proper evaluation of the head by designated authorities. Humans exposed to potentially rabid animals should be referred to their physician for appropriate postexposure prophylaxis. Postexposure prophylaxis, when performed early, is almost always effective in preventing rabies in people.

Suggested Readings

Fogelman V, Fischman HR, Horman JT, Grigor JK. Epidemiologic and clinical characteristics of rabies in cats. *J Am Vet Med Assoc* 1993;202(11):1829–1833.

Green CE, Dreesen DW. Rabies. In: Green CE, ed. Infectious diseases of the dog and cat. Philadelphia: WB Saunders, 1990;365–383.

National Association of State Public Health Veterinarians, Inc. Compendium of animal rabies control, 1995. In: Bonagura JD, ed. Current veterinary therapy XII: small animal practice. Philadelphia: WB Saunders, 1995;1422–1426.

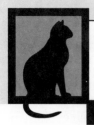

CHAPTER 107

Restrictive Cardiomyopathy

John-Karl Goodwin

Overview

Restrictive cardiomyopathy (RCM) is an uncommon cardiac disease characterized by myocardial or subendocardial fibrosis. There is no known cause, although myocarditis has been implicated as a precipitating condition. RCM may occur concurrently with hypertrophic cardiomyopathy or dilated cardiomyopathy.

Myocardial fibrosis may result in both diastolic dysfunction (loss of compliance) and systolic dysfunction (reduced contractility), features that have caused RCM to be classified as an intermediate cardiomyopathy.

Generalized congestive heart failure ensues, resulting in weakness and respiratory distress. Auscultatory abnormalities in order of incidence include gallop rhythm, arrhythmia, and murmur. Other physical findings may include ascites, hepatomegaly, muffled respiratory sounds (pleural effusion), and evidence of aortic thromboemboli.

Diagnosis

Primary Diagnostics

- **Radiography:** Thoracic radiographs reveal moderate-to-severe generalized cardiomegaly with variable pulmonary edema and/or pleural effusion.
- **ECG:** Ventricular premature complexes (VPCs), chamber-enlargement patterns, and intraventricular conduction defects are present.
- **Echocardiography:** Left atrial dilatation is consistently present. Other changes are variable and include ventricular dilatation, ventricular hypertrophy, and reduced fractional shortening (measure of contractility). Fibrosis is usually not evident by routine echocardiography.

Ancillary Diagnostics

- **Angiography:** An irregular left ventricular chamber with variable filling effects is found. Hypertrophy of the papillary muscles may be evident. Thrombi may be discernible.
- **Doppler echocardiography:** Mitral regurgitation is evident.

Diagnostic Notes

In cats over 6 years of age, hyperthyroidism should be ruled out.

Definitive diagnosis antemortem is difficult, as hallmark lesions (myocardial fibrosis) are not readily apparent during echocardiography. RCM cannot be differentiated from the other, more common, cardiomyopathies based on radiographs and ECG.

RCM is most often suspected when the degree of left atrial enlargement is greater than expected for the degree of left ventricular hypertrophy or dilatation. Cats with dilated cardiomyopathy usually have significantly lower indices of contractility (fractional shortening) than do cats with RCM.

 T r e a t m e n t

Primary Therapeutics

- **Reduce stress:** Take all measures to minimize any stress to cats exhibiting respiratory distress (e.g., delay radiographs and catheter placement).
- **Facilitate breathing:** Thoracocentesis should be performed in all dyspneic cats when pleural effusion is suspected (muffled lung sounds). With the cat placed sternally, place a 19–22-gauge butterfly catheter just into the pleural space (5th to 7th intercostal spaces, just cranial to the adjacent rib), and aspirate. Use a closed system and tap both sides of the chest. Use furosemide when pulmonary edema is present. In the crisis setting, use 2–4 mg/kg IV initially, then 1–2 mg/kg IV or IM every 4–6 hours until the edema has resolved. Furosemide is often continued as needed (6.25–12.5 mg SID-BID) to control edema formation. Apply nitroglycerin, 1/4 inch to a hairless area, every 4–6 hours until the edema has resolved.
- **Oxygen:** Administer via face mask, if tolerated, or oxygen cage (50% oxygen).

Secondary Therapeutics

- **Enalapril:** 0.25 mg/kg SID may be beneficial.
- **Digoxin:** Use if contractility is reduced: one-quarter of a 0.125-mg tablet every 24 to 48 hours.

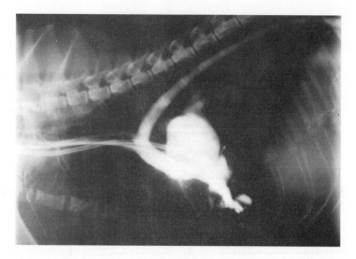

Figure 107.1. Restrictive cardiomyopathy (CM): Angiocardiogram showing irregular left ventricular chamber with filling defects that are often seen with restrictive cardiomyopathy.

- **Aspirin:** This drug may reduce the chance of thrombus formation: 81 mg every third day.
- **Diltiazem:** This drug may improve myocardial relaxation and control arrhythmias: 7.5 mg TID, or 30 mg daily of sustained release preparation.
- **Periodic centesis:** Thoracocentesis or abdominocentesis may be needed periodically.

Therapeutic Notes

- Monitor renal function if enalapril or digoxin is used.
- Warfarin (0.5 mg SID) may be used in lieu of aspirin but has a much greater chance of inducing a hemorrhagic crisis (see Chapter 117).
- The dosage of diuretics and need for antiarrhythmic agents may change during the course of the disease; frequent monitoring is recommended.

Prognosis

The prognosis of affected cats has not been objectively evaluated. In general, cats with preserved contractility are expected to have a more favorable prognosis, whereas those with more extreme left atrial enlargement usually develop life-threatening complications (arrhythmias, thromboembolic disease).

Suggested Readings

Pion, PD, Kienle RD. Feline cardiomyopathy. In: Miller MS, Tilley LP, eds. Manual of canine and feline cardiology, 2nd ed. Philadelphia: WB Saunders, 1995.

Stepien, RL. Restrictive cardiomyopathy in cats. In: Tilley LP, Smith FWK, eds. The 5-minute veterinary consult. Baltimore: Williams & Wilkins, 1997.

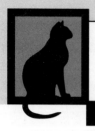

CHAPTER 108

Rodenticide Toxicosis

Mitchell A. Crystal

Overview

Next to insecticides, poison control centers receive more inquiries about rodenticide intoxicants than any other type of intoxicant. Several types of rodenticide intoxicants exist. Those commercially available are listed in Table 108.1.

TABLE 108.1.

Commercially Available Rodenticides That Cause Toxicity in Cats

Toxic Agent	Mechanism of Action	Toxic Dose (mg/kg of agent unless noted)	Onset	Clinical Signs
Bromethalin: Assault®, Trounce®, Vengeance®	Uncouples oxidative phosphorylation, leading to cerebral edema	300–1100 of bait	2–7 days, but can be as late as 2 weeks	Hind-limb ataxia, paresis or paralysis, depression, tremors, decerebrate posture, seizures
Cholecalciferol: Quintox®, Rampage®, Rat-B-Gone®	Hypervitaminosis D, leading to acute renal failure	Exact toxic dose is unknown < 1000 of bait < 10 of cholecalciferol	Within 24 hours	Vomiting with or without blood, anorexia, lethargy, PU/PD
Coumarins and indandiones: 1st generation: warfarin, pindone 2nd generation: bromadiolone,	Vitamin-K antagonism, leading to an acquired coagulopathy	Warfarin; Warfarin 5–50, Pindone 5–75, diphacinone 15, brodifacoum 25, bromadiolone 25	As early as 36–72 weeks, as late as 2–4 weeks	Variable depending on location of hemorrhage (ecchymosis, hematomas, dyspnea, lameness, etc.)

398

TABLE 108.1. CONT.

Commercially Available Rodenticides That Cause Toxicity in Cats

Toxic Agent	Mechanism of Action	Toxic Dose (mg/kg of agent unless noted)	Onset	Clinical Signs
brodifacoum, diphacinone				
Strychnine	Antagonizes the inhibitory neuro-transmitter glycine	2.0	Within 2 hours	Nervousness, stiffness, rigidity, seizures (spontaneous or induced by auditory stimulation), mydriasis, respiratory failure
Zinc Phosphide	Acid pH in stomach releases phosphine gas, leading to GI irritation and asphyxia	20–50	Within 1–4 hours	Anorexia, lethargy, hemorrhagic vomiting, abdominal pain, ataxia, seizures, dyspnea

Diagnosis

See Table 108.2 for diagnosis of rodenticide toxicosis.

Treatment

See Table 108.2 for treatment of toxicosis.

Prognosis

The prognosis for coumarins, indandiones, and strychnine is good to excellent for cure with early recognition and treatment. Most cats do not survive intoxication with bromethalin, cholecalciferol, or zinc phosphide.

TABLE 108.2.

Diagnostic Procedures and Therapy for Rodenticide Toxicosis in the Cat

Toxic Agent	Diagnosis (aside from exposure and clinical signs)	Treatment (aside from emesis and oral cathartic if within 8 hours of ingestion)
Bromethalin	Postmortem evidence of tissue residues	Control seizures if present (diazepam or barbiturates), maintain hydration, provide nutritional support
Cholecalciferol	Hypercalcemia with hyperphosphatemia with or without renal failure	NaCl diuresis (90 mL/kg/day IV), prednisone 1–2 mg/kg PO, SC BID, furosemide 1–2 mg/kg SC, IV BID, salmon calcitonin 4–6 IU/kg SQ every 2 to 3 hours; check serum calcium levels to assess effectiveness of overall therapy
Coumarins and indandiones	Increased activated clotting time, activated partial thromboplastin time, and one-stage prothrombin time; normal thrombin time; presence of proteins induced by vitamin K (PIVKA) in citrated plasma	Acute hemorrhage with significant anemia (PCV < 20%) is managed by transfusion with fresh whole blood (10–20 mL/kg IV). Vitamin-K antagonism is managed with vitamin K_1 (aquamephyton) at 5 mg/kg as an initial SQ loading dose followedby 2.5 mg/kg PO BID for 3 weeks. If the toxic agent is known to be a first-generation agent, therapy can be shortened to 1 week. Coagulation parameters should be checked 3 to 5 days following cessation of vitamin K_1 therapy.
Strychnine	Analysis of gastric contents, urine, and hepatic biopsies	Control tetany/seizures (diazepam or barbiturates); NaCl diuresis (70–80 mL/kg IV); endotracheal intubation; and artificial respiration if respiratory failure is present. Therapy is usually needed for 1 to 3 days.
Zinc phosphide	Analysis of gastric contents	Gastric lavage with bicarbonate within 8 hours of ingestion, NPO, maintain hydration, HCO_3- for acidosis if present

Suggested Readings

Grauer GF, Osweiler GD. Rodenticides. In: Morgan RV, ed. Handbook of small animal practice, 2nd ed. Philadelphia: WB Saunders, 1992;1305–1312.

Mount ME, Woody BJ, Murphy MJ. The anticoagulant rodenticides. In: Kirk RW, ed. Current veterinary therapy IX: small animal practice. Philadelphia: WB Saunders, 1986;156–165.

Nicholson SS. Toxicology. In: Ettinger SJ, Feldman EC, eds. Textbook of veterinary internal medicine, 4th ed. Philadelphia: WB Saunders, 1995;312–317.

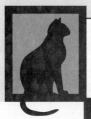

CHAPTER 109

Salmonellosis

Mitchell A. Crystal

Overview

S*almonella* spp. (most commonly *S. typhimurium*) are motile, nonspore-forming gram-negative rods of the family Enterobacteriaceae. *Salmonella* spp. may infect a wide variety of mammals, birds, reptiles, and insects, leading to gastrointestinal disease, systemic disease, or asymptomatic infection. *Salmonella* spp. may be isolated in up to 18% of normal cats. *Salmonella* spp. are acquired via ingestion of infected feces, infected prey, or contaminated food or water. Glucocorticoid therapy, obesity, and prolonged oral antibiotic administration may place cats at an increased risk of developing infection. *Salmonella* spp. can exist for prolonged periods in the environment and are often resistant to common disinfectants, making it a potential source for nosocomial infections. Clinical signs of feline salmonellosis include acute or chronic gastroenteritis, sepsis, chronic febrile illness without gastrointestinal signs, or localized tissue infections. Cats may also demonstrate no clinical illness. Cats with acute gastroenteritis may have mild-to-severe small and/or large bowel diarrhea, vomiting, abdominal pain, borborygmus, weight loss, and anorexia. Occasionally, cats may demonstrate only chronic diarrhea. Cats with sepsis may present with pyrexia or hypothermia, dehydration, weakness, or depression, and may or may not have accompanying gastrointestinal signs. Cats with *Salmonella* spp. have been reported to present for chronic fever and nonspecific signs of illness without gastrointestinal (GI) signs. *Salmonella* spp. have also been isolated from infected wounds and incisions. *Salmonella* spp. is considered of zoonotic importance, and appropriate handling of feces should be discussed with owners. Immunocompromised individuals should avoid contact with infected animals.

 D i a g n o s i s

Primary Diagnostics

- **Fecal culture and sensitivity:** The presence of *Salmonella* spp. does not necessarily indicate the organism is causing disease, as up to 18% of cats are asymptomatic carriers. Enrichment broth (selenite or tetrathionate) will help increase the chances of isolating *Salmonella* spp.

- **Blood or other (wound, urine, synovial fluid, etc.) culture and sensitivity:** Positive *Salmonella* spp. cultures from areas other than the GI tract indicate a definitive diagnosis of salmonellosis.

Ancillary Diagnostics

- **CBC:** Severe infections are associated with neutropenia with a left shift and toxic changes.
- **Chemistry profile:** Nonspecific changes such as hypoalbuminemia, liver enzyme elevation, hypoglycemia, and prerenal azotemia may be present.

Diagnostic Notes

- Negative cultures do not eliminate the possibility of infection, as *Salmonella* spp. is difficult to isolate in the presence of other organisms.
- Cats with *Salmonella* spp. should be screened for FeLV and FIV infections.

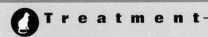 **T r e a t m e n t**

Primary Therapeutics

- **Enrofloxacin:** Administer 2.5 mg/kg BID PO for 7–10 days.
- **Norfloxacin:** Administer 22 mg/kg BID PO for 7–10 days.

Secondary Therapeutics

- **Trimethoprim/sulfa:** Administer 15 mg/kg BID PO for 7–10 days.
- **Chloramphenicol:** Administer 15–20 mg/kg TID-QID PO for 7–10 days.

Therapeutic Notes

- Mild infections may be self-limiting and thus may not require therapy. Antibiotic therapy has the potential to induce antibiotic-resistant strains and thus should be avoided if possible. Cats with moderate-to-severe clinical signs, chronic carriers, and cats that demonstrate neutropenia should receive therapy.
- Recent evidence suggests that fluoroquinolones are highly effective against active and chronic infections and may not induce antibiotic-resistant strains. Fluoroquinolone use in young, growing kittens has the potential to cause cartilage defects, though much less than in puppies.
- Parenteral fluid therapy and other supportive measures are needed for septicemic patients.
- Improve sanitation conditions to help prevent reinfection.
- In-vitro antibiotic sensitivity may not correlate with in-vivo activity.

P r o g n o s i s

The prognosis is generally good except for those with severe septicemia. Cats with underlying immunosuppressive diseases (FeLV- and FIV-induced) have a less favorable prognosis. The asymptomatic carrier state may be difficult to eliminate, so the zoonotic importance of this disease must be stressed to the owner. *Salmonella* spp. may also persist in the environment and lead to reinfection.

S u g g e s t e d   R e a d i n g s

Dow SW, Jones RL, Henik RA, Husted PW. Clinical features of salmonellosis in cats: six cases. *J Am Vet Med Assoc* 1989;194(10):1464–1466.

Kier AB. *Salmonellosis*. In Green CE, ed. Infectious diseases of the dog and cat. Philadelphia: WB Saunders, 1990;542–549.

Guilford WG, Strombeck DR. Gastrointestinal tract infections, parasites, and toxicoses. In: Strombeck's small animal gastroenterology, 3rd ed. Philadelphia: WB Saunders, 1996;411–432.

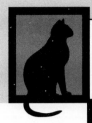

Skin Parasites

Sharon K. Fooshee

Overview

Flea infestation, notoedric mange, and cheyletiellosis are the three main ectoparasitic skin diseases of cats. Fleas and flea allergy are discussed in Chapters 58 and 59. Notoedric mange, caused by the sarcoptic mite *Notoedres cati*, is spread by direct contact between cats and is very contagious. Cheyletiellosis, also known as "walking dandruff," is caused primarily by *Cheyletiella blakei* mites. Like *Notoedres*, it is quite contagious. Both mites are obligate parasites; they may also infest humans, dogs, and rabbits. Notoedric mange is manifested as a pruritic, crusty dermatosis; initially, it involves primarily the head and neck. Scaling is the most consistent and important clinical sign of cheyletiellosis, although cats tend to scale less than dogs. Miliary lesions are sometimes present. Pruritus of acute onset is sometimes present, but this is not a reliable finding. Kittens are most often infested.

 D i a g n o s i s

Primary Diagnostics

- **Clinical signs:** Pruritic dermatitis, with or without crusting or scales, should be suspected of being due to mites.
- **Skin scraping:** When present, notoedric mites are usually easy to find on routine skin scrapings. *Cheyletiella* mites may, in addition to skin scrapings, require acetate tape preparations, flea combing, or fecal flotation to render a diagnosis. It is a large mite with characteristic hooks on the accessory mouthparts. Grooming habits of the cat may remove large numbers of mites from the hair.

Ancillary Diagnostics

If cheyletiellosis is suspected, but the mites cannot be demonstrated, it is acceptable to treat and monitor for a response to therapy.

Diagnostic Notes

- Many cats with scaling or pruritus due to *Cheyletiella* spp. infestation are misdiagnosed with other disorders.
- Some dermatologists suggest that flea combing is the most reliable method for detecting *Cheyletiella* mites.

 T r e a t m e n t

Primary Therapeutics

- **Topical:** Affected (as well as in-contact) dogs and cats should be clipped. Weekly dipping with lime sulfur or pyrethrin dips for a minimum of 6–8 weeks is safe and effective. *Cheyletiella* mites are susceptible to most parasiticidal agents, including lime sulfur, pyrethrins, and carbamates. In some cases, however, the mites may be difficult to eliminate. Also, topical therapy should not be looked to as the **sole** therapy for cheyletiellosis.

- **Systemic:** Ivermectin, although not approved for use in the cat, is very successful in eliminating both mites. For notoedric mange, a dose of 200 µg/kg is given subcutaneously, with the injections spread 2 weeks apart. For cheyletiellosis, a dose of 300 µg/kg subcutaneously is given for two to three treatments, 14 days apart.

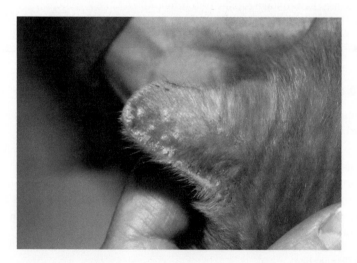

Figure 110.1. Skin parasites: Notoedric mange, caused by the sarcoptic mite *Notoedres cati*, results in the formation of a crusty dermatitis on the face, especially on the pinnae.

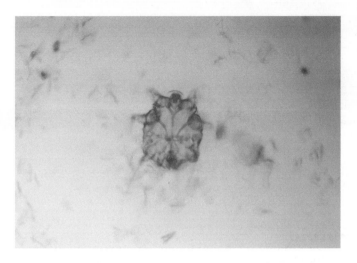

Figure 110.2. *Notoedres cati* can be recovered with a skin scraping and found microscopically at 100X magnification.

Secondary Therapeutics

- **Extended Control:** It is very important to treat all affected animals. The environment should be disinfected by vacuuming. Bedding should be washed where all pets sleep.

Therapeutic Notes

It is especially important that long-haired cats be clipped prior to topical therapy. This assists in dispersal of insecticide and also removes mite eggs, which cling to the hair.

Prognosi

The prognosis is good when appropriate therapy is instituted. All pets in the household, as well as the premises, must be treated for optimal outcome.

Suggested Reading

Moriello KA. Cheyletiellosis. In: Griffin CE, Kwochka KW, MacDonald JM, eds. Current veterinary dermatology. St. Louis: Mosby Yearbook 1993;90–95.

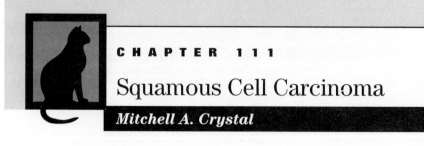

CHAPTER 111

Squamous Cell Carcinoma

Mitchell A. Crystal

Overview

Squamous cell carcinomas (SCC) make up 15% of feline skin tumors. Solar radiation is a contributing factor in tumor development. Affected cats usually have light or unpigmented skin, and thus white cats living in sunny climates are at greatest risk, and Siamese cats are under-represented. The mean age of cats with SCC is 12 years, with a range of 9–12.4 years. Common sites for tumor development are the nasal planum, pinnae, eyelids, and lips. Less common sites include the tongue and gingiva. SCC is locally invasive but slow to metastasize. It appears as a proliferative or ulcerative, plaque-like or cauliflower-like lesion with or without overlying crusts. About one-third of affected cats have multiple facial lesions. Differential diagnoses include basal cell tumor, melanoma, mast cell tumor, cutaneous hemangioma or hemangiosarcoma, hair follicle tumors, sebaceous gland tumors, and eosinophilic granuloma complex lesions.

A second form of SCC has recently been described: multiple squamous cell carcinoma in situ (MSCCI), also known as Bowen's disease. MSCCI is unrelated to sunlight. It occurs most commonly in thick-haired, pigmented areas over the head, neck, shoulder, and forelimbs. Lesions appear as multiple well-circumscribed, melanotic, hyperkeratotic plaques that progress to become crusted and ulcerated. Lesions are confined to the epidermis, and metastasis has not been reported.

Diagnosis

Primary Diagnostics

- **Clinical appearance:** Ulcerated areas on the pinnae, nasal planum, eyelids, and lips of white-haired cats should be highly suspect.
- **Surgical removal or incisional biopsy and histopathology:** This is the most definitive means of diagnosis.

Ancillary Diagnostics

- **Fine-needle aspiration/cytology:** This may reveal the diagnosis prior to surgery.
- **Lymph node aspiration/cytology:** Aspiration should be performed if regional lymphadenopathy is present.
- **Thoracic radiographs:** These should be performed to evaluate for metastasis.

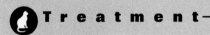 **T r e a t m e n t**

Primary Therapeutics

- **Surgery:** Cure rates vary from 17–66% depending on the stage of the tumor and aggressiveness of surgery. Control rates greater than 1–1.5 years or cure may be achieved in many cats with small, less-invasive tumors. Amputation of the margins of the pinnae can be curative.
- **Cryosurgery:** Cryosurgery in 102 cats with 163 lesions of the nasal planum, pinnae, and eyelids achieved a 1-year disease-free control rate of 82%.

Secondary Therapeutics

- **Radiation therapy:** In cats with small, less-invasive tumors, radiation (total dose of 40 Gray administered in 10 fractions over 3.5 weeks on a Monday-Wednesday-Friday schedule) has achieved a cure rate of 56% and progression-free 1 and 5 year survival rates of 60% and 10%.
- **Laser surgery:** Nd:YAG laser surgery was successful in treating a cat with nasal planum SCC. Four treatments were needed over 14 months.
- **Photodynamic therapy:** Laser excitation of an injected photosensitizing dye was successful in treating 12 of 19 cats with SCC of the nasal planum or pinnae. Success was related to minimal invasion and tumor size less than 5 cm.

Therapeutic Notes

- Oral chemotherapy has demonstrated inconsistent efficacy with low response rates of short duration.
- Other reported therapies with some success have included local hyperthermia and intralesional chemotherapy with cisplatin or 5-fluorouracil.

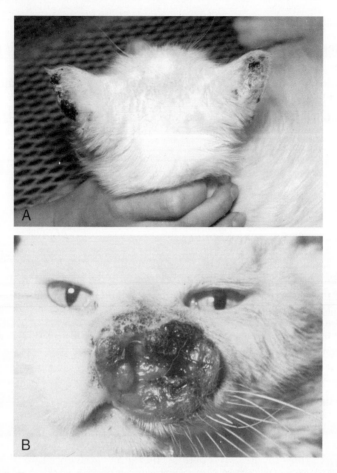

Figure 111.1. Squamous cell carcinoma: Squamous cell carcinoma occurs most commonly on the face of white-haired cats. It is commonly located on the pinnae (*A*) and the nasal planum (*B*).

Prognosis

Large, less-differentiated, invasive tumors have a worse prognosis. The prognosis is unrelated to the location of the tumor, although tumors of the pinna often allow a more aggressive therapy and thus may have a better outcome. A better prognosis is achieved with minimally invasive tumors less than 2 cm in diameter. See therapy above for specific prognosis details for the different therapies available.

Suggested Readings

Marks SL. Therapeutic options for solar-induced squamous cell carcinoma in dogs and cats. Proceedings of the Thirteenth Annual Veterinary Medical Forum 1995;272–275.

Vail DM, Withrow SJ. Tumors of the skin and subcutaneous tissues. In: Withrow SJ, MacEwen EG, eds. Small animal clinical oncology, 2nd ed. Philadelphia: WB Saunders, 1996;167–191.

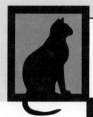

CHAPTER 112

Stud Tail

Gary D. Norsworthy

Overview

The supracaudal organ is a linear region on the dorsal surface of the tail that is rich in sebaceous and apocrine glands. Its secretions are used in scent marking. Stud tail is localized seborrhea due to hypersecretion of glands in the supracaudal organ. It results in oil accumulation and matting of the haircoat. Secondary bacterial folliculitis, comedones, localized furunculosis, and pruritus may occur. Although more common in intact males, it may occur in neutered or intact individuals of both genders. Persian, Siamese, and Rex breeds are predisposed to stud tail.

 D i a g n o s i s

Primary Diagnostics

- **Clinical signs:** The finding of seborrhea on the supracaudal region is diagnostic. The presence of folliculitis, comedones, and furunculosis are confirmatory.

 T r e a t m e n t

Primary Therapeutics

- **Clip hair:** Hair removal in the region will permit better penetration of medications.
- **Shampooing:** Cleanse the area with antiseborrheic shampoo.

Secondary Therapeutics

- **Antibiotics:** Secondary infections are generally caused by *Staphylococcus* spp. The use of a staph-effective antibiotic, i.e., enrofloxacin, amoxicillin and clavulanic acid, erythromycin, cephalosporins, etc., is indicated when infection is present.

Therapeutic Notes

- If infection is not present, this is a cosmetic problem that may not justify treatment.
- Surgical neutering may not be beneficial in all cases.

Prognosis

Treatment is generally successful, but recurrence is common.

Suggested Readings

Merchant SR. The skin: diseases of unknown or multiple etiology. In: Norsworthy GD, ed. Feline practice. Philadelphia: JB Lippincott, 1993;532–538.

Moriello KA. Diseases of the skin. In: Sherding RG, ed. The cat: diseases and clinical management, 2nd ed. Philadelphia: WB Saunders, 1994;1907–1968.

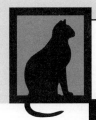

CHAPTER 113

Systemic Hypertension

John-Karl Goodwin

Overview

Systemic hypertension is defined as the sustained elevation of systolic (>180 mm Hg) or diastolic (> 120 mm Hg) arterial blood pressure. This disorder is common yet infrequently diagnosed due to limitations of accurately measuring blood pressure and spurious elevations secondary to stress and excitement.

Primary (essential) hypertension is the most common type of hypertension in humans but has not been documented in the cat. In cats, the most common causes of systemic hypertension are classified as diseases that increase cardiac output and those that cause increased peripheral resistance. Diseases in the first category include thyrotoxic cardiomyopathy due to hyperthyroidism and primary cardiomyopathy. The most common disease in the latter category is chronic renal failure (CRF). Incidence rates of systemic hypertension for cats with CRF and hyperthyroidism are reportedly 65% and 87%, respectively. Less common causes include hyperadrenocorticism, acromegaly, mineralocorticoid secreting tumors, and pheochromocytoma.

In CRF, salt and fluid retention, increased adrenergic tone, increased activity of renin-angiotensin-aldosterone, and stiffening of capacitance veins have been documented and are theorized to contribute to the development of systemic hypertension. In hyperthyroidism, elevations in heart rate, stroke volume, and beta-adrenergic receptors mediate increases in systemic blood pressure.

The mean age of affected cats is 15 years. Clinical features may include malaise, polyuria/polydipsia, acute blindness secondary to retinal hemorrhage and detachment, renomegaly (although kidneys may be small with CRF), hematuria, seizures, and congestive heart failure.

 D i a g n o s i s

Primary Diagnostics

- **Chemistry profile:** This will reveal azotemia and hyperphosphatemia (CRF) or moderate elevations in liver enzymes (hyperthyroidism).

- **Urinalysis:** urine specific gravity in isosthenuric range (CRF).
- **Thyroid screen:** Elevations in total and free T_4 are expected.
- **Ophthalmic examination:** Fixed and dilated pupils, retinal hemorrhage and detachment, and tortuosity of retinal vessels are commonly found.
- **Blood pressure determination:** Direct methods are very accurate but require expensive equipment and are associated with artifactually elevated pressures. Indirect methods include oscillometric and Doppler technology. These techniques employ a cuff that is inflated to obstruct blood flow through the radial or tarsal artery. The cat is placed in lateral recumbency and kept as calm as possible, preferably with the owner present. The oscillometric technique automates cuff inflation and pressure determination. For the Doppler technique, the evaluator notes the pressure that is associated with a return of the audible signal of blood flow. Doppler monitors* have been consistently more accurate in cats because of their small body weight. (*Pet Recovery Products, 1–800–484–6255 PIN 7778.)

Ancillary Diagnostics

- **Radiography:** Radiographs reveal variable cardiomegaly, with or without evidence of pulmonary congestion and edema, and small kidneys.
- **Echocardiography:** This may reveal left ventricular hypertrophy associated with hypertrophic cardiomyopathy or thyrotoxic cardiomyopathy.

Diagnostic Notes

A presumptive diagnosis is often made on the basis of characteristic clinical signs rather than on specific documentation of elevated blood pressure. If blood-pressure monitoring equipment is not available, cats that have sudden-onset retinal blindness, blood that is drawn extremely from peripheral veins, and a pounding heartbeat should be strongly suspected of hypertension. Early treatment (within 24 hours of blindness) yields the best chance of restoring vision, so cats fitting this protocol should be considered for antihypertensive therapy.

If measuring blood pressure, one should obtain seven measurements, discard the low and high values, and mean the remaining values.

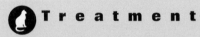 T r e a t m e n t

Primary Therapeutics

- **Low-sodium diet:** A diet moderately restricted in sodium should be offered.
- **Antihypertensive agent:** Administer one of the following agents: a) **diuretic**—furosemide (1–2 mg/kg q12–24 hr) or hydrochlorothiazide (1–2

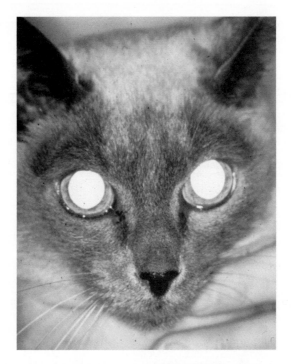

Figure 113.1. Systemic hypertension: Hypertension may cause acute blindness, resulting in fixed and dilated pupils.

mg/kg q12–24 hr); b) **ACE inhibitor**—enalapril (0.25–0.5 mg/kg q24–48 hr) or benazepril (0.25–0.5 mg/kg q24–48 hr); c) **beta-blocker**—atenolol (6.25–12.5 mg/cat q24hr) or propranolol (2.5–10 mg/cat q12hr); or d) **calcium channel blocker**—diltiazem (1.5–2.5 mg/kg q8hr) or amlodipine 0.625 mg/cat q24 hr).

Secondary Therapeutics

- Manage the hyperthyroid state if present.
- Treat aggressively for renal failure, if present. See Chapter 37.

Therapeutic Notes

- Amlodipine is currently the drug of choice. It should be tried first.
- Antihypertensive therapy usually is not needed long term when hyperthyroidism is successfully treated. However, such therapy may need to be part of long-term management of CRF.

P r o g n o s i s

Systemic hypertension can often be successfully controlled, especially when there is high owner compliance and cats are rechecked and medications adjusted as needed. The prognosis is best when hypertension is secondary to hyperthyroidism, as this disorder can often be reversed.

Suggested Readings

Labato MA, Ross LA. Diagnosis and management of hypertension. In: August JR, ed. Consultations in feline internal medicine. Philadelphia: WB Saunders, 1990;301–308.

Littman MP. Spontaneous systemic hypertension in 24 cats. *J Vet Intern Med* 1994;8:79–86.

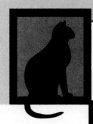

CHAPTER 114

Tapeworm Infections

Mitchell A. Crystal

Overview

Tapeworms are small intestinal cestode parasites that cause few, if any, clinical signs. *Dipylidium caninum* and *Taenia* spp. are the most common tapeworms seen in the cat. *D. caninum* is acquired via ingestion of infected fleas, and *Taenia* spp. are acquired via ingestion of infected small mammals. There is no extraintestinal migration, and transplacental and transmammary infections do not occur. The most common problem associated with tapeworm infection is the complaint of owners of seeing proglottid sections within the feces or on the perianal hair. Physical examination is normal. Rarely, in the southeast United States, infection with the tapeworm *Spirometra* spp. occurs. This cestode is acquired by ingestion of infected small mammals and can lead to diarrhea.

 D i a g n o s i s

Primary Diagnostics

- **Direct examination of feces:** Proglottid sections can be seen.
- **Examination of the perineum:** Dried proglottid sections can be seen on the perineal hair, and moving proglottid sections can be seen near the anus.

Ancillary Diagnostics

- **Proglottid squash preparation:** A proglottid can be squashed in a drop of water between two microscope slides. *D. caninum* eggs are organized into an egg basket containing 20 to 30 eggs. *Taenia* spp. are liberated as single eggs.
- **Fecal sedimentation and floatation:** Single eggs of *D. caninum or Taenia* spp. may be seen if the egg baskets have been ruptured. Single operculated eggs of *Spirometra* spp. may be seen.

Diagnostic Notes

The importance of identifying the specific type of tapeworm lies in prevention. If *D. caninum* is identified, flea control is needed. If *Taenia* spp. is identified, prevention of ingestion of small mammals is needed.

T r e a t m e n t

Primary Therapeutics

- **Praziquantel:** Administer 3–7 mg/kg PO or SC.
- **Epsiprantel:** Administer 2.75 mg/kg PO.
- **Praziquantel/pyantel pamoate (Drontal):** Administer according to label direction PO.

Secondary Therapeutics

- **Bunamidine:** Administer 25–50 mg/kg PO.

Therapeutic Notes

- Only one treatment is necessary for *D. caninum* and *Taenia* spp. because there is no tissue migratory phase. However, none of the drugs should be considered 100% efficacious.
- Treatment of *Spirometra* spp. requires higher doses (1.5 ×) of praziquantel and may require treatment for several days.

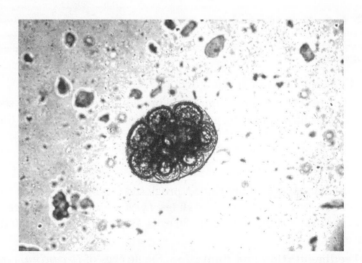

Figure 114.1. Tapeworm infection: The diagnosis of tapeworms is usually based on finding tapeworm segments on the surface of the stool or the perineal hair. However, occasionally the segments will rupture, releasing egg baskets, which may be found on a fecal floatation.

• Prevention (*D. caninum*—flea control, *Taenia* spp. and *Spirometra* spp.—predatory behavior/scavenging control) will help stop reinfection.

Prognosis

The prognosis is excellent because these worms are essentially nonpathogenic, and the anthelminthics are very effective.

Suggested Readings

Burrows CF, Batt RM, Sherding RG. Diseases of the small intestine. In: Ettinger SJ, Feldman EC, eds. Textbook of veterinary internal medicine, 4th ed. Philadelphia: WB Saunders, 1995;1198–1199.

Reinemeyer CR. Feline gastrointestinal parasites. In: Kirk RW, Bonagura JD, eds. Kirk's current veterinary therapy XI: small animal practice. Philadelphia: WB Saunders, 1992;626–630.

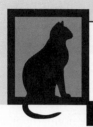

CHAPTER 115

Tetralogy of Fallot

John-Karl Goodwin

Overview

Tetralogy of Fallot is the most commonly occurring cyanotic heart disease in the cat. The components of tetralogy of Fallot include pulmonic stenosis, right ventricular concentric hypertrophy, a subaortic ventricular septal defect, and an overriding aorta. A right-to-left shunt results secondary to the right ventricular outflow obstruction caused by the pulmonic stenosis. Cyanosis is a blue discoloration of the mucous membranes that usually indicates a significant amount of desaturated hemoglobin (3–5 g/dl). Pulmonary atresia represents the exaggerated form of tetralogy of Fallot, inasmuch as the distal right ventricular outflow tract is atretic and the main pulmonary artery is a thin, useless vessel. A murmur of pulmonic stenosis is often absent in these cases.

Physical examination usually demonstrates a left basilar systolic ejection-type murmur. A soft systolic murmur associated with the ventricular septal defect may also be evident over the right hemithorax, although this finding is variable.

Diagnosis

Primary Diagnostics

- **Echocardiography:** The ECG reveals right ventricular concentric hypertrophy, subaortic ventricular septal defect, overriding of the aorta, high-velocity (>2 m/sec) turbulent systolic flow across the right ventricular outflow tract as demonstrated by spectral or color-flow Doppler, and right-to-left shunting as demonstrated by contrast echocardiography (bubble study). Aortic regurgitation, as demonstrated by Doppler echocardiography, may also be present.

Ancillary Diagnostics

- **Electrocardiography:** Right-axis deviation is commonly present, but findings may vary.

- **Thoracic radiography:** Right atrial and ventricular enlargement, dilated proximal pulmonary artery secondary to pulmonic stenosis, pulmonary vascular undercirculation, and an enlarged caudal vena cava may be present.
- **Nonselective angiography:** This procedure is useful in evaluating the pulmonary vascularity.
- **PCV:** Polycythemia is present in most cases.

Diagnostic Notes

Cardiac catheterization and selective angiocardiography are rarely needed to substantiate the diagnosis of tetralogy of Fallot.

 T r e a t m e n t

Primary Therapeutics

- **Surgical palliation:** The purpose of surgery is to create a systemic-to-pulmonary shunt to increase pulmonary flow, left atrial venous return, and arterial oxygen content.
- Specific procedures include the Blalock-Taussig (connection of the subclavian artery to the pulmonary artery) and Waterson-Cooley or Potts (connection of the aorta to a lobar or the main lobar pulmonary artery) operations.

Secondary Therapeutics

- Periodic phlebotomy with IV fluid replacement to maintain the PCV below 62% can be effective in some cats.
- Exercise restriction is encouraged. Beta blockade may reduce myocardial oxygen consumption, decrease heart rate, decrease right-to-left shunting by increasing left ventricular afterload, and provide a positive lusitropic effect (increased relaxation) of the right ventricle.

Therapeutic Notes

- Cats may tolerate the defect for years; however, chronic hypoxia, polycythemia and hyperviscosity syndrome, exercise intolerance, or seizure-like activity commonly occur.
- Sudden cardiac death is more likely to occur than congestive heart failure.
- Surgical palliation often reduces clinical signs and increases survival times.
- Surgical palliation is effective only if the pulmonary arteries are of sufficient diameter and available for anastomosis.
- The efficacy of beta blockers has not been proven in veterinary medicine in this scenario.

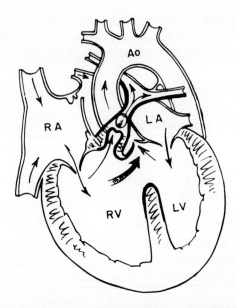

Figure 115.1. Tetralogy of Fallot: This drawing illustrates the blood flow patterns in a heart with tetralogy of Fallot.

Prognosis

The prognosis of tetralogy of Fallot is guarded-to-poor. Clinical signs may be palliated with surgery. However, few facilities routinely perform the surgical procedures, and significant complications are possible.

Suggested Reading

Abbott JA. Tetralogy of Fallot. In: Tilley LP, Smith FWK, eds. The 5-minute veterinary consult. Baltimore: Williams & Wilkins, 1997.

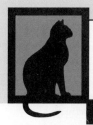

CHAPTER 116

Thiamine Deficiency

Gary D. Norsworthy

Overview

Thiamine deficiency occurs secondary to consumption of large quantities of uncooked fish that contain a thiaminase enzyme or diets that are thiamine-deficient due to improper processing. Cooking destroys the enzyme in fish. After about 2–4 weeks of a thiamine-deficient diet, cats salivate excessively, stand over the food bowl as if to eat, but eat only small amounts of food. After another 2–4 weeks, the cat experiences brief tonic seizures, cervical ventroflexion, and the loss of righting reflexes. Bradycardia, pronounced sinus arrhythmia, and retinal hemorrhages may also occur. If the cat is not treated at this stage, coma and death ensue.

 D i a g n o s i s

Primary Diagnostics

- **Dietary history:** A thiamine-deficient diet, especially consisting of large quantities of uncooked fish, is typical.
- **Clinical signs:** The clinical signs are listed in Overview, above. The most common sign on presentation is cervical ventroflexion. This differs from cervical ventroflexion due to organophosphate toxicosis or hypokalemic polymyopathy in that this disease causes a rigid paralysis of the cervical muscles. In the other two diseases mentioned, weakness due to flaccid paralysis occurs. The other mentioned clinical signs are indicative of this disease and others.
- **Response to therapy:** Cats treated with injectable thiamine return to normal within 24 hours. Such response is diagnostic.

Diagnostic Notes

Because thiamine is nontoxic, a test dose is indicated for cats, especially kittens, that are showing signs of cervical ventroflexion.

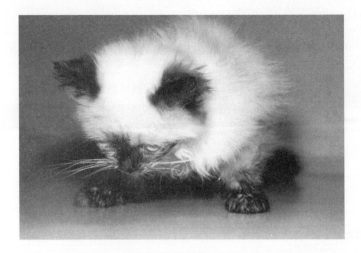

Figure 116.1. Thiamine deficiency: Thiamine deficiency usually occurs in kittens. The cats often present in cervical ventroflexion as a result of rigid paralysis of the cervical muscles.

T r e a t m e n t

Primary Therapeutics

- **Thiamine:** Cats suspected of having thiamine deficiency should be given 5 mg PO or 1 mg parenterally. Oral thiamine should be given for at least 1 week while the diet is being corrected.
- **Diet change:** Affected cats should be placed on a balanced feline diet.

P r o g n o s i s

The prognosis for thiamine-deficient cats is excellent if proper treatment is rendered and the cat's diet is changed to one with adequate thiamine.

S u g g e s t e d   R e a d i n g

Buffington CA. Nutritional diseases and nutritional therapy. In: Sherding RG, ed. The cat: diseases and clinical management, 2nd ed. Philadelphia: WB Saunders, 1994;161–190.

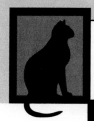

CHAPTER 117

Thromboembolic Disease

John-Karl Goodwin

Overview

Systemic thromboembolism is a frequent and life-threatening complication of cardiomyopathy (see Chapter 64 for a description of pulmonary thromboembolism). Stasis of blood within dilated cardiac chambers and increased platelet reactivity combine to predispose cardiomyopathic cats to systemic thromboembolism. Typically, a clot lodges at the aortic trifurcation (saddle thrombus), resulting in a severe ischemic insult to the rear limbs and tail. Systemic thromboembolism, however, can also affect other organs, including kidneys, gastrointestinal tract, and brain.

Vasoactive agents (prostaglandins, serotonin) released by platelets at the site of the thrombus result in constriction of collateral and regional vessels, further contributing to ischemia and reducing blood flow to terminal spinal cord segments.

Saddle thrombus results in a consistent constellation of physical abnormalities, including hind-leg paresis or paralysis, absent pulsations, cyanosis, and coolness of the skin. Hind-leg musculature is typically firm and painful. Organ dysfunction may occur depending upon the location of the thrombi.

Affected cats almost always have significant underlying cardiac disease, and congestive heart failure is often precipitated by the occurrence of systemic thromboembolism.

Diagnosis

Primary Diagnostics

- **Physical examination:** Posterior paralysis is the most common clinical sign. The rear feet are often cold and cyanotic.

Ancillary Diagnostics

- **Radiography:** Radiographs often reveal evidence of congestive heart failure including pulmonary edema, pleural effusion, and cardiomegaly. There should be an absence of spinal lesions.
- **Echocardiography:** This will demonstrate underlying heart disease.
- **Angiography:** This can be used to demonstrate the location of a thrombus. There will be an absence of contrast material in affected arteries.
- **Blood pressure determination of suspected limbs:** Impeded blood flow will result in no or very low blood pressure. It can replace Echocardigraphy, CBC, and/or chemistry profile. (Note: do not remove echocardiography, if possible.)

Diagnostic Notes

The diagnosis usually is based on characteristic physical examination abnormalities.

If not previously established, the underlying heart disease should be determined.

 T r e a t m e n t

Primary Therapeutics

- **Manage congestive heart failure:** See Chapters 6, 47, 74, and 107 for specific treatment guidelines.
- **Promote collateral circulation:** Acepromazine (0.1–0.4 mg/kg SC q8h as needed) is used to achieve evidence of tranquilization.
- **Heparin:** Give 200 IU/kg IV, followed by 200 IU/kg SC q8h for 48–72 hours.

Secondary Therapeutics

- **Provide warmth:** Use warm water bottles or gloves; avoid intense heat (lights, electrical pads), as limbs are very susceptible to thermal injury.
- **Sodium bicarbonate:** Give 1–2 mEq/kg IV slowly to correct metabolic acidosis and hyperkalemia. Administer with low-rate infusion of 0.45% saline/2.5% dextrose.
- **Analgesia:** Give pentazocine (0.2–0.5 mg/kg IM) or butorphanolol (0.2–0.4 mg/kg IM).
- **Aspirin:** Give 10 mg/kg PO twice weekly

Therapeutic Notes

The use of thrombolytic agents (streptokinase, tissue plasminogen activator) have been associated with high mortality rates.

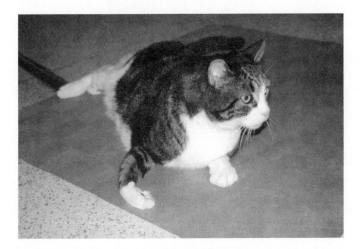

Figure 117.1. Thromboembolic disease: Cats with thromboembolic disease usually present with paralysis of the hind limbs owing to a saddle thrombus. This cat also has paralysis of the right front limb because another thrombus has affected the brachial artery.

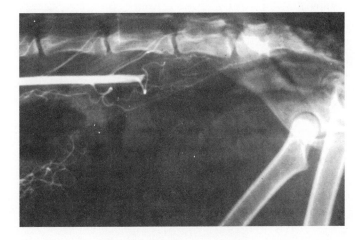

Figure 117.2. A nonselect angiogram shows the location of the aortic thrombus.

Anesthesia and surgical therapy (embolectomy) is also associated with a high mortality rate.

Nonselective beta-adrenergic blockers (e.g., propranolol) may impede the development of collateral circulation and should not be used when systemic thromboembolism is present.

P r o g n o s i s

Overall, the prognosis is guarded. Approximately 50% of affected cats survive the acute congestive heart failure and systemic thromboembolism crisis. Those surviving typically show steady improvement in limb function beginning within 24 to 72 hours of presentation. The prognosis is grave for cats showing no improvement over this time and in those developing gangrenous changes.

Cats surviving are at risk of recurrence (43% in one series).

S u g g e s t e d   R e a d i n g

Laste NJ, Harpster NK. A retrospective study of 100 cats with feline distal aortic thromboembolism: 1977–1993. *J Sm Anim Hosp Assoc* 1995;31:492–500.

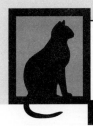

CHAPTER 118

Toxocara Infection

Mitchell A. Crystal

Overview

Toxocara are small intestinal nematode parasites that are also known as roundworms. There are two types of roundworms found in the cat: *Toxocara cati* (most common) and *Toxascaris leonina. T. cati* and *T. leonina* are acquired via ingestion of infected paratenic hosts (mice, birds, insects) or feces. Kittens may also acquire *T. cati* from ingestion of infected queen's milk during nursing. Roundworms have a 2–3 week life cycle. The life cycle of *T. cati* involves migration through the lungs and liver and in some cases through somatic tissues. The life cycle of *T. leonina* includes no extraintestinal migration. Transplacental infection does not occur with either *T. cati* or *T. leonina*. Clinical signs are more severe in kittens than in adult cats and include vomiting (with or without worms), diarrhea (with or without worms), abdominal distention and/or pain (kittens), weight loss or failure to gain weight (kittens), coughing (pneumonitis or pneumonia from *T. cati*), and, rarely, intestinal obstruction. Infections may also be asymptomatic. Physical examination may be normal, reveal evidence of abdominal distention and/or pain (kittens), weight loss (kittens), or diarrhea. Unlike *Toxocara canis, T. cati* has limited public health significance.

Diagnosis

Primary Diagnostics

- **History:** The owner may report seeing worms in vomitus or feces.
- **Fecal flotation:** Eggs are seen on microscopic examination.

Ancillary Diagnostics

- **Direct saline smear:** Eggs are sometimes seen on microscopic examination.
- **Chest radiographs:** These may suggest verminous pneumonia.

Diagnostic Notes

- Clinical signs may develop in kittens before eggs are detected in feces.
- The most common cause of coughing in kittens is due to pulmonary larval migration of *Toxocara*.

Treatment

Primary Therapeutics

- **Pyrantel pamoate:** Administer 20 mg/kg PO; repeat in 2–3 weeks.
- **Praziquantel/pyantel pamoate (Drontal):** Administer according to label directions; repeat in 2–3 weeks.

Secondary Therapeutics

- **Fenbendazole:** Administer 25 mg/kg PO for 3 days; repeat in 2–3 weeks.
- **Ivermectin:** Administer 200 µg/kg PO; repeat in 2–3 weeks.
- **Dichlorvos:** Administer 11 mg/kg PO; repeat in 2–3 weeks.

Therapeutic Notes

- Treat kittens routinely or if roundworm infection is suspected, even if fecal floatation is negative.
- A second treatment is needed 2 to 3 weeks following initial therapy to kill new adults arising from eggs and larva that were initially resistant to therapy.

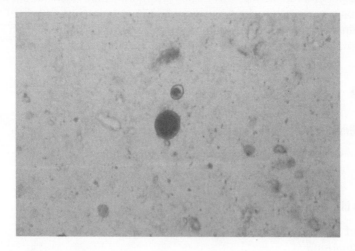

Figure 118.1. Toxocara: Eggs are found on a fecal floatation. *T. cati*, shown here, is much larger than the nearby *Isospora* oocyst.

Prognosis

The prognosis is excellent for cure, although roundworm eggs often persist in the environment for years and lead to reinfection. This may be a problem in outdoor cats.

Suggested Readings

Burrows CF, Batt RM, Sherding RG. Diseases of the small intestine. In: Ettinger SJ, Feldman EC, eds. Textbook of veterinary internal medicine, 4th ed. Philadelphia: WB Saunders, 1995;1196–1202.

Reinemeyer CR. Feline gastrointestinal parasites. In: Kirk RW, Bonagura JD, eds. Kirk's current veterinary therapy XI: small animal practice. Philadelphia: WB Saunders, 1992;626–630.

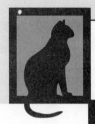

Toxoplasmosis

Gary D. Norsworthy

Overview

Toxoplasma gondii infects most warm-blooded animals, but domestic and wild Felidae are the only hosts in which the life cycle can be completed. There are three infectious stages: 1) tachyzoites, which live in body tissues, 2) bradyzoites, which live in body tissues, and 3) oocytes, which are excreted in feces. Although infections can be acquired in several ways, most cats become infected by eating the infected tissues of infected mammals. The most common life cycle begins with the ingestion of tissue cysts. These are digested, releasing bradyzoites, which penetrate the small intestinal wall. A series of asexual generations occurs, followed by a sexual cycle, finally producing oocytes. Oocysts pass in the feces; however, they are not infective until they are exposed to air and sporulate for at least 1 day. The entire life cycle can be completed within 3 days after ingestion of tissue cysts. If the life cycle begins with the ingestion of tachyzoites or oocysts, it requires about 3 weeks for completion.

Most cats infected with *T. gondii* show no clinical signs. However, following penetration of the small intestinal wall, the organism may spread to lymph nodes or to other organs via lymph and blood. If focal necrosis occurs in the target organs, clinical signs develop referable to the individual organ or organs. The lungs and liver are the most commonly affected organs. Anorexia, lethargy, and pneumonia-related dyspnea are the most common clinical signs. Uveitis and retinal hemorrhage are the second most common signs. Although some cats will die from the infection, most recover and develop immunity. It is unknown why some cats die and others remain asymptomatic.

Toxoplasmosis can be a serious disease in humans. Because of the cat's role in transmission, veterinarians should be aware of several important facts. Cats typically shed large quantities of oocysts for only 1 or 2 weeks and usually have only one shedding episode in their lifetime. If shedding recurs, the number of oocysts passed is almost insignificant. Oocyst shedding is heaviest in kittens 6 to 14 weeks of age. Once in the environment, oocysts resist disinfectants, freezing, and drying. They can be killed by temperatures of 70°C for 10 or more minutes.

An episode of shedding does not correlate with antibody production. A negative serologic test indicates lack of exposure and susceptibility to infection. A positive test indicates that a cat has probably shed oocysts in the past and is thus much less likely to be a future shedder than a seronegative cat.

 D i a g n o s i s

Primary Diagnostics

- **Radiographs:** The most commonly affected organ is the lungs. Radiographs reveal diffuse or patchy areas of pulmonary consolidation.
- **Liver enzymes:** Hepatic enzymes may be elevated when the liver is affected; however, this is a nonspecific finding that may occur in many feline diseases.
- **IgM antibody titers:** IgM antibodies appear early and are present for about 3 months. They correlate with recent or active infection. ELISA testing is preferred.*

Ancillary Diagnostics

- **IgG antibody titers:** IgG antibodies appear by the fourth week postinfection and are present for months or years. They generally represent a previous infection. Agglutination tests primarily detect these antibodies.
- **Response to therapy:** Clinical response to a 3-week course of clindamycin in conjunction with an elevated IgM titer and appropriate clinical signs is suggestive of a diagnosis of toxoplasmosis.
- **Cytology:** Impression smears or fine-needle aspirates (FNAs) of affected tissues can reveal *Toxoplasma* organisms when stained with a Wright's-type stain.
- **Histopathology:** The organism can be found in affected tissues. However, the presence of tissue cysts does not necessarily correlate with disease. It is necessary to find tachyzoites for confirmation of disease.

 T r e a t m e n t

Primary Therapeutics

- **Clindamycin:** This is the most effective drug for cats. It is dosed at 25 mg/kg BID PO for 2–3 weeks.
- **Sulfa plus pyrimethamine:** This combination has been used with success but sulfas need to be administered every 6 to 8 hours, so client compliance can be problematic.

* Available from the Toxoplasmosis Serology Laboratory, CVM, Colorado State University, and the Infectious Disease Laboratory, CVM, University of Georgia.

Therapeutic Notes

Because this is a potentially zoonotic disease, personnel involved in therapy should exercise caution in handling bodily fluids and secretions from the affected cat.

Prevention of Transmission

- **Meat handling:** Utensils and surfaces that contact uncooked meat should be washed with soap and water. Meat should be cooked at 70°C or frozen before cooking.
- **Pregnant women:** They should avoid contact with cat feces, litter box materials, soil, and raw meat. Cats should only be fed commercial cat food or food that has been cooked to 70°C or frozen. Litter boxes should be emptied daily. Cats should not be allowed to hunt, scavenge raw meat, or eat dead animals.

Prognosis

The prognosis is generally good if diagnosis and proper therapy begin early. The use of the ELISA IgM test is important in making an early diagnosis.

Suggested Reading

Dubey JP. Toxoplasmosis and other coccidial infections. In: Sherding RG, ed. The cat: diseases and clinical management, 2nd ed. Philadelphia: WB Saunders, 1994;565–581.

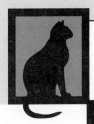

CHAPTER 120

Trichobezoars

Mitchell A. Crystal

Overview

Trichobezoars (hairballs) can be a cause of regurgitation or vomiting in the cat. Hairballs appear as hair with or without food and/or gastric secretions. Occasionally, a cat will attempt to regurgitate/vomit a hairball but will be unsuccessful and only produce gastric secretions. Cats accumulate hair as a result of normal grooming habits, although hairballs may accumulate as a result of behavioral/neurologic disorders (excessive grooming) and primary gastrointestinal diseases (motility disorders, infiltrative diseases). Therefore, in cats with normal grooming behaviors, regurgitation/vomiting of hairballs may be a normal phenomenon or may be an indicator of an underlying gastrointestinal disease.

The signalment of cats with trichobezoars varies (depending on whether the hairballs are normal or due to an underlying gastrointestinal or neurologic disease), although they tend to occur more frequently in long-haired young to middle-aged cats. Cats may also develop a problem from grooming other long-haired pets in the household. In the normal cat, no other clinical signs should be present aside from intermittent regurgitation/vomition of hairballs. If weight loss, diarrhea, anorexia, or other problems are present, a complete diagnostic evaluation should be performed to search for an underlying disease. Differential diagnoses should include diseases that cause regurgitation or vomiting. (See Chapter 23.)

Diagnosis

Primary Diagnostics

- **History:** Trichobezoars may have occurred in the past without other clinical signs.
- **Response to therapy:** See below.

Ancillary Diagnostics

- **Complete diagnostic evaluation:** If other clinical signs are present or the problem is frequent and nonresponsive to therapy, a complete workup is indicated. (See Chapter 23.)

Diagnostic Notes

Clients frequently want to blame hairballs on a variety of ailments. Although they may even cause intestinal obstruction, many cats pass them without clinical signs.

 T r e a t m e n t

Primary Therapeutics

- **Grooming:** Frequent grooming is needed to prevent exposure to excessive hair buildup.
- **Petroleum-based laxatives:** These should be administered orally to lubricate the material and facilitate normal aboral passage. Several preparations are commercially available. Most are in the form of a jelly. Doses vary but generally are suggested at 1–5 mL/cat/day to effect.

Secondary Therapeutics

- **Motility enhancers:** Cisapride (2.5–7.5 mg/cat PO SID-TID) or metoclopramide (0.2–0.4 mg/kg PO BID-QID) may provide support for those cats with motility disorders.

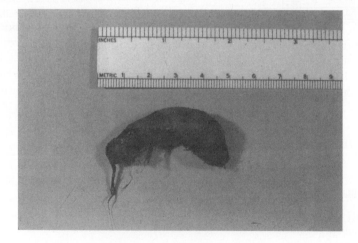

Figure 120.1. Trichobezoars are frequently vomited. If they pass into the small intestine, they may be the cause of intestinal obstruction and require surgical removal.

- **Shaving:** Long-haired cats can be shaved every 3–4 months to minimize hair ingestion.

Therapeutic Notes

Mineral oil should be avoided as it is tasteless and odorless and thus may lead to aspiration and lipid pneumonia.

Prognosis

Cats without underlying disease are not at risk of becoming ill and only create an inconvenience to the owner. Most of these cats can be controlled with therapy, although occasional episodes can be expected. The prognosis of cats with underlying disease varies depending on the disease.

Suggested Reading

Twedt DC. Diseases of the stomach. In: Sherding RG, ed. The cat: diseases and clinical management, 2nd ed. New York: Churchill Livingstone, 1994;1193–1195.

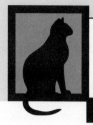

CHAPTER 121

Upper Respiratory Infections

Gary D. Norsworthy

Overview

T he causes of feline upper respiratory infections (URIs) include bacteria, fungi, and viruses. This chapter will concentrate on those diseases caused by the feline herpesvirus (rhinotracheitis virus), the feline calicivirus, and *Chlamydia psittaci*. However, recent evidence indicates that *Bordetella bronchiosepticum*, the cause of kennel cough in dogs, may also be a significant cause of feline URIs. The two aforementioned viruses account for about 80% of all feline URIs. These viruses are very contagious and often endemic to multicat households and catteries. Both are likely to produce a carrier state in which stress-induced intermittent viral shedding (herpesvirus) or continuous viral shedding (calicivirus) occurs. Maternal antibodies wane at about 5–7 weeks of age, so kittens in these environments are usually exposed before vaccine-induced immunity occurs. The most consistent clinical sign is sneezing; other common signs include fever, conjunctivitis, ocular and nasal discharge, corneal and oral ulceration, and hypersalivation. Anorexia occurs due to fever, oral ulceration, or nasal congestion and can lead to dehydration and death. Unusual signs caused by these viruses include abortion, footpad and interdigital ulceration, and arthritis. These organisms are not transmissible to humans.

Diagnosis

Primary Diagnostics

- **History and clinical signs:** Although there are several causes of sneezing, sneezing that persists over 48 hours is highly suggestive of URI. Some or many of the other aforementioned clinical signs are usually present.

Ancillary Diagnostics

- **Viral isolation:** Many veterinary reference laboratories can isolate and identify the herpesvirus and the calicivirus. This is best indicated for identifying chronic carriers.

- **Cytology:** Chlamydial inclusions may be identified in conjunctival scrapings stained with a modified Wright's stain. They are present for about 2 weeks following infection.

Diagnostic Notes

- The clinical signs of all of these infections are very similar. When secondary bacterial infections occur, these diseases are indistinguishable based on clinical signs.
- Because treatment of all of these infections are essentially identical, there are few instances in clinical practice in which differentiation is indicated.

Treatment

Primary Therapeutics

- **Antibiotics:** These infections are quickly complicated by bacteria. Although the viral infections are self-limiting in a few days, the bacterial infections can become life-threatening if not treated. The author's drugs of choice for mild-to-moderate infections are amoxicillin (12.5 mg/kg BID PO) or clavulanic acid/amoxicillin (15 mg/kg BID PO). If severe infections occur, clavulanic acid/amoxicillin plus enrofloxacin (15 mg/kg BID PO) is preferred for outpatients and amoxicillin (12.5 mg/kg BID SC) plus enrofloxacin (2 mg/kg BID SC) or gentamicin (2.2 mg/kg BID SC) is preferred for hospitalized cats.
- **Hydration:** Nasal and ocular secretions thicken when dehydration occurs. To prevent this added discomfort, cats should receive rehydrating and maintenance doses of balanced electrolyte fluids IV or SC.
- **Nutritional support:** Anorexia is very common and is the most serious complication of URIs. Nutritional support using orogastric or nasoesophageal tubes should begin as early as possible. Contraindications include dyspnea and severe depression. Nasal secretions should be removed before an orogastric tube is passed; severe nasal congestion and irritation contraindicates the use of nasoesophageal tubes.

Secondary Therapeutics

- **Ophthalmic antibiotics:** These are indicated when conjunctivitis exists. It is advisable not to use products containing corticosteroids because of the possibility of corneal ulcers.
- **Nasal decongestants:** Oxymetazoline hydrochloride (Afrin Pediatric Nasal Drops) is advocated by some. One drop is placed in one nostril once daily. However, most cats object to nasal drops; after-congestion may develop; and efficacy has not been clearly demonstrated.

Therapeutic Notes

- Tetracycline and chloramphenicol are efficacious for *Chlamydia psittaci*. However, this is a mild and uncommon infection, and these drugs have poor efficacy against the common secondary bacteria often present. In addition, they may contribute to fever and anorexia.

- Intranasal vaccination has not been shown to shorten clinical infection or to terminate the carrier state. However, immunity is developed quicker with intranasal vaccines than with injectable vaccines, so they have merit

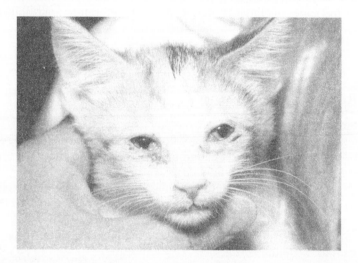

Figure 121.1. Upper respiratory infections: Sneezing with nasal and ocular discharge is common in cats with URIs.

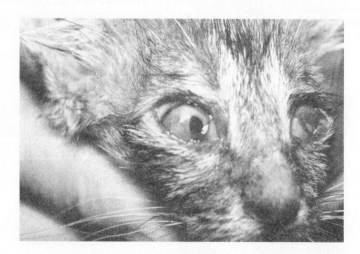

Figure 121.2. Some cats develop corneal ulcerations, which may become chronic if not treated aggressively.

in situations in which exposure is likely. Intranasal vaccines also may prevent the carrier state.

- Some cats receiving intranasal vaccine develop chronic sneezing.
- Injectable vaccines should be included in a cat's routine vaccination program.
- The author has used oral alpha interferon (2–4 IU/kitten PO) beginning at 3 weeks of age to control URI in kittens in endemic catteries and multicat households. It is given until the kitten leaves the contaminated facility.
- Cats should be treated in a hospital with isolation facilities when anorexia occurs or to prevent exposure of others cats in the household.

Prognosis

The prognosis is good if anorexia and dehydration do not occur or if they are treated aggressively. Cats that fail to respond to appropriate therapy within 4–6 days should be tested for the feline leukemia virus (FeLV) and the feline immunodeficiency virus (FIV), two viruses that can be immunosuppressive and prevent response to therapy .

Suggested Readings

Ford RB, Levy JK. In: Sherding RG, ed. The cat: diseases and clinical management, 2nd ed. Philadelphia: WB Saunders, 1994;489–500.

Norsworthy GD. Upper respiratory infections. In: Norsworthy GD, ed. Feline practice. Philadelphia: JB Lippincott, 1993;570–576.

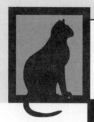

CHAPTER 122

Urolithiasis

Gary D. Norsworthy

Overview

A urolith is a rock-like mass found in the urinary tract. It is composed of a small amount of organic matrix (generally mucoid material) and a large amount of crystalline material. There are at least four types that have been found in cats. Struvite (magnesium ammonium phosphate hexahydrate) uroliths account for about 65% of those found; calcium oxalate uroliths are present about 20% of the time. The balance are calcium phosphate, urate, and of mixed composition. A small percent of struvite uroliths are induced by bacterial infections, usually *Staphylococci* spp. or *Proteus* spp. The remainder of struvite uroliths and the other types are typically unrelated to bacteria, and their pathogenesis is not understood, although dietary factors are important in some cases. Uroliths in the kidneys are generally asymptomatic. When found in the bladder, hematuria and dysruia result. Ureteral or urethral uroliths cause severe dysuria or obstruction.

Diagnosis

Primary Diagnostics

- **Clinical signs:** The clinical signs of hematuria, dysuria, or urethral obstruction are typical of urolithiasis; however, some cats are asymptomatic.

- **Radiography or ultrasound:** These imaging modalities are able to identify most uroliths. Very small size may elude detection; radiolucent uroliths may require contrast radiographic studies or ultrasound examination.

Ancillary Diagnostics

- **Palpation:** Because of their size, most uroliths in the urinary bladder are not palpable. However, this should be part of the physical examination.

Diagnostic Notes

- Many uroliths in the urinary bladder are very thin ("wafer-like"). High-definition radiographic technique may be necessary to identify them. Double-contrast (positive and negative) radiographic studies of the bladder are recommended, because some are radiolucent.

- Small uroliths may be passed through the urethra of females. They may lodge in the vagina or adhere to the perineal hair. These should be submitted for analysis so that appropriate treatment and preventative strategies can be formulated.

- Quantitative analysis of the urolith is strongly encouraged. The composition of the center of the stone is the most important aspect for planning preventive measures.

- If bacteria are noted within the center of the urolith, they should be cultured.

T r e a t m e n t

Primary Therapeutics

- **Surgical removal:** Uroliths within the bladder can be removed surgically via cystotomy. Uroliths lodged within the urethra may be backflushed into the bladder for surgical removal or medical dissolution or removed by perineal urethrostomy. Ureteral uroliths require surgical removal.

- **Medical dissolution:** Struvite uroliths located in the bladder may be dissolved with Feline Prescription Diet s/d (Hill's Pet Products, Topeka, KS). Two to 4 months of feeding s/d exclusively are required.

- **Antibiotic therapy:** Some struvite uroliths are induced by bacteria, especially staphylococcus and *Proteus* spp. When culture reveals their presence in urine or within the center of a urolith, appropriate antibiotics are indicated.

Secondary Therapeutics: Prevention

- **Struvite uroliths with infection:** Culture and sensitivity serve as the basis for antibiotic selection. If medical dissolution is used, appropriate antibiotics should be continued for 2 weeks past completion. If surgical removal is chosen, antibiotics should be given for no less than 4 weeks. The urine should be cultured monthly for 2 or 3 months, then again in 6 months. The urine should also be cultured any time the urine pH exceeds 7.5.

- **Struvite uroliths without infection:** Acidifying diets that are restricted in magnesium, phosphorus, and calcium are beneficial. Commercially available diets include UR-Formula Feline Diet (Ralston Purina, St. Louis,

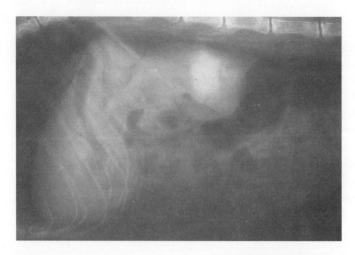

Figure 122.1. Urolithiasis: Renal uroliths are usually visible with radiography.

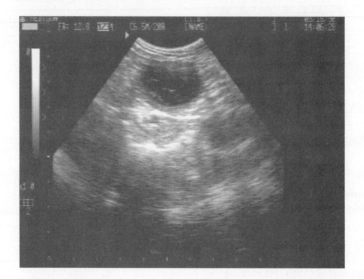

Figure 122.2. Uroliths in the urinary bladder may also be visible with radiography, but very small stones or those composed of calcium oxalate may be best seen with an ultrasound study.

MO) and Feline Prescription Diet c/d (Hill's). Alternatively, urinary acidifiers given with meals are also effective. DL-methionine or ammonium chloride are most effective and are each dosed at 1 g/cat/day.

- **Calcium oxalate uroliths:** Nonacidifying diets that have reduced sodium and protein but are not restricted in phosphorus or magnesium are recommended. Commercially available diets include NF-Formula Feline Diet (Ralston Purina) and Feline Prescription Diet k/d (Hill's). Unproved, but possibly effective, drugs include thiazide diuretics (hydrochlorothiazide: 2–4 mg/kg q12h PO), potassium citrate (50–75 mg/kg BID PO, and vitamin B6 (25 mg/cat q48h PO).

- **Urate uroliths:** An alkalinizing diet not containing liver is recommended. The effectiveness of allopurinol in the cat is unknown.

- **Cystine uroliths:** An alkalinizing diet is recommended.

- **Calcium phosphate uroliths:** An effective approach is not currently recognized, but the approach taken for calcium oxalate uroliths seems appropriate. If hypercalcemia is present, its cause should be diagnosed and treated, if possible.

Therapeutic Notes

- Successful medical dissolution requires that the stone be bathed in urine, so only uroliths in the bladder are amenable to this approach.

- Acidifying diets or acidifiers are contraindicated in cats with a history of renal failure or disease.

- Acidifying diets and urinary acidifiers should not be used concomitantly unless it is documented that such a practice is required to produce acid urine.

Prognosis

The prognosis for uroliths is good; however, recurrence is problematic. Identification of the crystal or urolith composition is essential so appropriate dietary therapy may be employed.

Suggested Reading

JA Barsanti, DR Finco, SA Brown. Diseases of the lower urinary tract. In: Sherding RG, ed. The cat: diseases and clinical management, 2nd ed. Philadelphia: WB Saunders, 1994;1769–1823.

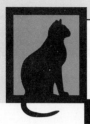

CHAPTER 123

Vaccinosarcoma (Vaccine-Related Sarcoma)

Sharon K. Fooshee

Overview

S ince 1992, a strong association has been recognized between administration of certain feline vaccines and development of connective tissue
tumors, primarily fibrosarcomas. Increased numbers of tumors were first
noticed following several changes in vaccine products. First, the modified live rabies vaccine was abandoned in favor of a killed product. In 1985, addition of aluminum as an adjuvant allowed rabies vaccine to be given subcutaneously. Vaccines
for leukemia virus (FeLV) were also introduced to the market during this time. The
mechanism of tumor induction remains unknown, but it is speculated that the local inflammatory response associated with certain vaccines may precipitate a de-
ranged fibrous connective tissue repair response, leading to neoplasia. The most
notable clinical finding is a soft-tissue swelling at the site of a previous vaccination:
hind limb or flank, dorsolateral thorax, interscapular space, or over the scapula.

 D i a g n o s i s

Primary Diagnostics

- **Clinical signs:** Any soft-tissue swelling near a vaccination site should
  raise one's index of suspicion.
- **Histopathology:** *Do not try to excise the mass prior to biopsy.* Local
  recurrence is likely to become increasingly aggressive with subsequent
  attempts at excision. A Tru-Cut biopsy or wedge (incisional) biopsy should
  be used to differentiate sarcoma from a vaccine-related granuloma.

Ancillary Diagnostics

- **Data base:** A minimum data base should be performed to determine
  overall health of the cat: CBC, biochemical profile, urinalysis, FeLV/FIV
  tests, and a T_4 in geriatric cats.

- **Radiographs:** The affected area should be radiographed to identify bone lysis and extension of tumor along tissue planes. The chest should also be radiographed for evidence of metastasis, although it is very unlikely.

Diagnostic Notes

Metastatic disease is uncommon. Local invasion is the primary concern.

 T r e a t m e n t

Primary Therapeutics

- **Triple approach:** Early investigations have suggested that trimodality therapy is likely to offer the most successful outcome.
- Surgery is recommended. Wide and deep surgical margins are essential because the tumors are quite aggressive and extend far beyond the palpable mass. When possible, any bone in the area of the tumor should also be removed.
- Radiation therapy may help to destroy a tumor that extends beyond the mass and into adjacent tissue. As such, a wide field of radiation is recommended. No clear-cut benefit has yet been found in comparing presurgical to postsurgical radiation. Further research is needed to investigate the role of radiation therapy.
- Chemotherapy is optional. Palliative therapy with doxorubicin may benefit some patients. A specific protocol has not yet been suggested by researchers.

Therapeutic Notes

- Because of the location, invasiveness, and aggression of these tumors, surgical excision alone is unlikely to offer a cure unless the *first* procedure is performed very aggressively.
- To decrease the chance of vaccine-related tumor induction, avoid previous vaccination sites when giving boosters. Vaccines should not be administered intramuscularly or in the interscapular space. Some practitioners have advocated subcutaneous vaccine administration on the limbs because of the potential to totally remove a tumor by amputation.
- Apparent vaccine-related granulomas that remain after one month should be removed and submitted for histopathology.
- Vaccine manufacturers, lot numbers, and sites of injection should be recorded in the medical record.
- Acemannan, a chemotherapeutic agent, has been touted as effective for fibrosarcomas; however, documented evidence is lacking.

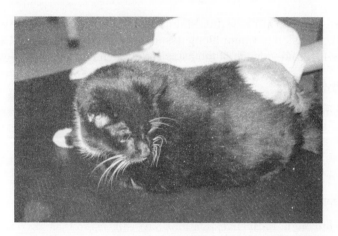

Figure 123.1. Vaccine-induced sarcomas: This rapidly-growing sarcoma occurred 2 months following vaccination.

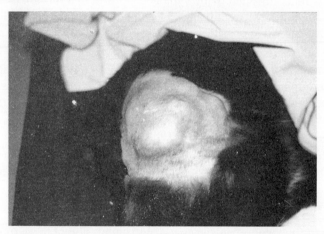

Figure 123.2. The sarcoma was removed with liberal excision but recurred within 30 days.

Prognosis

Prognosis is usually guarded because of local recurrence and the aggressive nature of these tumors.

Suggested Readings

Esplin DG, McGill LD, Meininger AC, Wilson SR. Postvaccination sarcomas in cats. *J Am Vet Med Assoc* 1993;202:1245–1247.

Macy D. Vaccine-associated sarcomas. Feline health topics for veterinarians. Cornell Feline Health Center, 1995;10:1–4.

Smith CA. Are we vaccinating too much? *J Am Vet Med Assoc* 1995;207:421–425.

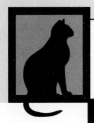

CHAPTER 124
Ventricular Septal Defects

John-Karl Goodwin

Overview

V entricular septal defects (VSDs) are among the most common congenital heart defects found in the feline (with atrioventricular valvular dysplasias being the most common). The interventricular septum separates the left and right ventricles and is divided into membranous and muscular components. Ventricular septal defects may occur in any area of the septum, but more commonly occur in the membranous portion near the base of the heart. Additionally, concurrent congenital defects may be present (i.e., tetralogy of Fallot). Intracardiac shunting of blood results when the defect is present.

Clinical significance of a VSD is determined by two factors: the size of the defect and the relative pressures in the ventricles, which influence the degree and direction of the shunt. Small defects (restrictive VSDs) often are of no hemodynamic significance, whereas large defects (nonrestrictive VSDs) are usually of significant hemodynamic consequence. When left and right ventricular pressures are normal, left-to-right shunting occurs and the left atrium and ventricle become volume-overloaded secondary to the increased venous return. If pulmonary vascular resistance is high either secondary to pulmonary hypertension as a result of chronic pulmonary venous hypertension or as a result of pulmonary arterial hypoplasia, right-to-left shunting may occur.

Physical examination usually reveals a holosystolic regurgitant-type murmur heard loudest over the right sternal border, a left apical systolic regurgitant-type murmur of mitral regurgitation, and a systolic ejection-type murmur at the left base consistent with relative pulmonic stenosis. Cyanosis may be present if a right-to-left shunt is present.

 ## Diagnosis

Primary Tests
- **Echocardiogram:** This will reveal evidence of a left-to-right shunt: left atrial and ventricular eccentric hypertrophy; ventricular septal defect,

449

most commonly located high in the septum. Contrast echocardiography (bubble study) demonstrates left-to-right shunting (i.e., no contrast enters the left ventricle). Ultrasound may also reveal evidence of a right-to-left shunt: right ventricular concentric hypertrophy; right atrial enlargement. Contrast echocardiography demonstrates right-to-left shunting (bubbles entering the left ventricle from the right ventricle).

Ancillary Diagnostics

- **Electrocardiogram:** There will be variable findings that are dependent on the severity of the shunt.
- **Thoracic radiography:** Variable findings are present that are dependent on the severity and direction of the shunt. Significant left-to-right shunts cause left atrial and ventricular enlargement, pulmonary vascular overcirculation, and possibly evidence of left-sided congestive heart failure. Right-to-left shunts are associated with right atrial and ventricular enlargement and pulmonary vascular undercirculation.

Diagnostic Notes

Ventricular septal defects may exist concurrently with other congenital heart defects.

Cardiac catheterization and selective angiocardiography are rarely needed to confirm the diagnosis.

 T r e a t m e n t

Primary Therapeutics

- **Medical:** Medical management of left-sided congestive heart failure is employed utilizing diuretics, vasodilators such as ACE inhibitors, digoxin, and moderate dietary salt restriction.
- **Surgery:** Banding of the pulmonary artery may be attempted in cats with large nonrestrictive VSD, left-to-right shunting, and congestive heart failure.
- Primary repair of the defect is costly, requires specialized equipment, and is associated with significant complications.

Secondary Therapeutics

- Exercise restriction.
- Periodic phlebotomy is indicated if significant polycythemia is present in right-to-left hunting VSDs.

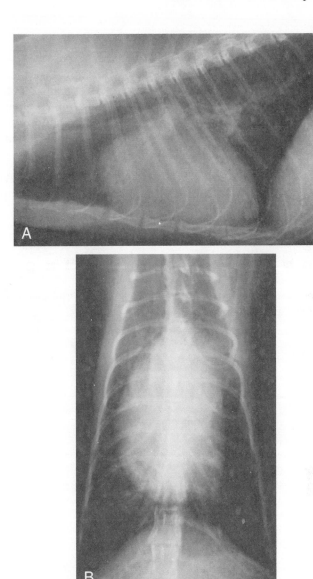

Figure 124.1. Ventricular septal defects: Extreme right-sided enlargement is characteristic of a ventricular septal defect. This can be seen on the lateral (*A*) and VD (*B*) views.

Therapeutic Notes

- The response to therapy may be quite variable.
- Digoxin therapy is indicated in selected cases with obvious systolic dysfunction and/or arrhythmias such as atrial fibrillation.

P r o g n o s i s

Cats with small-to-medium left-to-right shunting restrictive VSDs typically have a favorable prognosis, especially if they remain asymptomatic at 6 months of age. Most cats with significant lesions develop congestive heart failure within the first few weeks of life or reverse their shunt due to pulmonary hypertension. Patients with moderate-to-severe cardiomegaly have significant volume overload and are at risk for developing congestive heart failure.

Cats with a large nonrestrictive VSD or right ventricular hypertrophy, evidence of pulmonary hypertension and Eisenmenger's physiology have a poor prognosis similar to cats with tetralogy of Fallot.

S u g g e s t e d   R e a d i n g

Abbott JA. Ventricular septal defect. In: Tilley LP, Smith FWK, eds. The 5-minute veterinary consult. Baltimore: Williams & Wilkins, 1997.

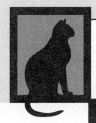

CHAPTER 125

Vestibular Syndrome

Mitchell A. Crystal

Overview

Feline idiopathic vestibular syndrome is a frequent disorder of unknown etiology. It results from dysfunction of either the peripheral vestibular receptors in the inner ear or the vestibulocochlear nerve (eighth cranial nerve). Adult cats of any age are affected, with one study of 75 cats reporting a median age of 4 years. There is no sex or breed predilection. The disease may be more prevalent in the summer and fall months. Clinical signs include an acute or peracute onset of rolling, falling, ataxia, tight circling, and/or head tilt. Cats will often assume a crouched position or lean to one side and are reluctant to move. Clinical signs are always toward the side of the lesion. Other less common accompanying signs include vomiting, anorexia, and vocalizing. Physical examination reveals a horizontal or rotary nystagmus with the fast phase away from the lesion and, aside from those described above, no other physical or neurologic abnormalities. Conscious proprioception is normal but may be difficult to assess due to patient struggle and disorientation. Rarely, bilateral disease is present. These cats present with a wide stance and wide head excursions, no nystagmus or head tilt, and they may fall to either side; many of these cats are deaf. Differential diagnoses to consider for peripheral vestibular signs include otitis interna, nasopharyngeal polyps, neoplasia of the eighth nerve or inner ear, trauma, toxicity (aminoglycosides, furosemide), and vascular disorders (heart disease, vasculitis, coagulopathy).

 Diagnosis

Primary Diagnostics

- **History:** The owner should be questioned about the possibility of trauma, any recent or current drug therapy, the rapidity of onset and progression of illness, and whether any other signs are present.

- **Examination:** Physical and neurologic examination should be normal aside from signs of peripheral vestibular disease (see above). A careful otic exam is needed to exclude inner ear disease (otitis, polyps, neoplasia).

Ancillary Diagnostics

- **Tympanic bulla radiographs:** These will help exclude otitis interna, polyps, and neoplasia.

Diagnostic Notes

A diagnosis of feline idiopathic vestibular syndrome is made by the presence of clinical signs, rapid improvement, and the exclusion of other differential diagnoses. Routine laboratory tests are within normal limits.

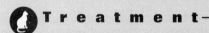 **T r e a t m e n t**

Primary Therapeutics

- **Supportive care:** The cat should be placed in a quiet area with minimal stimulation. If imbalance/disorientation/apprehension is severe, sedation with diazepam (0.1–0.5 mg/kg IV, PO BID-QID) may be helpful.

Secondary Therapeutics

- **Fluids and nutrition:** Fluid and/or nutritional support are occasionally initially needed in cats that are adipsic and/or anorexic.
- **Antiemetics:** Metoclopramide (0.2–0.4 PO, SQ, IM TID-QID or 1–2 mg/kg/day constant rate IV infusion), chlorpromazine (0.2–0.4 SQ, IM TID-QID) or prochlorperazine (0.2–0.4 SC, IM TID-QID) can be used if vomiting is present.

Therapeutic Notes

- Glucocorticoids do not speed recovery and are not recommended.
- Tranquilizers may help in control of severe clinical signs but do not speed recovery.

P r o g n o s i s

The prognosis for complete or near-complete recovery is excellent and usually occurs within 2–3 weeks, although occasional cats require several months to recover. Most cats show dramatic improvement in 72 hours and continue to gradually improve. The head tilt is often the last problem to resolve, and some cats retain a residual mild-to-moderate head tilt indefinitely. Recurrence is rare.

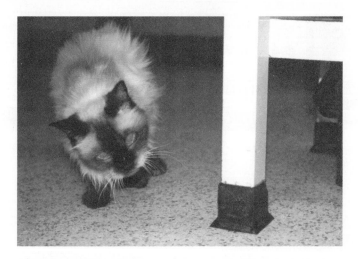

Figure 125.1. Vestibular syndrome: Acute onset of head tilt and circling without a history of trauma are characteristic of the feline vestibular syndrome.

S u g g e s t e d   R e a d i n g s

Burke EE, Moise NS, De Lahunta A, Erb HN. Review of idiopathic feline vestibular syndrome in 75 cats. *J Am Vet Med Assoc* 1985;187(9):941–943.

Chrisman CL. Head tilt, circling, nystagmus, and other vestibular deficits. In: Problems in small animal neurology, 2nd ed. Philadelphia: Lea & Febiger, 1991;268–294.

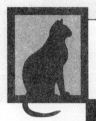

CHAPTER 126

Vitamin A Toxicosis

Gary D. Norsworthy

Overview

Vitamin A is a fat-soluble vitamin that accumulates if overdosed. It is found in large quantities in liver and cod liver oil. Cats fed large quantities of these products or given vitamin A supplements are subject to hypervitaminosis A. It is characterized by poor appetite, depression, a dull, dry haircoat, and exophthalmos that develop within 4 to 6 weeks. Kittens, but not adults, also develop gingivitis, and the teeth loosen. Within 1 year, skeletal lesions form. Affected cats develop cervical vertebral spondylosis and new periosteal bone formation. Ankylosis of cervical vertebrae and elbows are classic findings. The forelimbs become painful, causing affected cats to assume a kangaroo-like sitting posture. Eating becomes difficult because of the cat's inability to reach the food bowl. Grooming is also impaired, so the haircoat becomes oily and matted.

Diagnosis

Primary Diagnostics

- **Dietary history:** These cats typically have a diet that is high in liver or cod liver oil or are being supplemented heavily with vitamin A.
- **Clinical signs:** Inability to move the neck and forelimbs due to ankylosis is classic. The kangaroo-like sitting posture is typical. An unkempt haircoat is common.
- **Radiographs:** Radiographs of the cervical spine and forelimbs reveal exostoses and ankylosis after about 1 year of the toxicosis.

Treatment

Primary Therapeutics

- **Dietary change:** The cat must be removed from the liver or cod liver oil diet, and vitamin A supplements must be discontinued. The cat needs to be placed on a balanced feline diet.

- **Pain relief:** Anti-inflammatories and analgesics may be helpful.

Secondary Therapeutics

- **Feeding:** Placing the food and water bowls on a platform may make eating and drinking easier for the cat.

Therapeutic Notes

- Most bony changes are irreversible.
- Cat owners should be warned of the dangers of feeding diets and supplements with excessive vitamin A.
- Plasma levels of vitamin A will become normal within a few weeks of diet correction; however, liver vitamin A levels will be elevated for years.

Prognosis

The prognosis is guarded. Bony changes are generally irreversible. Other symptoms will resolve when a proper diet is fed.

Suggested Readings

Buffington CA. Nutritional diseases and nutritional therapy. In: Sherding RG, ed. The cat: diseases and clinical management, 2nd ed. Philadelphia: WB Saunders, 1994;161–190.

Goldman AL. Hypervitaminosis A in a cat. *J Am Vet Med Assoc* 1992;200:1970–1972.

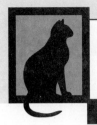

CHAPTER 127

Vitamin D Toxicosis

Gary D. Norsworthy

Overview

Hypervitaminosis D is an accumulation of toxic levels of vitamin D. It is almost always due to the ingestion of vitamin D-containing rodenticides or oversupplementation with this vitamin by the owner. It has also been called cholecalciferol toxicosis. It results in a pathologic increase in vitamin D from increased gastrointestinal (GI) absorption, bone resorption, and reabsorption of vitamin D by the renal tubules. The net result is hypercalcemia and dystrophic calcification. The typical clinical signs include polyuria, polydipsia, vomiting, diarrhea, anorexia, and depression. The kidneys may be painful on palpation, and gastrointestinal or pulmonary hemorrhage may occur.

 D i a g n o s i s

Primary Diagnostics

- **History:** The owner should be questioned carefully to determine if the cat has exposure to vitamin D-containing rodenticides or if vitamin D supplementation is occurring.
- **Biochemical profile:** The typical findings are hypercalcemia, hyperphosphatemia, hyperproteinemia, and azotemia. The serum calcium level may be normal for up to 24 hours following ingestion of a rodenticide.
- **Urinalysis:** The typical findings are hyposthenuria (SG = 1.001–1.007), proteinuria, and glucosuria.

Ancillary Diagnostics

- **Radiographs:** Radiographs of the kidneys, GI tract, and lung may reveal mineralization.
- **Electrocardiogram:** Bradycardia is often present.

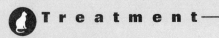

Treatment

Primary Therapeutics

- **Induction of vomiting:** This is appropriate for acute exposure to a rodenticide. Syrup of ipecac (3.3 mL/kg PO) and 3% hydrogen peroxide (1–5 mL/kg) are usually effective. If vomiting has not occurred in 15 minutes, administration of the drug should be repeated.
- **Activated charcoal:** This drug will prevent further absorption of the toxin.
- **Reduce serum calcium:** This may be accomplished by a) diuresis with normal saline solution; b) furosemide (2–5 mg/kg q8h); c) oral prednisolone (2 mg/kg q12h); or d) salmon calcitonin (4–6 IU/kg q2–3h SC until serum calcium is normal).

Secondary Therapeutics

- **Maintenance of furosemide and prednisolone:** These drugs should be continued for several days at 2–4 mg/kg q12h PO and 2 mg/kg q12h PO, respectively.

Therapeutic Notes

- Do not administer any calcium-containing fluids.
- Serum calcium levels should be monitored for several days or weeks. Many vitamin D-containing rodenticides require several weeks of treatment.

Prognosis

The prognosis is generally good if rapid, aggressive treatment is instituted. However, persistent hypercalcemia in spite of aggressive therapy warrants a grave prognosis.

Suggested Readings

Dorman DC. Anticoagulant, cholecalciferol, and bromethlin-based rodenticides. *Vet Clin North Am Sm Anim Pract* 1990;20:339–352.

Osweiler GD. Vitamin D toxicity. In: Smith FWK, Tilley LP, eds. The 5-minute veterinary consult. Baltimore: Williams & Wilkins, 1996:1156–1157.

Moore FM, Kudisch M, Richter K, Faggella A. Hypercalcemia associated with rodenticide poisoning in three cats. *J Am Vet Med Assoc* 1988;193:1099–1100.

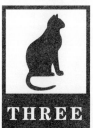

PART

THREE

APPENDICES

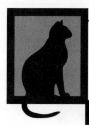

APPENDIX A

Feline Body Surface Area Conversion

Gary D. Norsworthy

Feline Body Surface Area Conversion*

Pounds	Kilograms	Meter²
1.1	0.5	0.063
2.2	1.0	0.100
4.4	2.0	0.159
6.6	3.0	0.208
8.8	4.0	0.252
11.0	5.0	0.292
13.2	6.0	0.330
15.4	7.0	0.366
17.6	8.0	0.400
19.8	9.0	0.433
22.0	10.0	0.464
24.2	11.0	0.494

* These values are slightly different than those for dogs. They are based on the following formula:

$$\text{BSA in } m^2 = [10 \times W^{2/3}] / 10^4$$

BSA = body surface area; m^2 = square meters;

W = weight in grams

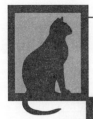

Chemotherapy for Lymphoma

Mitchell A. Crystal

Overview

Combination therapy allows for the killing of tumor cells by several mechanisms to try to prevent resistance, while minimizing side effects that would occur if larger doses of single agents were used. Chemotherapy drugs are administered by injection on an outpatient basis or orally at home. Cats should have food (but not water) withheld the morning of the day that they are scheduled for outpatient injectable chemotherapy.

Selected Protocols

Below are four chemotherapy protocols that have been successfully used in the treatment of lymphoma. Whereas specific lymphoma types may respond differently, overall first remission rates, durations, and survival times (when available) are listed.

COP (CYCLOPHOSPHAMIDE, VINCRISTINE [ONCOVIN], PREDNISONE)

- First remission rate: 80%
- First remission duration: 42–1260 days (median = 150 days)
- Survival time: not reported
- Vincristine: 0.75 mg/m^2 IV; weekly for 4 weeks (days 0,7,14,21), then every 3 weeks.
- Cyclophosphamide: 300 mg/m^2 PO; every 3 weeks beginning on day 0.
- Prednisone: 2 mg/kg/day PO; given continuously beginning day 0.
- Treatment is continued for 1 year

COPI (CYCLOPHOSPHAMIDE, VINCRISTINE [ONCOVIN], PREDNISONE, IDARUBICIN)

- First remission rate: 80%
- First remission duration: 30–825 days (median = 183 days)
- Survival time: not reported

- Vincristine: 0.75 mg/m^2 IV; weekly for 4 weeks on days 0, 7, 14, and 21.
- Cyclophosphamide: 300 mg/m^2 PO; two treatments 3 weeks apart on days 0 and 21.
- Prednisone: 2 mg/kg/day PO; given continuously beginning day 0 and ending day 28.
- Idarubicin: 2 mg/day PO or IV; given for 2 consecutive days every 3 weeks beginning on day 42.
- Treatment is continued for 1 year. Oral form of idarubicin has limited availability in the USA.

MADCOP (METHOTREXATE, L-ASPARAGINASE, DOXORUBICIN, CYCLOPHOSPHAMIDE, VINCRISTINE [ONCOVIN], PREDNISONE)

- First remission rate: 67%
- First remission duration: 0–2006 days (median = 148 days)
- Survival time: 16–2022 (median = 209)
- L-asparaginase: 400 IU/kg IM; given once on day 0.
- Vincristine: 0.75 mg/m^2 IV; given on days 0, 21, and 42, and then every 4 weeks.
- Cyclophosphamide: 250 mg/m^2 PO; given on days 7, 28, and 56, and then every 8 weeks.
- Doxorubicin: 20 mg/m^2 IV; given on days 14 and 35 over 15–20 minutes
- Methotrexate: 0.8 mg/kg IV; given every 8 weeks beginning on day 84.
- Prednisone: 2 mg/kg/day PO; given continuously beginning on day 0.
- Note that in this protocol, maintenance begins on day 42 as vincristine-cyclophosphamide-vincristine-methotrexate, with each agent given every 2 weeks.
- Treatment is continued for 1 year, then the maintenance therapy interval is increased to every 3 weeks (vincristine-cyclophosphamide-vincristine-methotrexate, with each agent given every 3 weeks) for 1 year.

COPA (CYCLOPHOSPHAMIDE, VINCRISTINE [ONCOVIN], PREDNISONE, DOXORUBICIN [ADRIAMYCIN])

- First remission rate: 80%
- First remission duration: 123–547 days (median = 259 days)
- Survival time: not reported
- Vincristine: 0.75 mg/m^2 IV; weekly for 4 weeks on days 0, 7, 14, and 21.
- Cyclophosphamide: 300 mg/m^2 PO; two treatments 3 weeks apart on days 0 and 21.
- Prednisone: 2 mg/kg/day PO; given continuously beginning day 0 and ending day 28.

- Doxorubicin: 25 mg/m^2 IV; given every 3 weeks beginning on day 42 for 6 months.
- Treatment ends when doxorubicin therapy is completed.

Potential Side Effects of Chemotherapy

CYCLOPHOSPHAMIDE (CYTOXAN) (given orally)

1. Anorexia/vomiting/diarrhea: This is less common in cats than in humans undergoing chemotherapy. Giving the drug with food may help prevent vomiting.
2. Low white-blood-cell count: The neutrophil count may drop below normal 6–10 days after therapy, then usually returns quickly to normal. The low count does not cause signs of illness unless infection/sepsis occurs.
3. Infection/sepsis: Neutropenia can occasionally result in serious infection 6–10 days after drug administration. Infections are potentially the most severe side effect of chemotherapy and are considered an emergency.
4. Hematuria: Cyclophosphamide may rarely cause a chemical irritation of the bladder, leading to a condition known as hemorrhagic cystitis. This is not an infection but must be differentiated from infectious cystitis by a urine culture. Cyclophosphamide-induced cystitis can be prevented in some cases by giving the drug in the morning, allowing opportunity for urination during the day, and maintaining adequate fluid intake. Prednisone will also help this condition.
5. Hair loss: Loss of hair is unusual in cats because their hair does not grow continuously throughout their life (as in people). Shaved hair is slow to regrow.

DOXORUBICIN (ADRIAMYCIN) (given intravenously)

1. Anorexia/vomiting/diarrhea: See Cyclophosphamide. Doxorubicin is more likely to cause anorexia, vomiting, and diarrhea than other drugs.
2. Infection/sepsis: See Cyclophosphamide.
3. Low white-blood-cell count: See Cyclophosphamide.
4. Itching or hives: A few cats may itch or develop hives as the drug is being given. This is a transient event. Drug administration should be stopped for 15–30 minutes and at that time administered at a slower rate.
5. Severe tissue necrosis at the injection site: This will occur if any drug contacts the perivascular area. This should be prevented by administering the drug via a secure IV catheter.
6. Renal failure: Nephrotoxicity is an uncommon side effect of therapy. Urine specific gravity, creatinine, and BUN should be assessed in cats prior to administering therapy.
7. Heart failure: Unlike the dog, cardiomyopathy after cumulative doses of greater than 180 mg/m^2 rarely occurs in the cat. Nevertheless, chemotherapy protocols try to avoid this by using this drug only infrequently to avoid excessive cumulative doses.

8. Red discoloration of the urine: This may occur after the drug is given. This is not abnormal and is merely from the color of the drug.
9. Hair loss: See Cyclophosphamide.

L-ASPARAGINASE (ELSPAR) (given intramuscularly)

1. Allergic reactions: cats may rarely experience a major allergic reaction to L-as-paraginase. Cats that have received the drug before should be observed at home or in the hospital after the injection. Reactions usually occur immediately.
2. Vomiting: extremely uncommon. Rarely, severe vomiting can occur from drug-induced acute pancreatitis.
3. Hair loss: very rare. See Cyclophosphamide.

METHOTREXATE (given intravenously)

1. Anorexia/vomiting/diarrhea: See Cyclophosphamide.
2. Low white-blood-cell count: See Cyclophosphamide.
3. Renal failure: uncommon. Seen only when very high doses are used.
4. The antidote for toxicity resulting from this drug is leucovorin (3 mg/m^2 Q 3 hours $\times$ 8 doses) and is effective if given within a few hours of toxicity.

PREDNISONE (given orally)

1. Few side effects occur as a result of prednisone therapy in the cat.

VINCRISTINE (ONCOVIN) (given intravenously)

1. Anorexia/vomiting/diarrhea: very uncommon with this drug. See Cyclophosphamide.
2. Low white-blood-cell count: uncommon with this drug. See Cyclophosphamide.
3. Severe tissue necrosis at the injection site: see Doxorubicin.
4. Constipation: an uncommon occurrence with this drug.
5. Neurologic abnormalities: Weakness is a common side effect in people but is very rare in cats.
6. Thrombocytophilia: The thrombocyte count may elevate to two- or threefold of normal. However, no ill effects are seen.

Approach to Common Chemotherapy Side Effects

Many chemotherapy reactions are listed in the literature and drug inserts. There are two common side effects to remember:
1. **Sepsis** (life threatening—most serious)
2. **Gastroenteritis** (self-limiting with support)

Neutropenia without illness is a nonserious problem that also will be addressed.

Sepsis

Sepsis occurs 7–10 days after chemotherapy.

- Clinical signs: anorexia, lethargy, vomiting, diarrhea, collapse, fever (not all animals have all of these)
- Diagnosis: clinical signs and neutropenia on a CBC
- Treatment: IV catheter

  IV fluids (usually requires shock fluids (50 mL/kg/hr) initially, then 1.5 × the maintenance fluids for 1 to 3 days

  IV antibiotics (broad-spectrum, such as cephalosporins; aminoglycosides can be added but only after dehydration and shock have been treated and resolved)

  NPO if vomiting; withhold food but not water if diarrhea occurs without vomiting.

- Prognosis: good if detected and treated early
- Prevention: Decrease the dose of the chemotherapy agent causing the neutropenia/sepsis by 10–20% for all subsequent doses of that drug.

How to Approach Sepsis

1. If the owner calls with a sick animal in the 7–10 day postchemotherapy window, instruct the client to bring in the patient immediately. This is a potentially life-threatening condition.
2. Once the cat is at the hospital, collect blood for a CBC, chemistry profile, and urinalysis.
3. Place an IV catheter, and begin fluid therapy.
4. Begin IV antibiotic therapy.
5. When the bloodwork returns, evaluate the neutrophil count and adjust fluids for electrolyte abnormalities if needed.

Gastroenteritis

Gastroenteritis occurs 2–5 days after chemotherapy.

- Clinical signs: anorexia, lethargy, vomiting, diarrhea, mild fever
- Diagnosis: clinical signs, timing of clinical signs and lack of neutropenia on a CBC (if one is run[this is not always necessary]).
- Treatment: NPO (if vomiting); withhold food but not water if the cat has diarrhea without vomiting. If there is suspicion of dehydration (severity of vomiting/diarrhea), subcutaneous fluids on an outpatient basis or hospitalization with IV fluids is appropriate.
- Prognosis: good
- Prevention: There is no need to decrease the dose of the chemotherapy agent causing the gastroenteritis unless the episode is severe or unless this has occurred from the same agent previously.

How to Approach Gastroenteritis

1. If the owner calls with a sick animal in the 2–5 day postchemotherapy window, ascertain from the client how sick is the patient (how much vomiting/diarrhea, the patient's attitude and appetite, etc.). If there is concern for the patient's hydration status, request that the patient be brought in for examination.
2. If the patient is not dehydrated (decision by phone or examination), instruct the client to make the patient NPO (if the cat is vomiting) or withhold food but not water if the cat has diarrhea without vomiting.
3. Slowly (with small amounts frequently) begin water and an easily digestible diet.
4. Return to normal diet gradually over 1–2 days.

A simple way to help determine if sepsis is a consideration for the borderline cases (5 to 7 days) when a client phones in from home is to ask the client to take the patient's body temperature. If there is a fever present, the animal should be seen immediately. If there is no fever present, conservative therapy can be attempted. Oral antibiotics should be utilized in these cases along with conservative therapy.

Neutropenia without Illness: 6–10 days after chemotherapy

How to Approach Neutropenia

Decrease the dose of the chemotherapy agent causing the neutropenia by 10–20% for all subsequent doses of that drug.

Suggested Readings

MacEwen GE. Feline lymphoma and leukemias. In: Withrow SJ, MacEwen EG, eds. Small animal clinical oncology, 2nd ed. Philadelphia: WB Saunders, 1996;479–495.

Mauldin GE, Mooney SC, Maleo KA, Matus RE, Mauldin GN. Chemotherapy in 132 cats with lymphoma: 1988–1994. Proceedings of the Veterinary Cancer Society 15th Annual Conference 1995;35–36.

Moore AS, Mahony OM. Treatment of feline malignant lymphoma. In: Bonagura JD, ed. Kirk's current veterinary therapy XII: small animal practice. Philadelphia: WB Saunders, 1995;498–502.

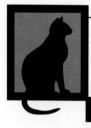

APPENDIX C

Echocardiographic Values in Normal Cats and Cats with Acquired Heart Disease

Larry P. Tilley

TABLE C.1.

Normal Echocardiographic Values in Cats (Six Studies)

Mensural	[N = 11]	[N = 25]	[N = 30]	NG	[N = 30]c	[N = 16]c
LVEDD (cm)	1.51 ± 0.21[a]	1.48 ± 0.26[a]	1.59 ± 0.19[a]	1.10–1.60[b]	1.40 ± 0.13[a]	1.28 ± 0.17[a]
LVESD (cm)	0.69 ± 0.22	0.88 ± 0.24	0.80 ± 0.14	0.60–1.00	0.81 ± 0.16	0.83 ± 0.15
Ao (cm)	0.95 ± 0.15	0.75 ± 0.18	0.95 ± 0.11	0.65–1.10	0.94 ± 0.11	0.94 ± 0.14
LA (cm)	1.21 ± 0.18	0.74 ± 0.17	1.23 ± 0.14	0.85–1.25	1.03 ± 0.14	0.98 ± 0.17
LA/Ao (cm)	1.29 ± 0.23	—	1.30 ± 0.17	0.80–1.30	1.10 ± 0.18	1.09 ± 0.27
IVSED (cm)	0.50 ± 0.07	0.45 ± 0.09	0.31 ± 0.04	0.25–0.50	0.36 ± 0.08	—
IVSES (cm)	0.76 ± 0.12	—	0.58 ± 0.06	0.50–0.90	—	—
LVWED (cm)	0.46 ± 0.05	0.37 ± 0.08	0.33 ± 0.06	0.25–0.50	0.35 ± 0.05	0.31 ± 0.11
LVWES (cm)	0.78 ± 0.10	—	0.68 ± 0.07	0.40–0.90	—	0.55 ± 0.88
RVED (cm)	0.54 ± 0.10	—	0.60 ± 0.15	—	0.50 ± 0.21	—
LVWA (cm)	0.50 ± 0.07	—	—	—	—	0.32 ± 0.11
EPSS (cm)	0.04 ± 0.07	—	0.02 ± 0.09	—	—	—
AA (cm)	0.36 ± 0.10	—	—	—	—	—
MVEFS (mm/sec)	54.4 ± 13.4	—	87.2 ± 25.9	—	—	83.78 ± 23.81
ΔD% (%)	55.0 ± 10.2	41.0 ± 7.3	49.8 ± 5.3	29–35	42.7 ± 8.1	34.5 ± 12.6
LVWT (%)	39.5 ± 7.6	—	—	—	—	—
IVST (%)	33.5 ± 8.2	—	—	—	—	—
HR (beats/min)	182 ± 22	167 ± 29	194 ± 23	—	255 ± 36	—
Wt (kg)	4.3 ± 0.5	4.7 ± 1.2	4.1 ± 1.1	—	3.91 ± 1.2	—

[a]Mean ± SD   [b]Usual range   [c]Cats anesthetized with ketamine

LVEDD = left ventricular end-diastolic diameter	LVWED = left ventricular wall at end-diastole	ΔD% = fractional shortening
LVESD = left ventricular end-systolic diameter	LVWES = left ventricular wall at end-systole	LVWT = left ventricular wall thickening
Ao = aorta	RVED = right ventricular diameter at end-diastole	IVST = interventricular septal thickening
LA = left atrium	LVWA = left ventricular wall amplitude	HR = heart rate
LA/Ao = left atrium to aortic root ratio	EPSS = E point-septal separation	Wt = weight
IVSED = interventricular septum at end-diastole	AA = aortic amplitude	N = number of animals in study
IVSES = interventricular septum at end-systole	MVEFS = mitral valve E-F slope	

Reprinted with permission from Moise NS. Echocardiography. In: Fox P, ed. Canine and feline cardiology. New York: Churchill Livingstone, 1989.

TABLE C.2.

M-Mode and 2-D Echocardiographic Alterations in Acquired Heart Disease

	RV Wall	RVID$_d$	IVS$_d$	LVPW$_d$	LVID$_d$	SF	Ao	LA	Additional M-mode or 2-D Findings
Dilated cardiomyopathy	N↓	↑	N↓	N↓	↑	↓	N↓	↑	Reduced wall thickening
Hypertrophic cardiomyopathy	N↑	N↓	N↑	N↑	N↓	N↑	N	↑	Focal septal hypertrophy may be present
Intermediate cardiomyopathy	N↑	N↑	N↑	N↑	N↑	N↓	N	↑	Focal septal hypertrophy may be present
Mitral regurgitation	N	N	N↑	N↑	↑	↑N↓	N↓	↑	Increased SF early in disease, N↓ later
Tricuspid regurgitation	N↑	↑	N↑	N	N	N	N	N	Usually accompanies mitral value insufficiency
Pericardial effusion	N	↓	N	N	↓	↓	↓	↓	Collapse of RA wall occurs with tamponade; Abnormal septal motion; echo-free space between pericardium and LVPW
Hypothyroidism	N	N	N	N	N*	↓	N	N	Prolonged PEP
Hyperthyroidism	N↑	N↑	N↑	N↑	N↑	N↑	N	N↑	Myocardial failure may develop with severe disease
Heartworm disease	↑	↑	↑	N	N↓	N↓	N	N	Echodense worm mass or linear echoes may be associated with TV; PSM may be present
Systemic hypertension	N	N	N↑	N↑	N↑	N↑	N	↑	Focal or diffuse septal hypertrophy may be present

Abbreviations: RV = right ventricle; RVID$_d$ = right ventricular internal dimension at end diastole; IVS$_d$ = interventricular septum at end diastole; LVPW$_d$ = left ventricular posterior wall at end diastole; LVID$_d$ = left ventricular internal dimension at end diastole; SF = shortening fraction; Ao = aortic root; LA = left atrium; RA = right atrial; PEP = pre-ejection period; TV = tricuspid value; PSM = paradoxical septal motion; N = normal; ↑ = increased; ↓= decreased.

*Systolic LVID increased

Reprinted with permission from Henick RA. Echocardiography and Doppler ultrasound. In: Miller MS, Tilley LP, eds. Manual of canine and feline cardiology. Philadelphia: WB Saunders, 1995.

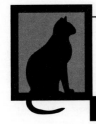

APPENDIX D

Feline Cardiac Chamber Enlargement— Electrocardiographic Features

Larry P. Tilley

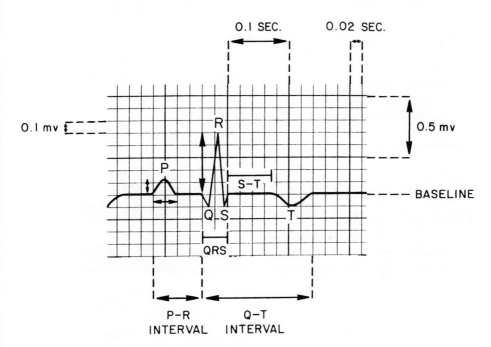

Close-up of a normal feline lead II P-QRS-T complex with labels and intervals.
Paper speed of 50 mm/sec; 1 cm = 1 mv.

Right Atrial Enlargement

1. The P wave is greater than 0.2 mv (two boxes) and is usually slender and peaked.
2. The T_a wave is sometimes present. This slight depression of the baseline following the P wave represents atrial repolarization.

Left Atrial Enlargement

The duration of the P wave is greater than 0.04 sec (two boxes). Notching of the P wave is abnormal when the wave is also wide.

Right Ventricular Enlargement

1. The electrocardiographic critieria for right ventricular enlargement in the cat have not been well established. Severe right ventricular enlargement produces some of the same electrocardiographic features observed in the dog. The most frequently observed electrocardiographic signs include the following:
   a. S waves in leads I, II, III, and aVF (usually 0.5 mv [five boxes] or greater).
   b. Mean electrical axis of the QRS complex in the frontal plane greater than +160° and clockwise, especially when serial electrocardiograms on the same animal are compared.
   c. Prominent S waves in leads CV_6LL and CV_6LU.
   d. Positive T wave in lead V_{10}.
   e. Right atrial enlargement (tall P waves).

Left Ventricular Enlargement

1. The R wave of the QRS complex exceeds 0.9 mv (nine boxes) in lead II. The R wave should not exceed 1.0 mv or 10 boxes in CV_6LU or CV_6LL. The amplitude of the R wave in V_{10} exceeds the Q wave amplitude ($R/Q > 1.0$).
2. The maximum width of the QRS is 0.04 sec (two boxes).
3. Displacement of the S-T segment occurs in a direction opposite the main QRS deflection. This causes the S-T segment to sag into the T wave (S-T coving).
4. Repolarization changes cause the T wave to be of increased amplitude (usually greater than 0.3 mv or three boxes in lead II).
5. A mean electrical axis deviation in the frontal plane of less than 0° may be present.

Reprinted with permission from Tilley LP. Essentials of canine and feline electrocardiography. Interpretation and treatment, 3rd ed. Baltimore: Williams & Wilkins, 1992.

TABLE D.1.

Normal Feline Electrocardiographic Values

Rate
 Range: 120 to 240 beats/min
 Mean: 197 beats/min
Rhythm
 Normal sinus rhythm
 Sinus tachycardia (physiologic reaction to excitement)
Measurements (lead II, 50 mm/sec, 1 cm = 1 mv)
 P wave
  Width: maximum, 0.04 sec (two boxes wide)
  Height: maximum, 0.2 mv (two boxes tall)
 P-R interval
  Width: 0.05 to 0.09 sec (two and one-half to four and one-half boxes)
 QRS complex
  Width: maximum, 0.04 sec (two boxes)
  Height of R wave: maximum, 0.9 mv (nine boxes)
 S-T segment
  No depression or elevation
 T wave
  Can be positive, negative, or biphasic; most often positive
 Maximum amplitude: 0.3 mv (three boxes)
 Q-T interval
  Width: 0.12 to 0.18 sec (six to nine boxes) at normal heart rate (range 0.07 to 0.20
   sec, three and one-half to ten boxes); varies with heart rate (faster rates, shorter
   Q-T intervals; and vice versa)
Electrical axis (frontal plane)
 0 to ± 160° (not valid in many cats)
Precordial chest leads
 CV_6LL (V_2): R wave <1.0 mv (ten boxes)
 CV_6LU (V_4): R wave not greater than 1.0 mv (ten boxes)
 V_{10}: T wave negative; R/Q <1.0 mv

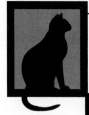

Veterinary Prescription Diets

Mitchell A. Crystal

The following section summarizes recommended veterinary prescription dietary therapies. All diets are listed in alphabetical order by disease categories in which they are recommended. All veterinary prescription diets, including each diet's characteristics, are listed by pet food company at the end of this section.

Cardiovascular Disease

- CNM-CV Formula
- CNM-NF Formula
- Feline Mature Formula
- Feline Modified Formula
- h/d
- k/d

Urologic Disease

Advanced Renal Disease (BUN > 80 mg/dL)

- CNM-NF Formula
- Feline Mature Formula
- Feline Modified Formula
- k/d
- Low Protein
- RenalCare Feline Liquid Diet

Lower Urinary Tract Disease

This excludes oxalate urolithiasis unless mentioned.
- CNM-UR Formula
- c/d

- Control pHormula Feline Control Formula (struvite and oxalate urolithiasis)
- Feline HiFiber Formula (struvite and oxalate urolithiasis)
- Feline Mature Formula (struvite and oxalate urolithiasis)
- Feline Modified Formula (FLUTD with oxalate urolithiasis)
- Feline Weight Formula (struvite and oxalate urolithiasis)
- r/d
- s/d
- w/d

Gastrointestinal Disease

Digestion/Absorption Diseases and Food Hypersensitivities/Intolerances

- c/d
- CNM-EN Formula
- d/d
- Limited Ingredient Diets—Feline, Protein source duck
- Feline Development Formula
- Feline Neutral Formula
- Limited Ingredient Diets—Feline, Protein source lamb
- Limited Ingredient Diets—Feline, Protein source rabbit
- Response Formula LB
- Selected Protein with Duck and Rice
- Selected Protein with Venison and Rice
- Limited Ingredient Diets—Feline, Protein source venison

Colonic Disease

- Calorie Control
- CNM-OM Formula
- Feline HiFiber Formula
- Restricted-Calorie Formula
- w/d

Obesity

- Calorie Control
- CNM-OM Formula
- Feline HiFiber Formula

- Feline Weight Formula
- r/d
- Restricted-Calorie Formula
- w/d

Diabetes Mellitus

- Calorie Control
- CNM-OM Formula
- Feline HiFiber Formula
- w/d

Increased Metabolic/Nutritional Demand

- a/d
- CNM-CV Formula
- CliniCare Feline Liquid Diet
- Feline Development Formula
- Nutritional Recovery Formula
- p/d
- RenalCare Feline Liquid Diet

Hepatic Disease

Hepatic Disease with Hepatoencephalopathy

- CNM-NF Formula
- Feline Mature Formula
- Feline Modified Formula
- h/d
- k/d
- Low Protein
- RenalCare Feline Liquid Diet

Hepatic Lipidosis

- a/d
- CliniCare Feline Liquid Diet
- CNM-CV Formula
- Feline Development Formula
- Nutritional Recovery Formula
- p/d

Food Hypersensitivity

- d/d
- Limited Ingredient Diets—Feline, Protein source duck
- Feline Neutral Formula
- Limited Ingredient Diets—Feline, Protein source lamb
- Limited Ingredient Diets—Feline, Protein source rabbit
- Response Formula LB
- Selected Protein with Duck and Rice
- Selected Protein with Venison and Rice
- Limited Ingredient Diets—Feline, Protein source venison

Diets Listed By Veterinary Prescription Pet Food Companies

Companies are listed alphabetically.

Hill's Feline Veterinary Prescription Diets

- a/d (canned): protein and energy-increased (including increased branched-chain amino acids), highly digestible, omega-3 fatty acids, B-complex vitamins, vitamin E, zinc, potassium, magnesium, glutamine and arginine-increased.
- c/d (canned and dry): magnesium and phosphorus-reduced, highly digestible, creates a urine pH of 6.2–6.4, high-fat content.
- d/d (canned): limited antigen (lamb and rice) protein source, highly digestible, magnesium-reduced, creates a urine pH of 6.2–6.4.
- h/d (canned): sodium and magnesium-reduced, taurine-increased, creates a urine pH of 6.2–6.4.
- k/d (canned and dry): sodium, magnesium, phosphorus, calcium, dietary acid load, and protein-reduced, creates a urine pH of 6.6–6.9.
- p/d (canned): increased protein, fat, and energy, decreased fiber
- r/d (canned and dry): energy, fat, and magnesium-reduced, fiber greatly increased, creates a urine pH of 6.2–6.4.
- s/d (canned and dry): sodium-increased, phosphorus, magnesium, and calcium-reduced, creates a urine pH of 5.9–6.1.
- w/d (canned and dry): energy, fat, and magnesium-reduced, fiber increased, creates a urine pH of 6.2–6.4.

Iam's Feline Eukanuba Veterinary Prescription Diets

- Nutritional Recovery Formula Nutrient (canned and dry): dense, protein and energy-increased, adjusted omega-6:omega-3 fatty acid ratio (between 5:1 and 10:1), highly palatable.

- Response Formula LB (canned): limited antigen (lamb) protein source, limited carbohydrate (barley) source, adjusted omega-6:omega-3 fatty acid ratio (between 5:1 and 10:1), highly palatable.
- Restricted-Calorie Diet (dry): energy and fat-reduced, adjusted omega-6:omega-3 fatty acid ratio (between 5:1 and 10:1), highly palatable.

Innovative Veterinary Diets: Feline Limited Ingredient Diets

- Limited Ingredient Diets—Feline, Protein source duck (dry): limited antigen (duck) protein source, limited carbohydrate (potato) source.
- Limited Ingredient Diets—Feline, Protein source lamb (canned and dry): limited antigen (lamb) protein source, limited carbohydrate (potato) source.
- Limited Ingredient Diets—Feline, Protein source rabbit (canned): limited antigen (rabbit) protein source, limited carbohydrate (potato) source.
- Limited Ingredient Diets—Feline, Protein source venison (canned and dry): limited antigen (venison) protein source, limited carbohydrate (potato) source.

Pet-Ag, Inc. Formula V Products Diets

- CliniCare Feline Liquid Diet: energy, B-complex vitamins, taurine, glutamine-increased, lactose-reduced, highly digestible, highly palatable.
- RenalCare Feline Liquid Diet: protein, phosphorus, and lactose-reduced, energy, B-complex vitamins, taurine, glutamine-increased, highly digestible.

Purina Feline Clinical Nutritional Management Diets

- CNM-CV Formula (canned): sodium-reduced, potassium, taurine, and carnitine-increased, highly digestible.
- CNM-EN Formula (dry): fiber-reduced, moderate fat, highly digestible, source of omega-3 fatty acids, creates an acid urine pH.
- CNM-NF Formula (dry): protein, phosphorus, and sodium-reduced, B-complex vitamins and potassium-increased, adjusted omega-6:omega-3 fatty acid ratio (7:1), creates a neutral urine pH.
- CNM-OM Formula (dry): fat and energy-reduced, fiber-increased, creates an acid urine pH.
- CNM-UR Formula (canned and dry): magnesium-reduced, taurine and potassium-increased, creates an acidic urine pH.

Vet's Choice Select Care Diets

- Feline Control Formula (canned and dry): magnesium and sodium-reduced, potassium citrate added to prevent oxalate uroliths, creates a urine pH < 6.6, adjusted omega-6:omega-3 fatty acid ratio (between 5:1 and 10:1).

- Feline Development Formula (canned and dry): protein, energy, phosphorus, and calcium-increased fructooligosaccharides and digestive enzymes added, adjusted omega-6:omega-3 fatty acid ratio (between 5:1 and 10:1).
- Feline HiFiber Formula (canned and dry): energy, fat, and magnesium-reduced, fiber greatly increased, potassium citrate added to prevent oxalate uroliths, creates a urine pH < 6.6, adjusted omega-6:omega-3 fatty acid ratio (between 5:1 and 10:1).
- Feline Mature Formula (canned and dry): sodium, magnesium, phosphorus, and protein-reduced anti-oxidant vitamins added, creates a urine pH < 6.6, potassium citrate added to prevent oxalate uroliths, adjusted omega-6:omega-3 fatty acid ratio (between 5:1 and 10:1).
- Feline Modified Formula (canned and dry): sodium, calcium, phosphorus and protein-reduced vitamin B6 and potassium-increased, creates a slightly alkaline urine pH, potassium citrate added to prevent oxalate uroliths, adjusted omega-6:omega-3 fatty acid ratio (between 5:1 and 10:1).
- Feline Neutral Formula (dry): limited antigen (duck) protein source, limited carbohydrate (potato and rice) source, fructooligosaccharides, digestive enzymes, and anti-oxidant vitamins added, adjusted omega-6:omega-3 fatty acid ratio (between 5:1 and 10:1).
- Feline Weight Formula (canned and dry): energy, fat, sodium, and magnesium-reduced, fiber-increased, potassium citrate added to prevent oxalate uroliths, creates a urine pH < 6.6, adjusted omega-6:omega-3 fatty acid ratio (between 5:1 and 10:1).

Waltham Veterinary Feline Diets

- Calorie Control (canned and dry): fat and energy-reduced, fiber-increased.
- Low Protein (canned and dry): protein, phosphorus, and sodium-reduced, energy, potassium, and B vitamins-increased, creates a urine pH > 6.5.
- Selected Protein with Duck and Rice (dry): limited antigen (duck) protein source, limited carbohydrate (rice) source, highly digestible.
- Selected Protein with Venison and Rice (canned): limited antigen (venison) protein source, limited carbohydrate (rice) source, highly digestible.
- Control pHormula (canned and dry): magnesium-reduced, moisture-increased, acidifies urine, highly digestible.

S u g g e s t e d   R e a d i n g s
a n d   C o n t a c t   N u m b e r s

Comprehensive Guide to Vet's Choice, Select Care, Vet's Choice, an affiliate of VCA, 1996. 1-800-494-7387

Eukanuba Veterinary Diets, The Iam's Company, 1996. 1-800-535-VETS (8387)

Formula V products, Pet-Ag, Inc., 1990. 1-800-323-0877

IVD Limited Ingredient Diets, Innovative Veterinary Diets, 1996. 1-800-359-4IVD (4483)

Purina CNM Veterinary Product Guide, Ralston Purina Company, 1994. 1-800-222-VETS (8387)

The Hill's Key To Clinical Nutrition, Hill's Pet Nutrition, 1996. 1-800-548-VETS (8387)

Waltham Veterinary Diets, Waltham Center for Pet Nutrition, 1996. 1-800-528-1838

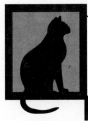

APPENDIX F

Testing Procedures

Gary D. Norsworthy

Formalin-Ether Sedimentation Technique

1. Suspend 1 g of feces in 25 mL of saline solution.
2. Filter the suspension through a small mesh screen.
3. Centrifuge at 1500 rpm for 5 minutes.
4. Pour off the supernatant.
5. Resuspend the sediment in 7 mL of 10% buffered formalin and incubate at room temperature for 10 minutes.
6. Add 3 mL of cold ether to the top of the suspension.
7. Resuspend the sediment at the bottom in a few drops of saline.
8. Place the suspension on a slide with a coverslip.
9. Examine at 100× (low power).

Glucose Curve

Indications

1. Initial regulation of diabetes mellitus
2. Dysregulation
3. To rule out or confirm rebound hyperglycemia

Objectives: To identify:

1. Time of peak insulin effect
2. Level of peak insulin effect (nadir)
3. If the maximum glucose is likely to be > 300 mg/dL

Technique

1. Give insulin for 3–5 days
2. Begin early in the morning
3. Have the owner feed the cat at home, and then bring it in immediately
4. Take an initial glucose reading immediately

5. Administer insulin subcutaneously **at the same dose as for the past 3–5 days**
6. If feeding was not done at home, feed the cat; it is essential that the cat eat or the results are not valid
7. Take a glucose reading every 1-1/2 to 2 hours until you can determine:
   a) The time of peak effect
   b) The nadir
   c) If the glucose is likely to rise above 300 mg/dL
8. 24-hour samples are desirable but usually not necessary; 6–10 hours is usually adequate if the cat is receiving BID dosing of insulin

Notes: a) Do not tranquilize the cat because most tranquilizers are insulin antagonists; b) When initial regulation is performed on a nonketoacidotic cat, the author begins insulin at 1/4 u/kg, a very conservative dose. The cat is treated for 3–5 days in the hospital or as an outpatient, then presented for a glucose curve. If the initial blood glucose reading is above 350 mg/dL, the author stops the glucose curve, increases the dose of insulin, and sends the cat home. The cat is returned after 3–5 days of the new dose for a curve. Only when the initial reading is below 350 mg/dL is the curve completed. This approach prevents the performance of several meaningless glucose curves and is especially helpful if the client's finances are limited.

T3 Suppression Test

Indication

This test is indicated when there are signs of hyperthyroidism (clinical signs, palpable thyroid lobe) but the T_4 is normal.

Technique

1. Collect a serum sample and freeze it.
2. Administer 25 μg of sodium liothyronine (T_3) every 8 hours for seven doses.
3. Collect a second serum sample 2–4 hours after the last dose.
4. Submit both serum samples to the laboratory for TT4 and T3.

Interpretation

A normal cat and a cat with nonthyroidal illness will have a post-test TT_4 value that suppresses below 1.5 μg/dL (20 nmol/L). A hyperthyroid cat will have a posttest TT_4 value that does not suppress and thus remains above 1.5 μg/dL (20 nmol/L). The results are considered extremely accurate. The T_3 values are measured only to confirm owner compliance of tablet administration. The second T_3 value should be above baseline. If the cost of performing this test is prohibitive, the T_3 values can be omitted because they are not involved in the interpretation. However, the owner must realize that improper administration of the tablets will invalidate the results.

TRH Response Test

Indication

This test is indicated when there are signs of hyperthyroidism (clinical signs, palpable thyroid lobe) but the T_4 is normal.

Technique

1. Administer thyrotropin-releasing hormone (TRH) at the dose of 0.1 mg/kg IV.
2. Collect a serum sample 4 hours later for T_4 determination.

Interpretation

- Normal cats and cats with nonthyroidal illness will have a 60% or more rise in serum T_4.
- Hyperthyroid cats will have a 50% or less rise in serum T4.
- A 50–60% rise is considered borderline (nondiagnostic).

Transient side effects of salivation, vomiting, tachypnea, and defecation may occur during the 4-hour testing period. The results are considered extremely accurate.

Note: The advantage of this test over the T_3 suppression test is the short testing time and the lack of reliance on owner compliance.

Trichogram

Indication

This test is to determine if hair loss is due to chewing, licking, or scratching versus hair loss due to hair falling out.

Technique

1. Pluck a tuft of hair within the area of alopecia.
2. Place the hair in a drop of mineral oil on a microscope slide. Attempt to keep the distal ends together.
3. Cover the mineral oil and hair with a cover slip.
4. Observe the distal ends of the hair under 100× magnification.

Broken hairs will be blunt on the end. This correlates with licking, chewing, or scratching. Normal distal ends are pointed.

S u g g e s t e d   R e a d i n g s

Bielsa LM, Greiner EC. Liver flukes (*Platynossomum concinnum*) in cats. *J Am Anim Hosp* 1985;21:2.

Miller WH. Symmetrical truncal hair loss in cats. *Compend Contin Educ Pract Vet* 1990;12: 461–465.

Norsworthy GD. A rational approach to feline blood glucose curves. *Vet Med J* 1995;90(11): 1064–1069.

Peterson ME, Graves TK, Gamble DA. Triiodothyronine (T_3) suppression test. An aid in the diagnosis of mild hyperthyroidism in cats. *J Vet Intern Med* 1990;4:233–237.

Sparkes AK, Jones BR, Gruffydd-Jones TJ, et al. Thyroid function in the cat: assessment by the TRH response test and the thyrotrophin stimulation test. *J Small Anim Pract* 1991; 32:59–64.

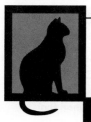

Drug Formulary

Mark G. Papich

D r u g   F o r m u l a r y

Only systemic drugs are listed; topicals, dermatologics, ointments, ophthalmic and otic treatments, vaccines, and nutritional supplements are not included.

Many of the drugs and doses listed are unapproved for veterinary use. Dosing information and indications for unapproved drugs are listed as a guide only. The author does not advocate use of unapproved drugs when equivalent approved veterinary drugs exist.

For many of the drugs listed in this formulary, adequate safety and efficacy studies have not been performed in cats. Doses and indications listed in this formulary were derived from the most current available information at the time of publication. The author is not responsible for adverse effects or toxicity occurring in patients when drugs are used according to the guidelines used in this formulary.

For drugs listed in this formulary, brand names may be listed as examples only. Other brand names may exist, and by listing a particular brand name, the author is not advocating one brand name over another.

Drug Name [Other Names]	Pharmacology and Indications	Dosage
Acepromazine (PromAce, many generics)	Phenothiazine tranquilizer. Inhibits action of dopamine as neurotransmitter. Used for sedation and preanesthetic purposes.	1.13–2.25 mg/kg IM, SC, IV PO for sedation; 0.05–0.1 mg/kg SC BID for thromboembolism or preanesthesia
Acetazolamide (Diamox)	Carbonic anhydrase inhibitor and diuretic. Used primarily to lower intraocular pressure. See dichlorphenamide.	5–10 mg/kg PO q8–12h Glaucoma: 4–8 mg/kg PO q8–12h

Drug Name (Other Names)	Pharmacology and Indications	Dosage
Acetylcysteine (Mucomyst)	Decreases viscosity of secretions. Used as a mucolytic agent in eyes and in bronchial nebulizing solutions. As a donator of sulfhydryl group, used as an antidote for intoxications (e.g., acetaminophen toxicosis).	Antidote: 140 mg/kg (loading dose) PO, IV, then 70 mg/kg q4h for five doses. Eyes: 2% solution topically q2h
Albendazole (Valbazen)	Benzimidazole antiparasitic drug. Inhibits glucose uptake in parasites.	25–50 mg/kg PO q12h for 10–21 days. Giardia: 25 mg /kg q12h for 2 days
Albuterol (Proventil, Ventolin)	Beta-2(β_2) adrenergic agonist. Bronchodilator. Stimulates β_2 receptors to relax bronchial smooth muscle. May also inhibit release of inflammatory mediators, especially from mast cells.	20–50 mcg/kg up to 4 times a day
Allopurinol (Lopurin, Zyloprim)	Decreases production of uric acid by inhibiting enzymes responsible for uric acid	10 mg/kg q8h, then reduce to 10 mg/kg q24h (questionable efficacy.)
Alumunium carbonate gel (Basalgel)	Antacid (neutralizes stomach acid) and phosphate binder in intestine.	10–30 mg/kg PO q8h (with meals)
Aluminium hydroxide gel (Amphogel)	Antacid (neutralizes stomach acid) and phosphate binder in intestine.	10–30 mg/kg PO q8h (with meals)
Amikacin (Amiglyde-V, Amikin)	Aminoglycoside antibacterial drug. Inhibits protein synthesis. See gentamicin.	6.5 mg/kg IV, IM, SC q8h or 20 mg/kg IV, IM, SC q24h
Aminopentamide (Centrine)	Antidiarrheal and antiemetic. Anticholinergic (blocks acetylcholine at parasympathetic synapse).	0.1 mg/cat IM, SC, PO q8–12h
Aminophylline	Bronchodilator	6.6 mg/kg PO q12h
Amitraz (Mitaban)	Antiparasitic drug for ectoparasites. Used for treatment of mites, including Demodex. Inhibits monoamine oxidase in mites.	10.6 mL per 7.5 L water (0.025% solution). Apply 3–6 topical treatments every 14 days
Amitriptyline (Elavil)	Tricyclic antidepressant drug. Used in humans to treat	5–10 mg/day PO

Drug Name [Other Names]	Pharmacology and Indications	Dosage
	anxiety and depression. Used to treat a variety of behavioral disorders. Action is via inhibition of uptake of serotonin at presynaptic nerve terminals.	
Amlodipine (Norvasc)	Calcium channel blocker. Antihypertensive drug.	0.625 mg/cat PO q24h
Ammonium chloride (generic)	Urine acidifier.	800 mg/cat (approx. 1/4 to 1/3 tsp) mixed with food daily.
Amoxicillin/clavulanic acid (Clavamox)	Beta-lactam antibiotic and betalactamase inhibitor (clavulanic acid)	62.5 mg/cat PO q12h
Amphotericin B (Fungizone)	Antifungal drug. Fungicidal for systemic fungi (damages fungal membranes).	0.5 mg/kg IV (slow infusion) q48h, to a cumulative dose of 4–8 mg/kg
Ampicillin (Omnipen, Principen)	Beta-lactam antibiotic. Inhibits bacterial cell wall synthesis.	20–40 mg/kg PO q8h, 10–20 mg/kg IV, IM, SC q6–8h (ampicillin sodium)
Ampicillin and Sulbactam (Uhasyn)	Same mechanism as ampicillin-clavulanate	10–20 mg/kg IV or IM q8h
Ampicillin trihydrate (Polyflex)	Beta-lactam antibiotic. Inhibit bacterial cell wall synthesis.	6.5–10 mg/kg IM, SC q12h
Amprolium (Amprol, Corid)	Antiprotozoal drug. Antagonizes thiamine in parasites. Used for treatment of coccidiosis, especially in kittens.	1.25 g of 20% amprolium powder to daily feed or 30 mL of 9.6% amprollum solution to 3.8 L of drinking water for 7 days
Ascorbic acid (vitamin C)	Vitamin. Used as acidifier but of questionable efficacy.	100–500 mg/animal/day (diet supplement); 100 mg/animal q8h (urine acidification)
L-asparaginase (Elspar)	Anticancer agent. Used in lymphoma protocols. Depletes cancer cells of asparagine and interferes with protein synthesis.	400 U/kg, IM, as part of a combination chemo protocol or every 1–2 weeks
Aspirin (Many generic and brand names [Bufferin, Ascriptin])	Nonsteroidal anti-inflammatory drug. Anti-inflammatory action is generally considered to be caused by inhibition of prostaglandins.	Anti-inflammatory: 10–20 mg/kg q72h Antiplatelet: 80 mg q72h

Drug Name [Other Names]	Pharmacology and Indications	Dosage
	Used as analgesic, anti-inflammatory, and anti-platelet drug.	
Atenolol (Tenormin)	Beta-adrenergic blocker. Relatively selective for β_1 receptor. Used primarily as an antiarrhythmic or in other cardiovascular conditions to slow sinus rate.	6.25–12.5 mg/cat q24h
Atracurium (Tracurium)	Neuromuscular blocking agent (nondepolarizing). Competes with acetylcholine at neuromuscular end plate. Used primarily during anesthesia or other conditions in which it is necessary to inhibit muscle contractions.	0.2 mg/kg IV initially, then 0.15 mg/kg every 30 minutes or IV infusion at 3–8 μg/kg/minute
Atropine (generic)	Anticholinergic agent (blocks acetylcholine effect at muscarinic receptor), parasympatholytic. Used primarily as adjunct to anesthesia or other procedures to increase heart rate and decrease respiratory and gastrointestinal secretion. Also used as antidote for or- ganophosphate intoxication.	0.02–0.04 mg/kg IV, IM, SC q6–8h; 0.2–0.5 mg/kg (as needed) for organophosphate and carbamate toxicosis
Aurothioglucose (Solganol)	For immune-mediated disease and L-P gingivitis/stomatitis.	0.5–1.0 mg/cat IM weekly until remission then monthly
Azathioprine (Imuran)	Thiopurine immunosuppressive drug. Inhibits T-cell lymphocyte function. This drug is metabolized to 6-mercaptopurine, which may account for immunosuppressive effects. Used to treat various immune-mediated disease.	1.5–3.125 mg/cat q48h
Azithromycin (Zithromax)	Azalide antibiotic. Similar mechanism of action as	5mg/kg PO every other day

Drug Name [Other Names]	Pharmacology and Indications	Dosage
	macrolides (erythromycin), which is to inhibit bacteria protein synthesis via inhibition of ribosome. Spectrum is primarily gram positive and gastric spiral bacteria.	
Benazapril (Lotensin)	ACE inhibitor. See captopril for details. Used for vasodilation, treatment of heart failure, and hypertension.	0.25–0.5mg/kg q24h PO
Betamethasone (Celestone)	Potent, long-acting corticosteroid. Anti-inflammatory and immunosuppressive effects are approximately 30 times more than cortisol. Anti-inflammatory effects are complex but primarily via inhibition of inflammatory cells and suppression of expression of inflammatory mediators. Used in treatment of inflammatory and immune-mediated disease.	0.1–0.2mg/kg PO q12–24h
Bethanechol (Urechloline)	Muscarinic, cholinergic agonist. Parasympathomimetic. Stimulates gastric and intestinal motility, but primarily used to increase contraction of urinary bladder.	1.25–5 mg/cat PO q8h
Bisacodyl (Dulcolax)	Laxative/cathartic. Acts via local stimulation of gastrointestinal motility, most likely by irritation of bowel. Used primarily as laxative or for procedures in which bowel evacuation is necessary.	5mg/cat PO q8–24M
Bismuth subsalicylate (Pepto-Bismol)	Antidiarrhea agent and gastrointestinal protectant. Precise mechanism of action is unknown, but antiprostaglandin action of	1–3 mL/kg/day (in divided doses) PO

Drug Name (Other Names)	Pharmacology and Indications	Dosage
	salicylate component may be beneficial for enteritis. Bismuth component is efficacious for treating infections caused by spirochaete bacteria (*Helicobacter* gastritis).	
Bleomycin (Blenoxane)	Anticancer antibiotic agent. Used for treatment of various sarcomas and carcinomas. Exact mechanism of action is unknown but may bind to DNA and prevent synthesis.	10 U/m^2 IV or SC for 3 days, then 10 U/m^2 weekly (maximum cumulative dose 200 U/m^2)
Bunamidine hydrochloride (Scolaban)	Used as anticestodal agent. Primarily to treat tapeworm infections. Mechanism of action is to damage integrity of protective integument on parasite.	20–50 mg/kg PO
Bupivacaine (Marcaine)	Local anesthetic. Inhibits nerve conduction via sodium channel blockade. Longer-acting and more potent than lidocaine or other local anesthetics.	0.22–0.3 mL epidural
Buprenorphine (Temgesic Buprenex)	Opioid analgesic. Partial μ-receptor agonist, κ-receptor antagonist. More potent than morphine (25–50 times).	0.005–0.01 mg/kg IV, IM q4–8h
Buspirone (BuSpar)	Antianxiety agent. Acts to block release of serotonin by binding to presynaptic receptors. In veterinary medicine, has been primarily used for treatment of inappropriate elimination in cats.	2.5–5 mg/cat PO q24h (may be increased to twice daily for some cats)
Busulfan (Myleran)	Anticancer agent. Bifunctional alkylating agent and acts to disrupt DNA of tumor cells. Used primarily for lymphoreticular neoplasia.	3–4 mg/m^2 PO q24h

Drug Name (Other Names)	Pharmacology and Indications	Dosage
Butorphanol (Torbutrol, Torbugesic)	Opioid analgesic. κ-receptor agonist and weak μ-receptor antagonist. Butorphanol is used for perioperative analgesia, for chronic pain, and as an antitussive agent.	Analgesia 0.4 mg/kg SC q4–6h; 0.2 mg/kg IV q4–6h
Calcitriol (Rocaltrol, Calcijex)	Used to treat calcium deficiency and diseases such as hypocalcemia associated with hypoparathyroidism. Not indicated as vitamin D supplement. Action is to increase calcium absorption in intestine.	2.5–3 ng/kg (0.0025–0.003 mcg/kg) PO q24h
Calcium carbonate (Titralac, Tums, generic)	Used as oral calcium supplement for hypocalcemia. Used as antacid to treat gastric hyperacidity and gastrointestinal ulcers. Neutralizes stomach acid. Also used as intestinal phosphate binder for hyperphosphatemia.	5–10 mL of oral solution PO q4–6h. Phosphate binder: 60–100 mg/kg/day PO in divided doses
Calcium chloride (generic 10% solution)	Calcium supplement. Used in acute situations to supplement as electrolyte replacement or as a cardiotonic.	0.1–0.3 mL/kg IV (slowly)
Calcium citrate (Citracal [OTC])	Calcium supplement. Used in treatment of hypocalcemia, such as with hypoparathyroidism.	10–30mg/kg PO q8h (with meals)
Calcium gluconate (Kalcinate, generic [10% solution])	Calcium supplement. Used in treatment of hypocalcemia, such as with hypoparathyroidism. Used in electrolyte deficiency.	0.5–1.5mL/kg IV (slowly)
Calcium lactate (generic)	Generally same comments as for other calcium supplements.	0.2–0.5 g/cat/day PO (in divided doses)

Drug Name [Other Names]	Pharmacology and Indications	Dosage
Captopril (Capoten)	Angiotensin-converting enzyme (ACE) inhibitor. Inhibits conversion of angiotensin I to angiotensin II. May have other vasodilating properties. Generally used to treat hypertension and congestive heart failure.	3.12–6.25 mg/cat PO q8h
Carbenicillin (Geopen, Pyopen)	Beta-lactam antibiotic. Inhibits bacterial cell wall synthesis. Active against *Pseudomonas* and other gram-negative bacteria.	40–50 mg/kg (up to 100 mg/kg IV, IM, SC q6–8h)
Carbenicillin indanyl sodium (Geocillin)	Same as for carbenicillin. Primary use is for treating infections of lower urinary tract.	10 mg/kg PO q8h
Carbimazole (Neomercazole)	Antithyroid drug similar to methimazole, but with perhaps fewer side effects	5 mg/cat PO q8h (Induction), followed by 5 mg/cat PO q12h
Carleoplatin (Paraplatin)	Interrupts replication of DNA in tumor cells by interstrand crosslinking. Used for SCC, melanoma, vaccino sarcomas, osteo sarcomas, transitional cell carcinomas.	200–250 mg/m^2 IV q4 wks
Cascara sagrada (many brands [e.g., Nature's Remedy])	Stimulant cathartic. Action is believed to be by local stimulation of bowel motility. Used as laxative to treat constipation or evacuate bowel for procedures.	0.5–1.5 mL/cat/day
Castor oil (generic)	Stimulant cathartic. Action is believed to be by local stimulation of bowel motility. Used as laxative to treat constipation or evacuate bowel for procedures.	4–10 mL/day PO
Cefaclor (Ceclor)	Cephalosporin antibiotic. Action is similar to other β-lactam antibiotics, which is to inhibit synthesis of bacterial cell wall leading to cell death. Cephalosporins are divided into first, sec-	4–20 mg/kg PO q8h

Drug Name [Other Names]	Pharmacology and Indications	Dosage
	ond, or third generation depending on spectrum of activity. Consult package insert or specific reference for spectrum of activity of individual cephalosporin. Cefaclor is a second-generation cephalosporin.	
Cefadroxil (Cefa-Tabs, Cefa-Drops)	See cefaclor. Cefadroxil is a first-generation cephalosporin.	22 mg/kg PO q24h
Cefazolin sodium (Ancef Kelzol, generic)	See cefadroxil. Cefazolin is a first-generation cephalo-sporin.	20–35 mg/kg IV, IM q8h. Perisurgical use: 22 mg/kg q2h (during surgery)
Cefixime (Suprax)	See cefaclor. Cefixime is a third-generation cephalosporin.	10 mg/kg PO q12h. Cysti-tis: 5 mg/kg PO q12–24h
Cefotaxime (Claforan)	See cefaclor. Cafotaxime is a third-generation cephalosporin.	20–80 mg/kg IV, IM q6h
Cefotetan (Cefotan)	See cefaclor. Cefotetan is a second-generation cephalo-sporin.	30 mg/kg IV, SC q8h
Cefoxitin sodium (Mefoxin)	See cefaclor. Cefoxitin is a second-generation cephalo-sporin. May have increased activity against anaerobic bacteria.	30 mg/kg IV q6–8h
Ceftiofur (Naxcel [Excenel in Canada])	See cefaclor. Ceftiofur is a unique cephalosporin that does not fit into a distinct generation, but some prop-erties are similar to 3rd generation class.	2.2–4.4 mg/kg SC q24h (for urinary tract infections)
Cephalexin (Keflex, generic forms)	See cefaclor. Cephalexin is a first-generation cephalosporin.	10–30 mg/kg PO q6–12h. Pyoderma: 22–35 mg/kg PO q12h
Cephalothin sodium (Keflin)	See cefaclor.	10–30 mg/kg IV, IM q4–8h
Cephapirin (Cefadyl)	See cefaclor. Cephapirin is a first-generation cephalosporin.	10–30 mg/kg IV, IM q4–8h
Cephradine (Velosef)	See cefaclor. Cephapirin is a first-generation cephalosporin.	10–25 mg/kg PO q6–8h
Charcoal, activated (ActaChar, Charcodote, Toxiban, generic)	Adsorbent. Used primarily to adsorb drugs and toxins in intestine to prevent their absorption.	1–4 gm/kg PO (granules); 6–12 mL/kg (suspension)

Drug Name (Other Names)	Pharmacology and Indications	Dosage
Chlorambucil (Leukeran)	Cytotoxic alkylating agent. Acts in similar manner as cyclophosphamide. Used for treatment of various tumors and immunosuppressive therapy.	$2–6$ mg/m^2 or $0.1–0.2$ mg/kg PO q24h initially, then q48h
Chloramphenicol and chloramphenicol palmitate (Chloromycetin, generic forms)	Antibacterial drug. Mechanism of action is inhibition of protein synthesis via binding to ribosome. Broad spectrum of activity.	$12.5–20$mg/kg PO q12h
Chloramphenicol sodium succinate (Chloromycetin, generic)	Injection form of chloramphenicol. Converted by liver to parent drug.	$12.5–50$ mg/cat IV, IM q12h
Chlorothiazide (Diuril)	Thiazide diuretic. Inhibits sodium reabsorption in distal renal tubules. Used as diuretic and antihypertensive. Because it decreases renal excretion of calcium, it also has been used to treat calcium-containing uroliths.	$20–40$ mg/kg PO q12h
Chlorpheniramine maleate (Chlortrimeton, Phenetron, others)	Antihistamine (H1 blocker). Blocks action of histamine on receptors. Also may have direct antiinflammatory action. Use most often to prevent allergic reactions. Used for pruritus therapy in dogs and cats.	2 mg/cat PO q12h
Chlorpromazine (Thorazine)	Phenothiazine tranquilizer/antiemetic. Inhibits action of dopamine as neurotransmitter. Most often used as central antiemetic. Also used for sedation and pre-anesthetic purposes.	0.5mg/kg IM, SC q6–8h
Chlortetracycline (generic)	Tectracycline antibacterial drug. Inhibits bacterial protein synthesis by interfering with peptide elongation by ribosome. Bacteriostatic agent with broad spectrum of activity.	25 mg/kg PO q6–8h

Drug Name (Other Names)	Pharmacology and Indications	Dosage
Cimetidine (Tagamet [OTC and prescription])	Histamine-2 antagonist (H_2 blocker). Blocks histamine stimulation of gastric parietal cell to decrease gastric acid secretion. Used to treat ulcers and gastritis.	10 mg/kg IV, IM, PO q6–8h (in renal failure, administer 2.5–5 mg/kg IV, PO q12h)
Ciprofloxacin (Cipro)	Fluoroquinolone antibacterial. Acts to inhibit DNA gyrase and inhibit cell DNA and RNA synthesis. Bactericidal. Broad antimicrobial activity.	5–15 mg/kg PO, IV q12h
Cisapride (Propulsid [Prepulsid in Canada])	Prokinetic agent. Stimulates gastric and intestinal motility by either acetylcholine action, activity on serotonin receptors, or direct effect on smooth muscle. Used for gastric reflux, gastroparesis, ileus, and constipation.	2.5–7.5 mg/cat PO q8–12h. (As much as 1 mg/kg q8h has been administered to cats.)
Clindamycin (Antirobe, Cleocin)	Antibacterial drug of the lincosamide class (similar in action to macrolides). Inhibits bacterial protein synthesis via inhibition ofbacterial ribosome. Bacteriostatic with spectrum of activity primarily against gram-positive bacteria and anaerobes.	5.5 mg/kg q12h or 11 mg/kg q24h (staphylococcal infections); 11 mg/kg q12h or 22 mg/kg PO q24h (anaerobic infections). Toxoplasmosis: 12.5 mg/kg PO q12h (in divided treatments) for 4 weeks
Clofazimine (Lamprene)	Antimicrobial agent used to treat feline leprosy. Slow bactericidal effect on *Mycobacterium leprae.*	1 mg/kg PO (up to a maximum of 4 mg/kg/day)
Clomipramine (Anafranil)	Tricyclic antidepressant (TCA). Used in humans to treat anxiety and depression. Used in cats to treat variety of behavioral disorders, including obsessive-compulsive disorders. Action is via inhibition of up-	1 mg/kg/day PO (up to a maximum dose of 3 mg/kg/day PO)

Drug Name (Other Names)	Pharmacology and Indications	Dosage
	take of serotonin at presynaptic nerve terminals.	
Clonazepam (Klonopin)	Benzodiazepine. Action is to enhance inhibitory effects of GABA in central nervous system. Used for anti- seizure action, sedation, and treatment of some behavioral disorders.	0.5 mg/kg PO q8–12h
Clorazepate (Tranxene)	Benzodiazepine. Action is to enhance inhibitory effects of GABA in central nervous system. Used for anti-seizure action, sedation, and treatment of some behavioral disorders.	2 mg/kg PO q12h
Cloxacillin (Cloxapen, Orbenin, Tegopen)	Beta-lactam antibiotic. Inhibits bacterial cell wall synthesis. Spectrum is limited to gram-positive bacteria, especially staphylococci.	20–40 mg/kg PO q8h
Colchicine (generic)	Anti-inflammatory agent. Used primarily to treat gout. In animals, used to decrease fibrosis and development of hepatic failure (possibly by inhibiting formation of collagen).	0.01–0.03 mg/kg PO q24h
Colony-stimulating factor (Amgen)	Stimulates granulocyte development in bone marrow. Used primarily to regenerate blood cells to recover from cancer chemotherapy or other therapy.	2.5 mcg/kg SC q12h
Corticotropin (ACTH) (Acthar)	Used for diagnostic purposes to evaluate adrenal gland function. Stimulates normal synthesis of cortisol from adrenal gland.	Response test: Collect pre-ACTH sample and inject 2.2 IU/kg IM. Collect post-ACTH sample in at 1 and 2 hours
Cosequin (Cosequin)	Cosequin is brand name for combination of glucosamine HCL and chondroitin sulfate.	1 RS capsule/day PO

Drug Name [Other Names]	Pharmacology and Indications	Dosage
	According to manufacturer these compounds stimulate synthesis of synovial fluid and inhibit degradation and improve healing of articular cartilage. Used primarily for degenerative joint disease.	
Cosyntropin (Cortrosyn)	Cosyntropin is a synthetic form of corticotropin (ACTH) used for diagnostic purposes only. In humans it is preferred over corticotropin because it is less allergenic.	Response test: Collect pre-ACTH sample and inject 0.125 mg IV. Collect post-ACTH sample at 30 and 60 minutes
Cyanocobalamin (vitamin B_{12}) (many)	Vitamin B analogue	50–100 μg/day PO
Cyclophosphamide (Cytoxan, Neosar)	Cytotoxic agent. Bifunctional alkylating agent. Disrupts base-pairing and inhibits DNA and RNA synthesis. Cytotoxic for tumor cells and other rapidly dividing cells. Used primarily as adjunct for cancer chemo-therapy and as immuno-suppressive therapy.	Immunosuppressive therapy: 6.25–12.5 mg/cat once daily 4 days per week
Cyclosporine (Sandim-mune, Optimmune [ophthalmic])	Immunosuppressive drug. Depresses T lymphocytes.	10 mg/kg PO q12h
Cyproheptadine (Periactin)	Phenothiazine with antihist-amine and antiserotonin properties. Used as appetite stimulant (probably by alter-ing serotonin activity in appetite center).	Appetite stimulant: 2 mg/cat PO
Cytarabine (cytosine arabinoside) (Cytosar)	Anticancer agent. Exact mech-anism is not known. Prob-ably inhibits DNA synthesis. Used for lymphoma and leukemia protocols.	100 mg/m^2 once daily for 2 days
Danazol (Danocrine)	Gonadotropin inhibitor. Sup-presses LH and FSH and	5–10 mg/kg PO q12h

Drug Name [Other Names]	Pharmacology and Indications	Dosage
	estrogen synthesis. In humans, used for endometriosis. May reduce destruction of platelets or RBC in immune-mediated disease.	
Dantrolene (Dantrium)	Muscle relaxant. Inhibits calcium leakage from sarcoplasmic reticulum. In addition to muscle relaxation, it has been used for malignant hyperthermia. Also has been used to relax urethral muscle in cats.	0.5–2 mg/kg PO q12h
Dapsone (generic)	Antimicrobial drug used primarily for treatment of mycobacterium. May have some immunosuppressive properties or inhibit function of inflammatory cells. Used primarily for dermatologic diseases in dogs and cats.	1.1 mg/kg PO q8–12h
Darbazine (prochlorperazine and isopropamide) (Darbazine)	Combination product. Prochlorperazine is a central-acting dopamine antagonist (antiemetic); isopropamide is an anticholinergic drug (atropine-like effects). Used primarily to control vomiting.	0.14–0.2 mL/kg SC q12h
Deferoxamine (Desferal)	Chelating agent with strong affinity for di- and trivalent cations. Used to treat acute iron toxicosis. Indicated in cases of severe poisoning. Deferoxamine also has been used to chelate aluminum and facilitate removal.	10 mg/kg IV, IM q2h for two doses, then 10 mg/kg q8h for 24 hours
Desmopressin acetate (DDAVP)	Synthetic peptide similar to antidiuretic hormone (ADH). Used as replacement therapy for patients with diabetes insipidus.	Diabetes insipidus: 2–4 drops (2 mg) q12–24h intranasally or in eye
Desoxycorticosterone pivalate (DOCP, DOCA pivalate)	Mineralocorticoid. Used for adrenocorticol insufficiency (hypoadrenocorticism). No glucocorticoid activity.	1.5–2.2 mg/kg IM every 25 days

Drug Name (Other Names)	Pharmacology and Indications	Dosage
Dexamethasone (Azium, generic)	Corticosteroid. Dexamethasone has approximately 30 times the potency of cortisol. Multiple anti-inflammatory effects. See betamethasone.	Anti-inflammatory: 0.1–0.2 mg/kg IV, IM, PO q12–24h. Shock, spinal injury: 2.2–4.4 mg/kg IV
Dextran (Dextran 70, Gentran 70)	Synthetic colloid used for volume expansion. High molecular weight fluid replacement. Primarily used for acute hypovolemia and shock.	10–20 mL/kg IV to effect
Dextromethorphan (Benylin, others)	Centrally-acting antitussive drug. Shares similar chemical structure as opiates but does not affect opiate receptors. Appears to directly affect cough receptor.	0.5–2 mg/kg PO q6–8h
Dextrose solution 5% (D5W)	Sugar added to fluid solutions. Isotonic.	40–50 mL/kg IV q24h
Diazepam (Valium, generic)	Benzodiazepine. Central-acting CNS depressant. Mechanism of action appears to be via potentiation of GABA-receptor mediated effects in CNS. Used for sedation, anesthetic adjunct, anti-convulsant, and behavioral disorders. Diazepam metabolized to desmethyl-diazepam (nor-diazepam) and oxazepam.	Preanesthetic: 0.5 mg/kg IV. Status epilepticus: 0.5 mg/kg IV, 1 mg/kg rectal, repeat if necessary. Appetite stimulant 0.2 mg/kg IV
Dichlorphenamide (Daranide)	Carbonic anhydrase inhibitor. Diuretic. Acts to inhibit enzyme that forms hydrogen and bicarbonate ions. Reduces plasma bicarbonate concentration, producing systemic metabolic acidosis and alkaline diuresis. Primarily used to treat glaucoma.	3–5 mg/kg PO q8–12h
Dichlorvos (Task)	Antiparasitic drug used primarily to treat hookworms,	11 mg/kg PO

Drug Name (Other Names)	Pharmacology and Indications	Dosage
	roundworms, and whipworms. Kills parasites by anticholinesterase action.	
Dicloxacillin (Dynapen)	Beta-lactam antibiotic. Inhibits bacterial cell wall synthesis. Spectrum is limited to gram-positive bacteria, especially staphylococci.	11–55 mg/kg PO q8h
Digoxin (Lanoxin, Cardoxin)	Cardiac glycoside.	Cats 2–3 kg: 0.0312 mg PO q48h. Cats 4–5 kg: 0.0312 mg PO q24h. Cats > 6kg: 0.0312 mg PO q12h
Dihydrotachysterol (vitamin D) (Hytakerol, DHT)	Vitamin D analogue. Used as treatment of hypocalcemia, especially that associated with hypoparathyroidism. Vitamin D promotes absorption and utilization of calcium.	0.01 mg/kg/day PO. Acute treatment administer 0.02 mg/kg initially, then 0.01–0.02 mg/kg PO q24–48h thereafter
Diltiazem (Cardizem, Dilacor)	Calcium-channel blocking drug. Blocks calcium entry into cells via blockade of slow channel. Produces vasodilation and negative chronotropic effects.	1.75–2.4 mg/kg PO q8h. Dilacor XR or Cardizem CD dose is 10 mg/kg PO q24h
Dimenhydrinate (Dramamine [Gravol in Canada])	Antihistamine drug. See chlorpheniramine.	12.5 mg PO, IM, IV q8h
Dimercaprol (BAL) (BAL in oil)	Chelating agent. Used to treat lead, gold, and arsenic toxicity.	4 mg/kg IM q4h
Diphenoxylate (Lomotil)	Opiate agonist. Stimulates smooth muscle segmentation in intestine as well as electrolyte absorption. Used for acute treatment of nonspecific diarrhea.	0.05–0.1 mg/kg PO q12h
Dipyridamole (Persantine)	Platelet inhibitor. Mechanism of action is attributed to increased levels of cAMP in platelet, which decreases platelet activation, indicated primarily to prevent thromboembolism.	4–10 mg/kg PO q24h

Drug Name (Other Names)	Pharmacology and Indications	Dosage
Dobutamine (Dobutrex)	Adrenergic agonist. Action is primarily to stimulate myocardium via action on cardiac beta-1 (β_1) receptors. Increases heart contraction without increase in heart rate. Some action may occur via alpha receptors. Primarily used for acute treatment of heart failure.	1–5 mcg/kg/min IV infusion
Docusate calcium (Surfak, Doxidan)	Stool softener (surfactant). Acts to decrease surface tension to allow more water to accumulate in the stool.	50 mg PO q12–24h
Docusate sodium (Colace, Doxan, Doss, many OTC brands)	See docusate calcium.	50 mg PO q12–24h
Domperidone (Motilium)	Motility modifier (similar to metoclopramide)	2–5 mg/cat PO
Dopamine (Intropin)	Adrenergic agonist. Action is primarily to stimulate myocardium via action on cardiac beta-1 (β_1) receptors. There is some suggestion that dopamine increases renal perfusion via action on renal dopaminergic receptors; however, clinical evidence for beneficial effect is lacking.	2–10 mcg/kg/min IV infusion
Doxapram (Dopram)	Respiratory stimulant via action on carotid chemoreceptors and subsequent stimulation of respiratory center. Used to treat respiratory depression or to stimulate respiration postanesthesia. May also increase cardiac output.	5–10 mg/kg IV. Neonate: 1–5 mg SC, sublingual, or via umbilical vein
Doxorubicin (Adriamycin)	Anticancer agent. Acts to intercalate between bases on DNA, disrupting DNA, and RNA synthesis in tumor	20–25 mg/m^2 IV every 21 days

Drug Name [Other Names]	Pharmacology and Indications	Dosage
	cell. Doxorubicin also may affect tumor cell membranes. Used for treatment of various neoplasia, including lymphoma.	
Doxycycline (Vibramycin, generic forms)	Tetracycline antibiotic. Mechanism of action of tetracyclines is to bind to 30S ribosomal subunit and inhibit protein synthesis. Usually bactericidal. Broad spectrum of activity, including bacteria, some protozoa and *Rickettsia*.	3–5 mg/kg PO, IV q12h, or 10 mg/kg PO q24h
Edetate calcium disodium ($CaNa_2EDTA$) (Calcium disodium versenate)	Chelating agent. Indicated for treatment of acute and chronic lead poisoning. Sometimes used in combination with dimercaprol (BAL).	25 mg/kg SC, IM, IV q6h for 2–5 days
Edrophonium (Tensilon, others)	Cholinesterase inhibitor. Causes cholinergic effects by inhibiting metabolism of acetylcholine. Very short acting and ordinarily is only used for diagnostic purposes (e.g., for myasthenia gravis). Also has been used to reverse neuromuscular blockade of nondepolarizing agents (pancuronium).	2.5 mg/cat IV
Enalapril (Enacard, Vasotec)	ACE inhibitor. See captopril for details. Used for vasodilation and treatment of heart failure.	0.25–0.5 PO mg/kg q12–24h
Enflurane (Ethrane)	Inhalant anesthetic	Induction: 2–3% Maintenance: 1.5–3%
Enilconazole (Imaverol, ClinaFarm-EC)	Azole antifungal agent (for topical use only). Like other azoles, inhibits membrane synthesis (ergosterol) in fungus. Highly effective for dermatophytes.	Nasal aspergillosis: 10 mg/kg q12h instilled into nasal sinus for 14 days (10% solution diluted 50/50 with water). Dermatophytes: Dilute 10% solution to

Drug Name (Other Names)	Pharmacology and Indications	Dosage
		0.2% and wash lesion with solution four times at 3–4-day intervals
Enrofloxacin (Baytril)	Fluoroquinolone antibacterial drug. Acts via inhibition of DNA gyrase in bacteria to inhibit DNA and RNA synthesis. Bactericidal. Broad spectrum of activity.	2.5 mg/kg PO, IM q12h (up to 10 mg/kg q24h) and 20 mg/kg for MIC of 5 μg/mL
Ephedrine (many, generic)	Adrenergic agonist. Agonist on alpha and beta-1 adrenergic receptors but not beta-2 receptors. Used as vasopressor (e.g., administered during anesthesia). Central nervous system stimulant. Also has been used to treat urinary incontinence because of action on bladder sphincter muscle.	Urinary incontinence 2–4 mg/kg. Vasopressor: 0.75 mg/ kg IM, SC (repeat as needed)
Epinephrine (Adrenaline, generic forms)	Adrenergic agonist. Nonselectively stimulates alpha (α) and beta (β) adrenergic receptors. Used primarily for emergency situations to treat cardiopulmonary arrest and anaphylactic shock.	Cardiac arrest: 10–20 μg/kg IV or 200 μg/kg intratracheal (may be diluted in saline before administration). Anaphylactic shock: 2.5–5 μg/kg IV or 50 μg/kg intratracheal (may be diluted in saline)
Epsiprantel (Cestex)	Anticestodal agent (similar to praziquantel)	2.75 mg/kg PO
Ergocalciferol (vitamin D_2) (Calciferol, Drisdol)	Vitamin D analogue. Used for vitamin D deficiency and as treatment of hypocalcemia, especially that associated with hypothyroidism. Vitamin D promotes absorption and utilization of calcium.	500–2000 U/kg/day PO
Erythromycin (many brands, generic)	Macrolide antibiotic. Inhibits bacteria by binding to 50S ribosome and inhibiting protein synthesis. Spectrum of activity limited primarily to gram-positive aer-	10–20 mg/kg PO q8–12h

Drug Name [Other Names]	Pharmacology and Indications	Dosage
	obic bacteria. Used for skin and respiratory infections.	
Erythropoietin (Epogen, epoetin alfa)	Hematopoietic growth factor that stimulates erythro-poiesis. Human recombinant erythropoietin. Used to treat nonregenerative anemia due to renal failure.	35 U/kg, SC three times per week (adjust dose to hematocrit of 0.30–0.34)
Estradiol cypionate (ECP, Depo-Estradiol, generic)	Semisynthetic estrogen compound. Used primarily to induce abortion.	250 µg/cat IM between 40 hours and 5 days of mating
Ethanol	Inhibits alcohol dehydrogen-ase to prevent breakdown of ethylene glycol into toxic meta-bolites. For antifreeze toxicity.	5 mL/kg IV q6h × 5 treat-ments then q8h × 4 treat-ments
Etidronate disodium (Didronel)	Bisphosphonate drug. Used to treat osteoporosis and hypercalcemia. Decreases bone turnover, inhibits os-teoclast activity, retards bone resorption, and de-creases rate of osteoporosis.	10 mg/kg/day PO
Etretinate (Tegison)	Used for treatment of idio-pathic seborrhea. Normal-izes epidermal differentiation.	2 mg/kg/day
Famotidine (Pepsid)	H$_2$ receptor antagonist. See cimetidine for details.	0.5 mg/kg PO q12– 24h
Fenbendazole (Panacur, SafeGuard)	Benzimidazole antiparasite drug. See albendazole.	25 mg/kg/day PO for 3 days
Fentanyl, transdermal (Duragesic)	Transdermal fentanyl incorporates fentanyl into adhesive patches applied to skin. Studies have determined that patches release sus-tained levels of fentanyl for 72–108 hours. One 100 µg/ hr patch is equivalent to 10 mg/kg of morphine IM every 4 hours.	25 µg patch q72h
Ferrous sulfate (many OTC brands)	Iron supplement	50–100 mg/cat PO q24h
Fluconazole (Diflucan)	Azole antifungal drug. Similar mechanism as other azole	50 mg/cat PO q12h

Drug Name (Other Names)	Pharmacology and Indications	Dosage
	antifungal agents. Inhibits ergosterol synthesis in fungal cell membrane. Fungistatic. Efficacious against dermatophytes and variety of systemic fungi.	
Flucytosine (Ancobon)	Antifungal drug. Used in combination with other antifungal drugs for treatment of cryptococcosis. Action is to penetrate fungal cells and is converted to fluorouracil, which acts as antimetabolite.	25–50 mg/kg PO q6–8h (up to a maximum dose of 100 mg/kg PO q12h)
Fludrocortisone (Florinef)	Mineralocorticoid. Used as replacement therapy in animals with adrenal atrophy/adrenocortical insufficiency. Has high potency of mineralocorticoid activity compared with glucocorticoid activity.	0.1–0.2 mg PO q24h
Flumethasone (Flucort)	Potent glucocorticoid anti-inflammatory drug. Potency is approximately 15 times that of cortisol. See dexamethasone for additional details.	0.03–0.125 mg/day IV, IM, SC, PO. Anti-inflammatory: 0.15–0.3 mg/kg IV, IM, SC, PO q12–24h
Flumazenil (Romazicon)	Benzodiazepine receptor antagonist. Used as reversal agent after benzodiazepine administration in humans (not commonly used in veterinary medicine).	0.2 mg IV (total dose) as needed
Flunixin meglumine (Banamine)	NSAID. Acts to inhibit cyclooxygenase enzyme (COX) that synthesizes prostaglandins. Other anti-inflammatory effects may occur (such as effects on leukocytes) but have not been well characterized. Used primarily for short-term treatment of moderate pain and inflammation.	1.1mg/kg IV, IM, SC 7d x 3 or 1.1 mg/kg/day PO 3 days per week. Ophthalmic: 0.5 mg/kg IV once

Drug Name (Other Names)	Pharmacology and Indications	Dosage
Fluoxetine hydrochloride (Prozac)	Antidepressant drug. Used to treat behavioral disorders such as obsessive-compulsive disorders. Mechanism of action appears to be via selective inhibition of serotonin reuptake and down regulation of 5-HT1 receptors.	Dose not established (approx. 1 mg/kg PO q24h)
Furazolidone (Furoxone)	Oral antiprotozoal drug with activity against *Giardia.* May have some activity against bacteria in intestine. Not used for systemic therapy.	4 mg/kg PO q12h for 7–10 days
Furosemide (Lasix, generic)	Loop diuretic. Inhibits sodium and water transport in ascending loop of Henle, which produces diuresis. Also may have vasodilating properties, increasing renal perfusion and decreasing preload.	1–4 mg/kg IV, IM, SC, PO q8–24h
Gentamicin (Gentocin)	Aminoglycoside antibiotic. Action is to inhibit bacteria protein synthesis via binding to 30S ribosome. Bactericidal. Broad spectrum of activity (except streptococci and anaerobic bacteria).	3 mg/kg IV, IM, SC q8h or 9 mg/kg q24h
Glipizide (Glucotrol)	Sulfonylurea oral hypoglycemic agent. Used as oral treatment in the management of diabetes mellitus. Increases secretion of insulin from pancreas, probably by interacting with sulfonylurea receptors on beta-cells.	0.25–0.5 mg/kg PO q12h
Glyburide (Diabeta, Micronase, Glynase)	Sulfonylurea hypoglycemic agent. See glipizide.	0.2 mg/kg PO daily
Glycopyrrolate (Robinul-V)	Anticholinergic drug. For mechanism, see atropine. Glycopyrrolate may have less effect on central ner-	0.005–0.01 mg/kg IV, IM, SC

Drug Name (Other Names)	Pharmacology and Indications	Dosage
	vous system compared with atropine because of lower CSF levels. May have longer duration of action than atropine.	
Gonadorelin (Gn-RH, LH-RH) (Factrel)	Stimulates synthesis and release of luteinizing hormone (LH) and to a lesser degree, follicle-stimulating hormone (FSH). Used to induce luteinization.	25 μg/cat IM once
Gonadotropin, chorionic (hCG) (Profasi, Pregnyl, generic, APL)	Action of hCG is identical to that of luteinizing hormone (LH). Used to induce luteinization.	250 U/cat IM once
Gonadotropin-releasing hormone	See gonadorelin.	
Griseofulvin (microsize) (Fulvicin U/F)	Antifungal drug. Incorporates into skin layers and inhibits mitosis of fungi. Antifungal activity is limited to dermatophytes.	50 mg/kg PO q24h (up to a maximum dose of 110–132 mg/kg/day in divided treatments)
Griseofulvin (ultramicrosize) (Fulvicin P/G, Gris-PEG)	Same as above	30 mg/kg/day PO in divided treatments
Growth hormone (hGH)	Growth hormone. Used to treat growth hormone deficiencies.	0.1 U/kg 3 times per week for 4–6 weeks
Halothane (Fluothane)	Inhalant anesthetic. Exact mechanism of action unknown.	Induction: 3%. Maintenance: 0.5–1.5%
Heparin sodium (Liquaemin [United States], Hepalean [Canada])	Anticoagulant. Potentiates anticoagulant effects of antithrombin III. Used primarily for prevention of thrombosis (efficacy questionable).	100–200 U/kg IV loading dose, then 100–300 U/kg SC q6–8h. Low dose prophylaxis: 70 U/kg SC q8–12h
Hydralazine (Apresoline)	Vasodilator. Antihypertensive. Used to dilate arterioles and decrease afterload. Primarily used for treatment of congestive heart failure and other cardiovascular disorders characterized by high peripheral vascular resistance.	2.5 mg/cat PO q12–4h

Drug Name [Other Names]	Pharmacology and Indications	Dosage
Hydrochlorothiazide (HydroDIURIL, generic)	Thiazide diuretic. Inhibits sodium reabsorption in distal renal tubules. Used as diuretic and antihypertensive. Because they decrease renal excretion of calcium, they also have been used to treat calcium-containing uroliths.	1–2 mg/kg PO q12h
Hydrocortisone (Cortef)	Glucocorticoid anti-inflammatory drug. Hydro-cortisone has weaker anti-inflammatory effects and greater mineralocorticoid effects compared with pred-nisolone or dexamethasone. See dexamethasone for further details. Also used for replacement therapy.	Replacement therapy: 1–2 mg/kg PO q12h. Anti-inflammatory: 2.5–5 mg/kg PO q12h
Hydrocortisone sodium succinate (Solu-Cortef)	Same as hydrocortisone, except that this is a rapid-acting injectable product	Shock: 50–150 mg/kg IV. Anti-inflammatory: 5 mg/kg IV q12h
Hydroxyethyl starch (HES) (HES, Hetastarch)	Synthetic colloid volume expander (used in same manner as dextran). Used primarily to treat acute hypovolemia and shock.	10–20 mL/kg IV to effect
Hydroxyurea (Hydrea)	Antineoplastic agent. Used in combination with other anticancer modalities for treatment of certain tumors. Has been used to treat polycythemia vera.	25 mg/kg PO once daily, 3 days per week
Imipenem (Primaxin)	Beta-lactam antibiotic with broad-spectrum activity. Action is similar to other beta-lactams. See amoxicillin. Imipenem is the most active of all beta-lactams. Used primarily for serious, multi-ply-resistant infections.	3–10 mg/kg IV, IM q6–8h
Imipramine (Tofranil)	Tricyclic antidepressant (TCA). Used in humans to treat anxiety and depression.	2–4 mg/kg q12–24h

Drug Name (Other Names)	Pharmacology and Indications	Dosage
	Used in animals to treat variety of behavioral disorders, including obsessive-compulsive disorders. Action is via inhibition of up-take of serotonin at presynaptic nerve terminals.	
Insulin, regular crystalline	Insulin has multiple effects associated with utilization of glucose. Used to treat diabetes mellitus in dogs and cats.	Ketoacidosis: 0.2 U/kg IM initially, then 0.1 U/kg IM q1h until blood glucose is < 300 mg/dl then 0.25–0.4 U/kg SC qbh
Insulin, lente	Same as above	Same as for NPH insulin
Insulin, NPH isophane	Same as above	0.25–0.5 U/kg q12h
Insulin, protamine zinc	Same as above	Same as for NPH insulin
Insulin, ultra lente	Same as above	Same as NPH insulin ex cept administer q24h in some cats
Interferon (interferon α, HuIFN-α) (Roferon)	Human interferon. Used to stimulate the immune sys-tem in patients.	10,000 U/kg SC q12h or 30 U PO once daily for 7 days and repeated every other week
Ipecac syrup (Ipecac)	Emetic drug. For emergency treatment of poisoning. Active ingredient is thought to be emetine.	2–6 mL PO
Isoflurane (Aerrane)	Inhalant anesthetic. See halothane.	Induction: 5%. Maintenance: 1.5–2.5%
Isoproterenol (Isuprel)	Adrenergic agonist. Stimu-lates both beta-1 (β_1) and beta-2 (β_2) adrenergic re-ceptors. Used to stimulate heart (inotropic and chronotropic). Also used to relax bronchial smooth muscle for acute treatment of broncho-constriction.	10 μg/kg IM, SC q6h or di-lute 1 mg in 500 mL of 5% dextrose or Ringer's solution and infuse IV 0.5–1 mL/min (1–2 μg/ min) or to effect
Isosorbide dinitrate (Isordil, Isorbid, Sorbitrate)	Nitrate vasodilator. Causes vasodilation via generation of nitric oxide. Relaxes vas-cular smooth muscle, es-	2.5–5 mg/cat PO q12h or 0.22–1.1 mg/kg PO q12h

Drug Name (Other Names)	Pharmacology and Indications	Dosage
	pecially venous. Reduces preload in patients with congestive heart failure. In humans, it is primarily used to treat angina.	
Itraconazole (Sporanox)	Azole (triazole) antifungal drug. See ketoconazole for mechanism of action. Active against derma- tophytes and systemic fungi, including *Blastomyces* and *Coccidioides*, and histoplasma.	5 mg/kg PO q12h
Ivermectin (Heartgard for cats, Ivomec)	Antiparasitic drug. Neurotoxic to parasites by potentiating effects of inhibitory neuro- transmitter GABA.	Heart worm preventative: 24 micrograms/kg q30d
Kanamycin (Kantrim)	Aminoglycoside antibiotic. See gentamicin and amikacin for details.	10 mg/kg IV, IM, SC q6–8h
Kaopectate (kaolin and pectin) (Kaopectate)	Antidiarrheal compound. Kaolin may act as adsorbent for endotoxins and pectin may protect intestinal mucosa.	1–2 mL/kg PO q2–6h
Ketamine (Ketalar, Ketavet, Vetalar)	Anesthetic agent. Exact mechanism of action is not known but appears to act as dissociative agent. Ke- tamine has little analgesic activity. Rapidly metabolized and eliminated in most cats.	2–25 mg/kg IV, IM (recom- mend adjunctive sedative or tranquilizer treatment)
Ketoconazole (Nizoral)	Azole (imidazole) antifungal drug. Similar mechanism of action as other azole anti- fungal agents. Inhibits er- gosterol synthesis in fungal cell membrane. Fungistatic. Efficacious against dermato- phytes and variety of sys- temic fungi.	5–10 mg/kg PO q8–12h
Ketoprofen (Orudis-KT [OTC tablet], Ketofen [injection])	Nonsteroidal anti-inflammatory drug. See flunixin meglu- mine.	1 mg/kg PO q24h (up to 5 days)

Drug Name (Other Names)	Pharmacology and Indications	Dosage
Lactated Ringer's solution	Fluid solution for replacement. IV administration.	Maintenance: 60–70 mL/kg IV per 24 hrs
Lactulose (Chronulac, generic)	Laxative. Produces laxative effect by osmotic effect in colon. Lactulose also has been used for treatment of hyperammonemia (hepatic encephalopathy) because it decreases blood ammonia concentrations via lowering pH of colon; thus ammonia in colon is not as readily absorbed.	Constipation: 1 mL per 4.5 kg PO q8h to effect. Hepatic encephalopathy: 2.5–5 mL/cat PO q8h or 20–30 mL/kg of a 30% solution given as a retention enema
Leucovorin (folinic acid) (Wellcovorin, generic)	Reduced to folic acid, which is available for purine and thymidine synthesis. Used as an antidote for folic acid antagonists.	With methotrexate administration: 3 mg/m^2 IV, IM, PO. Antidote for pyrimethamine toxicosis: 1 mg/kg PO q24h
Levamisole (Levasole, Tramisol, Ergamisol)	Antiparasitic drug of the imidazothiazole class. Mechanism of action a result of neuromuscular toxicity to parasites. In humans, levamisole is used as immunostimulant to aid in treatment of colorectal carcinoma and malignant melanoma.	4.4 mg/kg PO once. Lungworms: 20–40 mg/kg PO q48h five treatments
Levodopa (L-dopa) (Larodopa, L-dopa)	Converted to dopamine after crossing blood-brain barrier. Stimulates CNS dopamine receptors. In humans, used for treating Parkinson's disease. In cats, has been used for treating hepatic encephalopathy.	Hepatic encephalopathy: 6.8 mg/kg initially, then 1.4 mg/kg q6h
Levothyroxine sodium (Soloxine, Thyro-Tabs, Synthroid)	Replacement therapy for treating cats with hypothyroidism. Levothyroxine is T$_4$, which is converted in most patients to the active T$_3$.	10–20 µg/kg/day PO (adjust dose via monitoring)
Lidocaine (Xylocaine)	Local anesthetic. See bupivacaine for mechanism of action. Lidocaine is also used	0.25–0.75 mg/kg IV slowly or 10–40 mg/kg/min constant rate infusion

Drug Name (Other Names)	Pharmacology and Indications	Dosage
	commonly for acute treatment of cardiac arrhythmias. Class I antiarrhythmic. Decreases phase 0 depolarization without affecting conduction. Not useful for supraventricular arrhythmias.	
Lincomycin (Lincocin)	Lincosamide antibiotic. Similar in mechanism to clindamycin and erythromycin. Spectrum includes primarily gram-positive bacteria. Used for pyoderma and other soft-tissue infections.	15–25 mg/kg PO q12h. Pyoderma: Doses as low as 10 mg/kg q12h have been used
Liothyronine (Cytomel)	Liothyronine is equivalent to T_3. Used for thyroid testing.	For T_3 suppression test: see Appendix F
Lisinopril (Prinivil, Zestril)	ACE inhibitor. See captopril for details. Used for treatment of congestive heart failure and hypertension.	No dose established
Loperamide (Imodium)	Opiate agonist. Stimulates smooth muscle segmentation in intestine as well as electrolyte absorption. Used for acute treatment of nonspecific diarrhea.	0.08–0.16 mg/kg PO q12h
Lufenuron (Program)	Antiparasitic. Used for controlling fleas in animals. Inhibits development in hatching fleas.	30 mg/kg PO, q30 days
Magnesium citrate (Citroma, CitroNesia [Citro-Mag in Canada])	Saline cathartic. Acts to draw water into small intestine via osmotic effect. Fluid accumulation produces distension, which promotes bowel evacuation. Used for constipation and bowel evacuation before certain procedures.	2–4 mL/kg PO
Magnesium hydroxide (Milk of Magnesia)	Same as magnesium citrate. Magnesium hydroxide also is used as oral antacid to	Antacid: 5–10 mL/kg PO q4–6h. Cathartic: 2–6 mL/ cat PO q24h (cats)

Drug Name (Other Names)	Pharmacology and Indications	Dosage
	neutralize stomach acid.	
Magnesium sulfate (Epsom salts)	Same as magnesium citrate	2–5 g/cat PO q24h
Mannitol (Osmitrol)	Hyperosmotic diuretic. Increases plasma osmolality, which draws fluid from tissues to plasma. Antiglaucoma agent. Used for treatment of edema and reducing intraocular pressure. Mannitol also has been used to promote urinary excretion of certain toxins.	Diuretic: 1 g/kg IV 5–25% solution to maintain urine flow. Glaucoma or CNS edema: 0.25–2 g/kg IV 15–25% solution over 30–60 minutes (repeat in 6 hours if necessary)
Meclizine (Antivert, generic)	Antiemetic and antihistamine. Used for treatment of motion sickness. Action may be caused by central anticholinergic actions. Also may suppress chemoreceptor trigger zone (CRTZ).	12.5 mg PO q24h
Medroxyprogesterone acetate (Injection [Depo-Provera]; tablets [Provera])	Progestin hormone. Derivative of acetoxyprogesterone. In cats, used as progesterone hormone treatment to control estrus cycle. Also used for management of some behavioral and dermatologic disorders (such as urine spraying and alopecia).	1.1–2.2 mg/kg IM every 7 days. Behavioral disorders: 10–20 mg/kg SC
Megestrol acetate (Ovaban)	See medroxyprogesterone acetate.	Proestrus: 2 mg/kg PO q24h for 8 days. Anestrus: 0.5 mg/kg PO q24h for 30 days. Behavioral disorders: 2–4 mg/kg q24h for 8 days (reduce dose for maintenance). Dermatologic therapy or urine spraying: 2.5–5 mg/cat PO q24h for 1 week, then reduce to 5 mg once or twice per week. Suppress estrus: 5 mg/cat/day for 3 days, then 2.5–5 mg once per week

Drug Name [Other Names]	Pharmacology and Indications	Dosage
		for 10 weeks
Melphalan (Alkeran)	Anticancer agent. Alkylating agent, similar in action to cyclophosphamide.	1.5 mg/m^2 or 0.1–0.2 mg/kg PO q24h for 7–10 days (repeat every 3 weeks)
Meperidine (Demerol)	Synthetic opioid agonist with activity primarily at the μ-opiate receptor. Similar in action to morphine, except with approximately one seventh the potency (75 mg IM or 300 mg PO has similar potency as 10 mg morphine).	3–5 mg/kg IV, IM (as needed or every 2–4 hours)
Mepivacaine (Carbocaine)	Local anesthetic. See bupivacaine. Medium potency and duration of action compared to bupivacaine.	Variable dose for local infiltration or epidural injection
6-mercaptopurine (Purinethol)	Anticancer agent. Antimetabolite agent that inhibits synthesis of purines in cancer cells.	50 mg/m^2 PO q24h
Mesalamine (Asacol, Mesasal, Pentasa)	5-aminosalicylic acid. Used as treatment of colitis. Action is not precisely known, but suppresses inflammation in colon. Component of sulfasalazine.	Veterinary dose has not been established. The usual human dose is 400–500 mg q6–8h. See sulfasalazine
Methazolamide (Neptazane)	Carbonic anhydrase inhibitor. Produces less diuresis than others. See dichlorphenamide and acetazolamide.	2–4 mg/kg (to a maximum dose of 4–6 mg/kg) PO q8–12h
Methenamine hippurate (Hiprex)	Urinary antiseptic. Converted to formaldehyde in acidic urine to produce an antibacterial/antifungal effect. Active against a wide range of bacteria. Resistance does not develop. Less effective against *Proteus*, which produces an alkaline urine pH. Not effective for systemic infections.	250 mg/cat PO q12h
Methenamine mandelate (Mandelamine)	Urinary antiseptic. See methenamine hippurate.	10–20 mg/kg PO q8–12h

Drug Name (Other Names)	Pharmacology and Indications	Dosage
Methimazole (Tapazole)	Antithyroid drug. Used for treating hyperthyroidism. Action is to serve as substrate for thyroid peroxidase and decrease incorporation of iodide into thyrosine molecules.	2.5–5 mg/cat PO q8–12h for 1–4 wks for induction, then 2.5–10 mg/cat PO 12h according to T4 level
Methocarbamol (Robaxin-V)	Skeletal muscle relaxant. Depresses polysynaptic reflexes. Used for treatment of skeletal muscle spasms.	44 mg/kg PO q8h on the first day, then 22–44 mg/kg PO q8h
Methohexital (Brevital)	Barbiturate anesthetic. See thiopental for details. Methohexital is about 2–3 times more potent than pentothal, but with shorter duration.	3–6 mg/kg IV (give slowly to effect)
Methotrexate (MTX, Mexate, Folex, Rheumatrex, generic)	Anticancer agent. Used for various carcinomas, leukemia, and lymphomas. Action is via antimetabolite action. Analogue of folic acid that binds dihydrofolate reductase. Inhibits DNA, RNA, and protein synthesis. In humans, methotrexate is also commonly used for autoimmune diseases such as rheumatoid arthritis.	2.5–5 mg/m² PO q48h (dose depends on specific protocol). 0.8 mg/kg IV every 2–3 weeks
Methoxamine (Vasoxyl)	Adrenergic agonist. Sympathomimetic alpha-1 (α_1) adrenergic agonist. Specific for alpha-1 receptors.	200–250 μg/kg IM or 40–80 μg/kg IV
Methoxyflurane (Metofane)	Inhalant anesthetic. See halothane.	Induction: 3%. Maintenance: 0.5–1.5%
Methylene blue 0.1% (generic, new methylene blue)	Antidote for intoxication. Used to treat methemoglobinemia. Acts as reducing agent to reduce methemoglobin to hemoglobin.	1.5 mg/kg IV slowly
Methylprednisolone (Medrol)	Glucocorticoid anti-inflammatory drug. See betamethasone.	See doses for prednisolone. (Methylprednisolone has potency that is 1.25 times prednisolone.)

Drug Name (Other Names)	Pharmacology and Indications	Dosage
Methylprednisolone acetate (Depo-Medrol)	Depot form of methylprednisolone. Slowly absorbed from IM injection site, producing glucocorticoid effects for 3–4 weeks in some cats. Used for intralesional therapy, intra-articular therapy, and inflammatory conditions.	10–20 mg/cat IM every 1–3 weeks
Methylprednisolone sodium succinate (Solu-Medrol)	Same as methylprednisolone, except that this is a water-soluble formulation intended for acute therapy when high IV doses are needed for rapid effect. Used for treatment of shock and CNS trauma.	Emergency use: 30 mg/kg IV and repeat at 15 mg/kg in 2–6 hours. Replacement or anti-inflammatory therapy: See prednisolone
Methyltestosterone (Android, generic)	Anabolic androgenic agent. Used for anabolic actions or testosterone hormone replacement therapy (androgenic deficiency). Testosterone has been used to stimulate erythropoiesis.	2.5–5 mg/cat PO q24–48h
Metoclopramide (Reglan, Maxolon [Maxeran in Canada])	Prokinetic drug. Antiemetic. Stimulates motility of upper gastrointestinal tract and centrally-acting antiemetic. Action is to inhibit dopamine receptors and enhance action of acetylcholine in gastrointestinal tract. Used primarily for gastroparesis and treatment of vomiting.	0.2–0.5 mg/kg IV, IM, PO q6–8h (or 1–2 mg/kg/day via continuous IV infusion)
Metoprolol tartrate (Lopressor)	Adrenergic blocking agent. Beta-1 (β_1) adrenergic blocker. Similar properties to propranolol, except that metroprolol is specific for β_1 receptor. Used to control	2–15 mg/cat PO q8h

Drug Name [Other Names]	Pharmacology and Indications	Dosage
	tachyarrhymias and slow heart rate.	
Metronidazole (Flagyl, generic)	Antibacterial and antiprotozoal drug. Disrupts DNA in organism via reaction with intracellular metabolite. Action is specific for anaerobic bacteria. Resistance is rare. Active against someprotozoa, including *Giardia*.	Anaerobes: 10–25 mg/kg PO q24h; *Giardia:* 17 mg/kg (1/3 of a 250-mg tablet per cat) q24h for 8 days
Midazolam (Versed)	Benzodiazepine. Action is similar to other benzodiazepines. See diazepam. Used as anesthetic adjunct.	0.1–0.25 mg/kg IV, IM or 0.1–0.3 mg/kg/hour IV infusion
Milbemycin oxime (Interceptor)	Antiparasitic drug. Action is similar to ivermectin. Acts as GABA agonist in nervous system of parasite. Used as heartworm preventative.	Heartworm prevention: 500 micrograms/kg q30d
Mineral oil (generic)	Lubricant laxative. Increases water content of stool. Used to increase passage of feces for treatment of impaction and constipation.	10–25 mL/cat PO q12h
Minocycline (Minocin)	Tetracycline antibiotic. Similar to doxycycline in pharmacokinetics. See doxycycline.	5–12.5 mg/kg PO q12h
Misoprostol (Cytotec)	Prostaglandin E_2 analogue. Prostaglandins provide a cytoprotective role in the gastrointestinal mucosa. Misoprostol is used to prevent gastritis and ulcers associated with NSAID (aspirin drug) therapy.	Dose not established
Mitotane (o, p'-DDD) (Lysodren, o, p'-DDD)	Adrenocortical cytotoxic agent. Causes suppression of adrenal cortex. Used to	PDH: 50 mg/kg/day PO (In divided doses) for 5–10 days, then 50–70 mg/kg/

Drug Name [Other Names]	Pharmacology and Indications	Dosage
	treat adrenal tumors and pituitary-dependent hyper-adrenocorticism (PDH). Cats rarely respond.	week PO. Adrenal tumor: 50–75 mg/kg/day PO for 10 days, then 75–100 mg/ kg/week
Mitoxantrone (Novantrone)	Anticancer antibiotic. Similar to doxorubicin in action. See doxorubicin. Used for leukemia, lymphoma, and carcinomas.	6.5 mg/m^2 IV every 21 days
Morphine (generic)	Opioid agonist and analgesic. Prototype for other opioid agonists. Action of morphine is to bind to μ-and κ-opiate receptors on nerves and inhibit release of neurotrans-mitters involved with trans-mission of pain stimuli (such as substance P). Morphine also may inhibit release of some inflammatory media-tiors. Central sedative and euphoric effects related to mu-receptor effects in brain.	0.1 mg/kg IM, SC (as needed)
Nalorphine (Nalline)	Opiate antagonist. Used to reverse effects from opiate agonists (such as mor-phine). See naloxone.	0.44 mg/kg IV, IM, SC (1 mg for every 10 mg of mor-phine)
Naloxone (Narcan)	Opiate antagonist. Used to reverse effects from opiate agonists (such as morphine). Naloxone may be used to reverse sedation, anesthe-sia, and adverse effects caused by opiates.	0.01–0.04 mg/kg IV, IM, SC, as needed to reverse opiate
Naltrexone (Trexan)	Opiate antagonist. Similar to naloxone except that it is longer acting and adminis-tered PO. Used in humans for treatment of opiate de-pendence. In cats, it has been used for treatment of some obsessive-compulsive behavioral disorders.	Behavioral disorders: 2.2 mg/kg PO q12h

Drug Name [Other Names]	Pharmacology and Indications	Dosage
Nandrolone deconate (Deca-Durabolin)	Anabolic steroid. Derivative of testosterone. Anabolic agents are designed to maximize anabolic effects while minimizing androgenic action. See methyl-testosterone. Anabolic agents have been used to reverse catabolic conditions, increase weight gain, increase muscle, and stimulate erythropoiesis.	1 mg/kg/week IM
Neomycin (Biosol)	Aminoglycoside antibiotic. For mechanism and other effects see gentamicin and amikacin. Neomycin differs from other aminoglycosides because it is only administered topically or orally. Systemic absorption is minimal from oral absorption.	10–20 mg/kg PO q6–12h
Neostigmine bromide and neostigmine methylsulfate (Prostigmin, Stiglyn)	Anticholinesterase drug. Cholinesterase inhibitor. Inhibits breakdown of acetylcholine at synapse. Antimyasthenic drug. Used primarily for treatment of myasthenia gravis or as an antidote for neuromuscular blockade caused by nondepolarizing neuromuscular blocking drugs.	Antimyasthenic: 2 mg/kg/day PO (in divided doses, to effect). 10 μg/kg IM, SC, as needed. Antidote for curiform block: 40 μg/kg IM, SC. Diagnostic aid for myasthenia gravis: 40 μg/kg IM or 20 μg/kg IV
Nitrofurantoin (Furadantin, Macrodantin)	Antibacterial drug. Urinary antiseptic. Action is via reactive metabolites that damage DNA. Therapeutic concentrations are reached only in the urine.	4 mg/kg PO q8h
Nitroglycerin (Nitrol, Nitrobid, Nitrostat)	Nitrate. Nitrovasodilator. Used in heart failure to reduce preload or decrease pulmonary hypertension.	2–4mg (1/4 inch of ointment per cat) topically q12h

Drug Name (Other Names)	Pharmacology and Indications	Dosage
Nitroprusside (Nitropress)	Nitrate vasodilator. See nitroglycerin.	1–10 µg/kg/min IV infusion
Nizatidine (Axid)	Histamine H_2 blocking drug. See cimetidine. Same as cimetidine, except up to 10 times more potent.	5 mg/kg PO q24h
Norfloxacin (Noroxin)	Fluoroquinolone antibacterial drug. Same action as cipro-floxacin, except spectrum of activity is not as broad as with ciprofloxacin and enrofloxacin.	22 mg/kg PO q12h
Omeprazole (Prilosec)	Antacid and for gastric spirochetes.	0.7 mg/kg PO q24h
Ondansetron (Zofran)	Antiemetic drug. Ondanse-tron's action is to inhibit action of serotonin (blocks $5\text{-}HT_3$ receptors). Used pri-marily to inhibit vomiting associated with chemo-therapy.	0.5–1.0 mg/kg 30 minutes before administration of cancer drugs
Orbifloxacin (Orbax)	Antibacterial drug.	2.5–7.5 mg/kg PO q24h
Oxacillin (Prostaphilin, generic)	Beta-lactam antibiotic. In-hibits bacterial cell wall synthesis. Spectrum is limited to gram-positive bacteria, especially staphy-lococci.	22–40 mg/kg PO q8h
Oxazepam (Serax)	Benzodiazepine. Central-acting CNS depressant. Mechanism of action ap-pears to be via potentiation of GABA-receptor mediated effects in CNS. Used for sedation and to stimulate appetite.	Appetite stimulant: 2.5 mg/cat PO
Oxymetholone (Anadrol)	Anabolic steroid. See nan-drolone. There are no differ-ences in efficacy among the anabolic steroids.	1–5 mg/kg/day PO
Oxymorphone (Numorphan)	Opioid agonist. Action is similar to morphine, except that oxymorphone is 10–15	0.1–0.2 mg/kg IV, SC, IM (as needed); redose with 0.05–0.1 mg/kg q1–2h

Drug Name (Other Names)	Pharmacology and Indications	Dosage
	times more potent than morphine.	Preanesthetic: 0.025–0.05 mg/kg IM, SC
Oxytetracycline (Terramycin)	Tetracycline antibiotic. See tetracycline.	7.5–10 mg/kg IV q12h; 20 mg/kg PO q12h
Oxytocin (Pitocin, Syntocinon [nasal solution], generic)	Stimulates uterine muscle contraction via action on specific oxytocin receptors. Used to induce or maintain normal labor and delivery in pregnant cats. Does not increase milk production, but will stimulate contraction leading to milk ejection.	2.5– 5.0 U/cat IM,IV. Can be repeated q30–60min up to 3 times
Pancrelipase (Viokase)	Pancreatic enzyme. Used to treat pancreatic exocrine insufficiency. Provides lipase, amylase, and protease.	Mix 1/2 tsp powder with food per 5 kg body weight or 1–3 tsp per 0.45 kg of food
Pancuronium bromide (Pavulon)	Nondepolarizing neuromuscular blocker. See atricurium.	0.1 mg/kg IV or start with 0.01 mg/kg and additional 0.01 mg/kg doses every 30 minutes
Paregoric (Corrective mixture)	Paregoric (opium tincture) is an outdated product used to treat diarrhea. Paregoric contains 2 mg of morphine in every 5 mL of paregoric.	0.05–0.06 mg/kg PO q12h
D-penicillamine (Cuprimine, Depen)	Chelating agent for lead copper, iron, and mercury. Used primarily in animals for treatment of copper toxicity and hepatitis associated with accumulation of copper. It also has been used to treat cystine calculi. Penicillamine has been used in humans to treat rheumatoid arthritis.	10–15 mg/kg PO q12h
Penicillin G benzathine (Benza-Pen and other names)	All benzathine penicillin G is combined with procaine penicillin G in commercial formulation.	24,000 U/kg IM q48h
Penicillin G potassium and penicillin G sodium (many)	Beta-lactam antibiotic. Action is similar to other penicillins (see amoxicillin). Spectrum	20,000–40,000 U/kg IV, IM q6–8h

Drug Name [Other Names]	Pharmacology and Indications	Dosage
	of penicillin G is limited to gram-positive bacteria and anaerobes.	
Penicillin G procaine (generic)	Same as other forms of penicillin G, except procaine penicillin is absorbed slowly, producing concentrations for 12–24 hours after injections.	20,000–40,000 U/kg IM q12–24h
Penicillin V (Pen-Vee)	Oral penicillin. Otherwise same as other penicillins.	10 mg/kg PO q8h
Pentazocine (Talwin-V)	Synthetic opiate analgesic. Partial agonist (similar to buprenorphine or butorphanol).	2.2–3.3 mg/kg IV, IM, SC
Pentobarbital (Nembutal, generic)	Short-acting barbiturate anesthetic. Pentobarbital is used as an immediate acting anticonvulsant and as an IV anesthetic. Duration of action may be 3–4 hours.	25–30 mg/kg IV
Phenobarbital (Luminal, generic)	Long-acting barbiturate. See other barbiturates (thiopental). Phenobarbital's major use is as an anticonvulsant in which it potentiates in-hibitory actions of GABA.	1–2 mg/kg PO q12h. Status epilepticus: 15–200 mg/ animal IV (to effect)
Phenoxybenzamine (Dibenzyline)	Alpha-1 (α_1) adrenergic antagonist. Binds alpha-1 receptor on smooth muscle, causing relaxation. Potent vasodilator. Used primarily to treat peripheral vasoconstriction. In some cats, it has been used to relax urethral smooth muscle.	2.5 mg/cat PO q8–12h or 0.5 mg/kg q12h
Phentolamine (Regitine [Rogitine in Canada])	Nonselective alpha (α) adrenergic blocker. Vasodilator. Blocks stimulation of alpha receptors on vascular	0.02–0.1 mg/kg IV

Drug Name [Other Names]	Pharmacology and Indications	Dosage
	smooth muscle. Primarily used to treat hypertension.	
Phenylephrine (Neo-Synephrine)	Specific adrenergic agonist. Specific for alpha-1 receptor. Same as methoxamine.	0.01 mg/kg IV every 15 minutes: 0.1 mg/kg IM, SC every 15 minutes
Phenylpropanolamine (Dexatrim, Propagest, others)	Adrenergic agonist. Used as decongestant, bronchodilator, and to increase tone of urinary sphincter.	1.5–2 mg/kg PO q12h
Physostigmine (Antilirium)	Cholinesterase inhibitor. Antidote for anticholinergic intoxication, especially intoxication that exhibits CNS signs.	0.02 mg/kg IV q12h
Piperazine (many)	Antiparasitic compound. Produces neuromuscular blockade in parasite through inhibition of neurotransmitter, which causes paralysis of worms. Used primarily for treatment of helminth (ascarids) infections.	44–66 mg/kg PO once
Plicamycin (mithramycin) (Mithracin)	Anticancer agent. Action is to combine with DNA in presence of divalent cations and inhibit DNA and RNA synthesis. Lowers serum calcium. Used to treat carcinomas and hypercalcemia.	Antineoplastic: 25–30μg/kg/day IV (slow infusion) for 8–10 days. Antihyper calcemic: 25 μg/kg/day IV (slow infusion) over 4 hours
Polyethylene glycol electrolyte solution (Golytely)	Saline cathartic. See magnesium citrate. Nonabsorbable compounds that increase water secretion into bowel via osmotic effect. Used for bowel evacuation before surgical or diagnostic procedure.	25 mL/kg PO; repeat in 2–4 hours
Potassium bromide	Mechanism uncertain. Believe to hyperpolarize neurons. Used for chronic seizure disorders.	10–40 mg/kg PO q12h
Potassium chloride (generic)	Potassium supplement. Used for treatment of hypokalemia. Usually added to	0.5 mEq potassium/kg/day or supplement 10–40 mEq/500 mL of fluids, depend-

Drug Name [Other Names]	Pharmacology and Indications	Dosage
	fluid solutions.	ing on serum potassium concentration
Potassium citrate (generic, Urocit-K)	Alkylinizes urine to prevent calcium oxalate urolithiasis.	2.2 mEq per 100 kiloCalories of energy per day PO or 50–75 mg/kg PO q12h
Potassium gluconate (Kaon, Tumil-K, generic)	Same as potassium chloride	2–6 mEq/day
Potassium phosphate	For hypophosphatemia due to diabetic ketoacidosis.	0.03–0.12 mmol/kg/h IV
Pralidoxime chloride (2-PAM) (Protopam chloride)	Used for treatment of organophosphate toxicosis	20 mg/kg q8–12h (initial dose IV slow or IM)
Praziquantel (Droncit)	Antiparasitic drug. Used primarily to treat infections caused by tapeworms.	5 mg/kg IM, SC. Cats < 1.8 kg: 6.3 mg/kg PO once. Cats > 1.8 kg: 5 mg/kg PO once. Paragonimus: 25 mg/kg q8h for 2 days
Prednisolone (Delta-cortef, many others)	Glucocorticoid antiinflammatory drug. Potency is approxmately 4 times that of cortisol.	Anti-inflammatory: 0.5–1 mg/kg IV, IM, PO q12–24h initially, then taper to q48h. Immunosuppressive: 2.2–6.6 mg/kg/day IV, IM, PO initially, then taper to 2–4 mg/kg q48h
Prednisolone sodium succinate (Solu-Delta-Cortef)	Same as prednisolone, except that this is a water-soluble formulation intended for acute therapy when high IV doses are needed for rapid effect. Used for treatment of shock and CNS trauma. See also methylprednisolone sodium succinate.	Shock: 15–30 mg/kg IV; repeat in 4–6 hours. CNS trauma: 15–30 mg/kg IV; taper to 1–2 mg/kg q12h
Prednisone (See prednisolone.)	Same as prednisolone, except that after administration, prednisone is converted to prednisolone	Same as prednisolone
Primidone (Mylepsin, Neurosyn [Mysoline in Canada])	Anticonvulsant. Primidone is converted to phenylethylmalonamide and phenobar-bital, both of which haveanticonvulsant	8–10 mg/kg PO q8–12h as initial dose, then adjust via monitoring to 10–15 mg/kg q8h Note: May be hepatotoxic. Dose and efficacy not

Drug Name (Other Names)	Pharmacology and Indications	Dosage
	activity, but most of activity (85%) is probably a result of phenobarbital. See phenobarbital for more details.	well established
Primor (ormetoprim and sulfadimethoxine)	Antibacterial drug. Ormetoprim inhibits bacterial dihydrofolate reductase; sulfon-amide competes with PABA for synthesis of nucleic acids.Bactericidal/bacteriostatic. Broad antibacterial spectrum and active against some coccidia.	27 mg/kg PO on first day, followed by 13.5 mg/kg q24h
Prochlorperazine (Compazine)	Phenothiazine. Central-acting dopamine (D2) antagonist. Used for sedation, tranquilization, and as antiemetic. Antiemetic action also may be related to alpha-2 and muscarinic blocking effects.	0.1–0.5 mg/kg q6–8h IM SC
Promethazine (Phenergan)	Phenothiazine with strong antihistamine effects. Used for treatment of allergy and as antiemetic (motion sickness).	0.2–0.4 mg/kg IV, IM, PO q6–8h (up to a maximum dose of 1 mg/kg)
Propiopromazine (Tranvet, Largon)	Phenothiazine sedative. Also has antiemetic and anti-histaminic actions.	1.1–4.4 mg/kg q12–24h
Propofol (Diprivan) (Rapinovet)	Anesthetic. Used for induction or producing short-term general anesthesia. Mechanism of action is not well defined but may be barbiturate-like	6.5 mg/kg IV (slowly)
Propranolol (Inderal)	Beta (β) adrenergic blocker. Nonselective for beta-1 and beta-2 adrenergic receptors.	0.4–1.2 mg/kg (2.5–5 mg/cat) PO q8h

Drug Name (Other Names)	Pharmacology and Indications	Dosage
	Class II antiarrhythmic. Used primarily to decrease heart rate, cardiac conduction, tachyarrhythmias, and blood pressure.	
Propylthiouracil (PTU) (Generic, Propyl-Thyracil)	Antithyroid drug. See methimazole. Compared to methimazole PTU inhibits conversion of T_4 to T_3.	11 mg/kg PO q12h
Prostaglandin $F_{2\alpha}$ (Lutalyse)	Prostagindin induces leutolysis. Has been used to treat open pyometra in animals. Use for inducing abortion has been questioned.	Pyometra: 0.1–0.25 mg/kg SC once daily for 5 days; Abortion: 0.5–1 mg/kg IM for 2 injections
Psyllium (Metamucil, Vetasyl, others)	Bulk-forming laxative. Used for treatment of constipation and bowel evacuation. Action is to absorb water and expand to provide increased bulk and moisture content to the stool, which encourages normal peristalsis and bowel motility.	1 tsp per 5–10 kg (added to each meal)
Pyrantel pamoate (Nemex, Strongid)	Antiparasitic drug. Acts to block ganglionic neurotransmission via cholinergic action.	20 mg/kg PO once
Pyridostigmine bromide (Mestinon, Regonol)	Anticholinesterase. Same as neostigmine, except that pyridostigmine has longer duration of action.	Antimyasthenic: 0.02–0.04 mg/kg IV q2h or 0.5–3 mg/kg PO q8–12h. Antidote (curariform): 0.15–0.3 mg/kg IM, IV.
Pyrimethamine (Daraprim)	Antibacterial, antiprotozoal drug. Acts to antagonize dihydrofolate reductase enzyme to inhibit synthesize reduced folate and nucleic acids. Activity of pyrimethamine is greater against protozoa than bacteria.	0.5–1 mg/kg PO q24h for 14–28 days.
Quinacrine (Atabrine)	Outdated antimalarial drug. Used occasionally for treatment of protozoa (Giardia). Inhibits nucleic acid synthesis in parasite.	11 mg/kg PO q24h for 5 days.

Drug Name [Other Names]	Pharmacology and Indications	Dosage
Racemethionine (dL-methionine) (generic tablets)	Urinary acidifier. Lowers urinary pH. Also has been used to protect against acetaminophen overdose.	1–1.5 g/cat PO (added to food each day)
Ranitidine (Zantac)	H$_2$ antagonist. See cimetidine for details. Same as cimetidine except 4–10 times more potent and longer acting.	2.5 mg/kg IV q12h; 3.5 mg/kg PO q12h
Rifampin (Rifadin)	Antibacterial. Spectrum of action includes staphylococci, mycobacteria, and streptococci.	10–20 mg/kg PO q24h
Ringer's solution (generic)	IV solution for replacement	40–50 mL/kg/day IV, SC, IP
Rutin (OTC)	Benzopyrone drug for chylothorax.	50 mg/kg PO q12h
Senna (Senokot)	Laxative. Acts via local stimulation or via contact with intestinal mucosa.	5 mL/cat q24h (syrup); 1/2 tsp per cat q24h with food (granules)
Spironolactone (Aldactone)	Potassium-sparing diuretic.	1–2 mg/kg PO q12h
Sodium bicarbonate (generic, baking soda, soda mint)	Alkalizing agent. Antacid. Used to treat systemic acidosis or to alkalize urine. Increases plasma and urinary concentrations of bicarbonate.	Acidosis:0.5–1 mEq/kg IV. Renal failure: 10 mg/kg PO q8–12h. Alkalization of urine: 50 mg/kg PO q8–12h, (1 tsp = 2 g.)
Sodium chloride (0.9%) (generic)	Sodium chloride is used for IV infusion for maintenance.	40–50 mL/kg/day IV, SC, IP
Sodium chloride (7.5%) (generic)	Concentrated sodium chloride used for acute treatment of hypovolemia.	2–8 mL/kg IV
Sodium iodide (20%) (Iodopen, generic)	Used for iodine deficiency	20–40 mg/kg PO q8–12h
Stanozolol (Winstrol-V)	Anabolic steroid. See nandrolone. (There are no established differences in efficacy among the anabolic steroids.)	1 mg/cat PO q12h; 25 mg/cat/week IM
Sucralfate (Carafate [Sulcrate in Canada])	Gastric mucosa protectant. Antiulcer agent. Action of sucralfate is to bind to ulcer-	0.25 g PO q8–12h

Drug Name (Other Names)	Pharmacology and Indications	Dosage
	ated tissue in gastrointestinal tract to aid healing of ulcers. There is some evidence that sucralfate may act as a cyto-protectant (via prostaglandin synthesis). Used to treat or prevent ulcers.	
Sufentanil citrate (Sufenta)	Opiod agonist. Action of fentanyl derivatives is via μ-receptor. Sufentanil is 5–7 times more potent than fentanyl (13–20 μg of sufentanil produce analgesia equal to 10 mg of morphine).	2 μg/kg IV, (up to a maximum dose of 5 μg/kg)
Sulfadiazine (generic)	Sulfonamides compete with PABA for enzyme that synthesizes dihydrofolic acid inbacteria. Synergistic with trimethoprim. Broad spectrum of activity, including some protozoa. Bacteriostatic.	100 mg/kg IV, PO (loading dose), followed by 50 mg/kg IV, PO q12h. See trimetho-prim
Sulfadimethoxine (Albon, Bactrovet, generic)	See sulfadiazine.	55 mg/kg PO (loading dose), followed by 27.5 mg/kg PO q12h
Sulfamethazine (many brands [e.g., Sulmet])	See sulfadiazine.	100 mg/kg PO (loading dose), followed by 50 mg/kg PO q12h
Sulfamethoxazole (Gantanol)	See sulfadiazine.	100 mg/kg PO (loading dose), followed by 50 mg/kg PO q12h
Sulfasalazine (sulfa-pyridine and mesalamine) (Azulfidine [Salazopyrin in Canada])	Sulfonamide and anti-inflammatory drug. Used for treatment of colitis. Sulfon-amide has little effect; sali-cylic acid (mesalamine) has anti-inflammatory effects. See mesalamine.	10–30 mg/kg PO q12–24h. See mesalamine
Sulfisoxazole (Gantrisin)	See sulfadiazine. Sulfisoxizole	Urinary tract infections: 50

Drug Name (Other Names)	Pharmacology and Indications	Dosage
	is primarily used only for treating urinary tract infections.	mg/kg PO q8h
Tamoxifen (Nolvadex)	Nonsteroid estrogen receptor blocker. Also has weak estrogenic effects. Tamoxifen also may also increase release of Gn-RH. Used as adjunctive treatment for certain tumors.	10 mg PO q12h (human dose)
Taurine (generic)	Nutritional supplement for cats. Used in prevention and treatment of ocular and cardiac disease (cardiomyopathy) caused by taurine deficiency.	250 mg/cat PO q12h
Terbutaline (Brethine, Bricanyl)	Beta-adrenergic agonist. Beta-2 (β_2) specific. Used primarily for bronchodilation. See albuterol for further details.	0.1 mg/cat SC q12h or 0.625 mg/cat PO q12–24h
Testosterone cypionate (Andro-Cyp, Andronate, Depo-Testosterone, other forms)	Testosterone ester. See methyltestosterone. Testosterone esters are administered PO to avoid first-pass effects.	1–2 mg/kg IM every 2–4 weeks. See methyltestosterone
Testosterone propionate (Testex [Malogen in Canada])	Testosterone injection. See methyltestosterone.	0.5–1 mg/kg IM 2–3 times per week
Tetracycline (Panmycin)	Tetracycline antibiotic. Mechanism of action of tetracyclines is to bind to 30S ribosomal subunit and inhibit protein synthesis. Usually bactericidal. Broad spectrum of activity, including bacteria, some protozoa, *Rickettsia*, and *Ehrlichia*.	15–20 mg/kg PO q8h; 4.4–11 mg/kg IV, IM q8h
Theophylline (many brands, generic)	Methytxanthine bronchodilator. Mechanism of action is unknown but may be related to increased cyclic AMP or antagonism of adenosine. There appears to be anti-	4 mg/kg PO q8–12h

Drug Name [Other Names]	Pharmacology and Indications	Dosage
	inflammatory action as well as bronchodilating action.	
Theophylline, sustained-release (Theo-Dur, Slo-Bid Gyrocaps)	Same as theophylline. Also for AU blocks.	25 mg/kg PO q24h at night (Theo-Dur and Slo-Bid)
Thiabendazole (Omnizole, Equizole)	Benzimidazole anthelmintic. See fenbendazole and albendazole.	Strongyloides: 125 mg/kg q24h for 3 days
Thiacetarsamide	Arsenical used for treatment of heartworm infections and Hemobartonellosis.	HW: 2.2 mg/kg IV twice daily for 2 days. FIA: 2.2 mg/kg q24h for two doses
Thiamine (vitamin B_1) (Bewon and others.)	Vitamin B_1 is used for treatment of vitamin deficiency.	5–30 mg/cat/day PO (up to a maximum dose of 50 mg/cat/day)
Thiamylal sodium (Surital, Bio-Tal)	Ultra-short-acting barbiturate. See thiopental. Thiamylal is the thiobarbiturate analog of secobarbital.	8–10 mg/kg IV in incremental doses up to 20 mg/kg (2% solution)
Thioguanine (6-TG) (generic)	Anticancer agent. Antimetabolite of purine analog type. Inhibits DNA synthesis in cancer cells.	25 mg/m² PO q24h × 1–5d then repeat q30d PRN
Thiopental sodium (Pentothal)	Ultra-short-acting barbiturate. Used primarily for induction of anesthesia or for short duration of anesthesia (10–15 minutes). Anesthesia is produced by central nervous system depression, without analgesia. Anesthesia is terminated by redistribution in the body.	5–10 mg/kg IV (to effect)
Thiotepa (generic)	Anticancer agent. Alkylating agent of the nitrogen mustard type (similar to cyclophosphamide). Used for various tumors, especially malignant effusions.	0.2–0.5 mg/m² weekly or daily for 5–10 days IM, intracavitary, or intratumor
Thyroid releasing hormone (TRH, Thypinone)	Used to test for hyperthyroidism when TT4 is not elevated.	Collect baseline TT4; Give 0.1 mg/kg IV. Collect port-TRH TT4 sample at 4 hours

Drug Name [Other Names]	Pharmacology and Indications	Dosage
Ticarcillin (Ticar, Ticillin)	Beta-lactam antibiotic. Action similar to ampicillin/amoxicillin. Spectrum similar to carbenicillin. Ticarcillin is primarily used for gram-negative infections, especially those caused by *Pseudomonas.*	33–50 mg/kg IV, IM q4–6h
Ticarcillin and clavulanate (Timentin)	Same as ticarcillin, except clavulanic acid has been added to inhibit bacterial beta-lactamase and increase spectrum.	Same as ticarcillin (dose according to ticarcillin component.)
Tiletamine and zolazepam (Telezol, Zoletil)	Anesthetic.Combination of tiletamine (dissociative anesthetic agent similar in action to ketamine) and zolazepam (benzodiazepine similar in action to diazepam). Produces short duration (30 minutes) of anesthesia.	6–12 mg/kg IM
Tobramycin (Nebcin)	Aminoglycoside antibacterial drug. Similar mechanism of action and spectrum as amikacin and gentamicin.	2–4 mg/kg IV, IM, SC q8h
Triamcinolone (Aristocort, generic)	Glucocorticoid anti-inflammatory drug. See betamethasone for details. Triamcinolone's potency approximates methylprednisolone (about 5 times cortisol and 1.25 times prednisolone).	Anti-inflammatory: 0.5–1 mg/kg PO q12–24h; taper dose to 0.5–1 mg/kg PO q48h
Triamcinolone acetonide (Vetalog)	Same as triamcinolone, except that injectable suspension is slowly absorbed from IM or intralesional injection site. Used for intralesional therapy of tumors and similar purposes as methylprednisolone acetate.	0.1–0.2 mg/kg IM, SC; repeat in 7–10 days. Intralesional: 1.2–1.8 mg (or 1 mg for every cm diameter of tumor) every 2 weeks.
Trientine hydrochloride (Syprine)	Chelating agent. Used to chelate copper when penicillamine cannot be tolerated in a patient.	10–15 mg/kg PO q12h

Drug Name (Other Names)	Pharmacology and Indications	Dosage
Triflupromazine (Vesprin)	Phenothiazine. Similar action as other phenothiazines (see acepromazine), except triflupromazine may have stronger antimuscarinic activity than other phenothiazines. Used for antiemetic action.	0.1–0.3 mg/kg IM, PO q8–12h
Trimeprazine tartrate (Temaril [Panectyl in Canada])	Phenothiazine with antihistamine activity (similar to promethazine). Used for treating allergies and motion sickness.	0.5 mg/kg PO q12h
Trimethoprim sulfonamides (sulfadiazine or sulfamethoxazole) (Tribrissen, others)	Combination antibacterial drug. For action of sulfonamide, see sulfadiazine. Together, the combination is synergistic with a broad spectrum of activity.	15 mg/kg PO q12h or 30 mg/kg PO q12–24h. Toxoplasma: 30 mg/kg PO q12h.
Tripelennamine (Pelamine, PBZ)	Antihistamine (H1) blocker. Similar in action as other antihistamines. See chlorpheniramine. Used to treat allergic disease.	1 mg/kg PO q12h
Ursodiol (ursodeoxycholate) (Actigall)	Anticholelithic. Used for treatment of liver diseases. Increases bile flow. In humans, used to prevent or treat gallstones.	10–15 mg/kg PO q24h
Vasopressin (ADH) (Pitressin)	Antidiuretic hormone. Vasopressin is used for treatment of polyuria caused by central diabetes insipidus. Not effective for polyuria caused by renal disease.	Aqueous: 10 U IV, IM.
Verapamil (Calan, Isoptin)	Calcium-channel blocking drug. Blocks calcium entry into cells via blockade of slow channel. Produces vasodilation and negative chronotropic effects.	1.1–2.9 mg/kg PO q8h.

Drug Name (Other Names)	Pharmacology and Indications	Dosage
Vinblastine (Velban)	Similar to vincristine. Sometimes used as an alternative to vincristine. Do not use to increase platelet numbers (may actually cause thrombocytopenia).	2 mg/m^2 IV (slow infusion) once per week
Vincristine (Oncovin, Vincasar, generic)	Anticancer agent. Vincristine causes arrest of cancer cell division by binding to microtubules and inhibiting mitosis. Used in combination chemotherapy protocols. Vincristine also increases numbers of functional circulating platelets and is used for thrombocytopenia.	Antitumor: 0.5–0.7 mg/m^2 IV or 0.025–0.05 mg/kg once per week. Thrombocytopenia: 0.02 mg/kg IV once per week
Vitamin A (retinoids) (Aquasol-A)	Used to treat vitamin A deficiency.	625–800 U/kg PO q24h
Vitamin B$_1$	See thiamine.	
Vitamin B$_2$ (riboflavin) (Riboflavin)	Used to treat vitamin B$_2$ deficiency	5–10 mg/day PO
Vitamin B$_{12}$ (cyanocobalamin) (Cyanocobalamin)	Vitamin B$_{12}$ is used to treat deficiencies. Conditions caused by deficiency may include anemia.	50–100µg/day PO, SC
Vitamin C (ascorbic acid) (See ascorbic acid.)	Used to treat vitamin C deficiency and occasionally used as urine acidifier. Insufficient data to show that ascorbic acid is effective for preventing cancer or cardiovascular disease.	100–500 mg/day
Vitamin E (alphatocopherol) (Aquasol E, generic)	Vitamin considered as antioxidant. Used as supplement and treatment of some immune-mediated dermatoses.	100–400 U PO q12h. Immune-mediated skin disease: 400–600 U PO q12h
Vitamin K$_1$ (phytonadione, phytomenadione) (AquaMEPHYTON (injection), Mephyton (tablets), Veta-K1 (tablets))	Vitamin K$_1$ used to treat coagulopathies caused by anticoagulant toxicosis (warfarin or other rodenticides). Anticoagulants deplete vitamin K in the body, which is essential for synthesis of clotting factors.	Short-acting rodenticides: 1 mg/kg/day, IM, SC, PO for 10–14 days. Long-acting rodenticides: 2.5–5 mg/kg/day, IM, SC, PO for 3–4 weeks

Drug Name (Other Names)	Pharmacology and Indications	Dosage
Warfarin (Coumadin, generic)	Anticoagulant. Depletes vitamin K, which is responsible for generation of clotting factors. Used to treat hypercoagulable disease and prevent thromboembolism.	Thromboembolism: start with 0.5 mg per day and adjust dose based on clotting time assessment. (Maintain prothrombin time 2–2.5 $\times$ normal.)
Xylaxine (Rompun)	Alpha-2 (α_2) adrenergic agonist. Used primarily for anesthesia and analgesia.	1.1 mg/kg IM (emetic dose is 0.4–0.5 mg/kg IV).
Yohimbine (Yobine)	Alpha-2 (α_2) adrenergic antagonist. Used primarily to reverse actions of xylazine or detomidine.	0.11 mg/kg IV or 0.25–0.5 mg/kg SC, IM
Zidovudine (AZT) (Retrovir)	Antiviral drug. In humans, used to treat AIDS. In animals, has been experimentally used for treatment of FeLV and FIV viral infection in cats.	5–10 mg/kg PO, SC q12h (doses as high as 30 mg/kg/day also have been used)

Modified with permission from Papich MG. Drug formulary. In: Tilley LP, Smith FWK Jr. The 5-Minute Veterinary Consult Canine and Feline. Baltimore: Williams & Wilkins, 1997.

Key to abbreviations: IM: intramuscular; IP: intraperitoneal; IV: intravenous; OTC: over the counter (without prescription); PO: per os (orally); SC: subcutaneous; U: units.

Gary D. Norsworthy

ABCD: Airway, breathing, circulation, drugs (steps for resuscitation)
ACE: Angiotensin-converting enzyme
AChE: Acetylcholinesterase
ACT: Activated clotting time
ACTH: Adrenocorticotrophic hormone
A:G: Albumin to globulin
AIDS: Acquired immunodeficiency syndrome
ALT: Alanine aminotransferase
ANA: Antinuclear antibody
APC: Atrial premature complex
APTT: Activated partial thromboplastin time
ASH: Asymmetric septal hypertrophy
AST: Aspartate aminotransferase
ALP: Alkaline phosphatase
AV: Atrioventricular
AZT: Azidothymidine
BAL: Bronchoalveolar lavage
BCP: Buffy coat preparation
BID: Two times per day
BSA: Body surface area
BUN: Blood urea nitrogen
CBC: Complete blood count
CHF: Congestive heart failure
CHT: Cholangiohepatitis
CLO: *Campylobacter*-like organism
CND: Chronic nasal discharge
CNS: Central nervous system
CO_2: Carbon dioxide
CPA: Cardiopulmonary arrest
CRF: Chronic renal failure
CRT: Capillary refill time
CRTZ: Chemoreceptor trigger zone
CSD: Cat scratch disease
CSF: Cerebrospinal fluid
CT: Computerized tomography
CVM: College of Veterinary Medicine
DCM: Dilated cardiomyopathy
DEET: Fenvalerate plus diethyltoluamide
DH: Diaphragmatic hernia
DLH: Domestic long-hair
DM: Diabetes mellitus
DMH: Domestic medium-hair
DMSO: Dimethyl sulfoxide
DNA: Deoxyribonucleic acid
DSH: Domestic short-hair
DV: Dorsoventral
DX: Diagnosis
DZ: Disease
ECG: Electrocardiogram
EDTA: Ethylenediaminetetra-acetic acid
EEG: Electroencephalogram
EGC: Eosinophilic granuloma complex
ELISA: Enzyme-linked immunosorbent assay

EPI: Exocrine pancreatic insufficiency
ET: Endotracheal
FCoV: Feline coronavirus
FECV : Feline enteric coronavirus
FeLV: Feline leukemia virus
FHS : Feline hypereosinophilic syndrome
FIA: Feline infectious anemia
FIE: Feline infectious enteritis or feline ischemic encephalopathy
FIP: Feline infectious peritonitis
FIPV: Feline infectious peritonitis virus
FIV: Feline immunodeficiency virus
FLUTD: Feline lower urinary tract disease
FNA: Fine-needle aspirate
FNB: Fine-needle biopsy
EOD: Every other day
FT_4: Free thyroxine
FUO: Fever of unknown origin
FUS: Feline urologic syndrome
GBF: Glomerular blood flow
GFR: Glomerular filtration rate
GGT: γ-glutamyltransferase
GGPT: γ-glutamyltranspeptidase
GI: Gastrointestinal
GIS: Gastrointestinal smooth muscle
Gr.: Grain
GSPC: Gingivitis-stomatitis-pharyngitis complex
H&E: Hematoxylin and eosin
Hb: Hemoglobin
HB: Heinz body
HBHA: Heinz body hemolytic anemia
HCO_3: Bicarbonate
HCM: Hypertrophic cardiomyopathy
HCT: Hematocrit
^{131}I: Radioactive iodine
IBD: Inflammatory bowel disease
IC: Intercostal
ICP: Intracranial pressure
IDDM: Insulin-dependent diabetes mellitus
IFA: Indirect fluorescent antibody
IgA: Immunoglobulin A
IgG: Immunoglobulin G
IGR: Insect growth regulator
IM: Intramuscular
IT: Intrathoracic or intratracheal
IU: International unit
IV: Intravenous
KCl: Potassium chloride
kg: Kilogram
L: Liter
LAT: Latex agglutination test
LE: Lupus erythematosus
LN: Lymph node
LRS: Lactated Ringer's solution
LSA: Lymphosarcoma
^{99m}Tc: Pertechnetate thyroid
m^2: meter squared

mEq: Milliequivalents
MCT: Medium-chain triglycerides
MCV: Mean corpuscular volume
mL: Milliliter
MRI: Magnetic resonance imaging
MSCCI: Multiple squamous cell carcinoma in situ
MVD: Mitral valve dysplasia
NaCl: Sodium chloride
$NaHCO_3$: Sodium bicarbonate
NIDDM: Non-insulin-dependent diabetes mellitus
NPO: Nothing per os (orally)
OD: One time per day; referring to the right eye
OP: organophosphates
2-PAM: Pralidoxime
PAS: Periodic acid-Schiff
PBS: Phosphate buffered saline
PCR: Polymerase chain reaction
PCV: Packed cell volume
PD: Polydipsia
PDA: Patent ductus arteriosis
PE: Pemphigus erythematosus
PF: Pemphigus foliaceus
PO: Per os, orally
PP: Polyphagia
PRN: As needed
PS: Pulmonic stenosis
PSS: Portosystemic shunt
PT: Prothrombin time
PTT: Partial thromboplastin time
PTU: Propylthiouracil
PU: Polyuria
QOD: Every other day
RAST: Radioallergosorbent test
RBC: Red blood cell
RCM: Restrictive cardiomyopathy
RX: Treatment or prescription
SA: Sinoatrial
SAM: Systolic anterior motion
SC: Subcutaneous
SCC: Squamous cell carcinoma
SG: Specific gravity
SID: One time per day
SLE: Systemic lupus erythematosis
SX: Surgery
T_3: Triiodothyronine
T_4: Thyroxine
TAP: Trypsinogen activation peptides
TCO_2: Total carbon dioxide
TID: Three times per day
TLI: Trypsin-like Immunoreactivity
TRH: Thyrotropin-releasing hormone
TT_4: Total T_4
UA: Urinalysis
UC: Urine culture
URI: Upper respiratory infection(s)
US: Ultrasound
VC: Vomiting center
VD: Ventrodorsal
VPC: Ventricular premature complex
VSD: Ventricular septal defect
WL: Weight loss

NORMAL LABORATORY VALUES

Gary D. Norsworthy

Complete Blood Count

Test	Range
WBC	$5.5–19.5 \times 10^3/mm^3$
RBC	$5.5–10.0 \times 10^6/mm^3$
HGB	8.0–14.0 g/dL
HCT	24–45%
MCV	$39–55 \ \mu m^3$
MCH	12.5–19.0 µg
MCHC	30–36%
Segs	35–75%
Bands	0–3%
Eos	0–15%
Lymphs	20–55%
Monos	1–4%
Basos	0–2%
Platelets	$250–700 \times 10^3$

Chemistry Profile

Test	Range
Albumin	1.8–3.6 g/dL
Alk Phos	8–55 µ/L
Amylase	500–1200 µ/dL
Bil - Tot	0–1.0 mg/dL
Bil - Dir	0–0.3 mg/dL
Bil - Indir	0.1–0.44 mg/dL
BUN	20–35 mg/dL
Calcium	7.8–11.8 mg/dL
Chloride	96–127 mEq/L
Cholesterol	97–207 mg/dL
CO_2	16–25 mEq/L
Creatinine	0.6–1.8 mg/dL
CPK	32–311 µ/L
Gamma GT	0–33 µ/L
Glucose	60–175 mg/dL
LDH	38–116 µ/L
Lipase	0–190 µ/L
Phosphorus	2.5–7.5 mg/dL
Potassium	3.8–5.8 mEq/L
SGOT - AST	6–41 µ/L
SGPT - ALT	6–74 µ/L
Sodium	141–155 mEq/L
Total Protein	5.4–8.9 g/dL
Globulin	1.8–7.1 g/dL
A/G Ratio	0.3–2.0
Sod/Pot Ratio	24.3–40.8
$Ca \times P$ Product	20–60
T_3	40–182 ng/dL
Total T_4	1.0–4.8 µg/dL
Free T_4	3–9 pmol/L
Cortisol (Baseline)	0.5–5.4 µg/dL
Bile Acid	0–5 mmol/L

Urinalysis

Test	Range
Color	Light yellow
pH	5.0–7.0
Specific gravity*	1.001–1.080
Specific gravity **	1.018–1.050
Creatinine	110–280 mg/dL
Urea	1.0–3.0 g/dL
Glucose	0
Ketones	0
Bilirubin	0
Protein	0–20 mg/dL

*Absolute limits   **Expected range

Miscellaneous

Test	Range
TLI	17–49 µg/L
Electrophoresis	
Total protein	5.2–7.9 g/dL
Albumin	2.1–3.3 g/dL
Globulin	
Alpha 1	0.2–1.1 g/dL
Alpha 2	0.4–0.9 g/dL
Beta	0.9–1.9 g/dL
Gamma	1.7–4.4 g/dL

Hemostatic Values

Test	Range
Activated clotting time	< 65 sec
Bleeding time	105 min
Whole blood coag time (glass)	8 min
Whole blood coag time (cap tb)	5.0–5.4 min
Activated coag of whole blood at room temp	60–125 sec
Prothrombin time	8.1–9.1 sec
Russell's viper venom time	9 sec
Prothrombin consumption	20 sec

These values are courtesy of IDEXX Veterinary Services. They are the normal reference values for this laboratory. However, there is variation between various laboratories and hospital laboratory machines. The reader is encouraged to consult his or her laboratory or machine's operating manual for values that are relevant to his or her situation.

Subject Index

Note: Page numbers in *italics* indicate figures; numbers followed by t indicate tables.